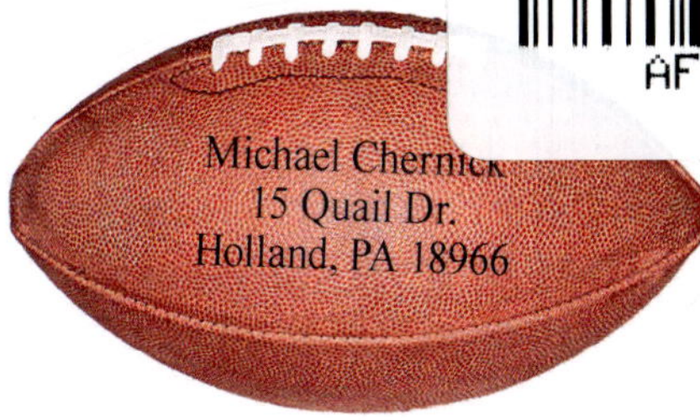
Michael Chernick
15 Quail Dr.
Holland, PA 18966

CLASSICAL AND ADAPTIVE CLINICAL TRIAL DESIGNS USING EXPDESIGN STUDIO™

CLASSICAL AND ADAPTIVE CLINICAL TRIAL DESIGNS USING EXPDESIGN STUDIO™

Mark Chang
Millennium Pharmaceuticals, Inc.

WILEY

A JOHN WILEY & SONS, INC., PUBLICATION

Published by John Wiley & Sons, Inc., Hoboken, New Jersey.
Published simultaneously in Canada.

Library of Congress Cataloging-in-Publication Data:

Chang, Mark.
Classical and adaptive clinical trial designs using ExpDesign Studio™ / Mark Chang.
p. ; cm.
Includes bibliographical references and index.
ISBN 978-0-470-27612-9 (cloth/cd)
1. Drugs–Testing–Computer simulation. 2. Adaptive sampling (Statistics) 3. Clinical trials–Data processing. I. Title.
[DNLM: 1. Drugs, Investigational. 2. Research Design. 3. Clinical Trials as Topic–methods. 4. Software. QV 771 C4565c 2008]
RM301.27.C47 2008
615′.190113—dc22

2008001358

Printed in the United States of America

10 9 8 7 6 5 4 3 2 1

CONTENTS

PREFACE

Drug development is shifting from the classical approaches to more dynamic or adaptive approaches. The pharmaceutical industry and the U.S. Food and Drug Administration (FDA) has been seeking efficient methods of drug development as indicated in the FDA's critical path document. Many people believe that the innovative approach of adaptive design is a major pathway to success in drug development in today's challenging drug development environment.

In a book that I co-authored, *Adaptive Design Methods in Clinical Trials* (Chow and Chang, 2006), various adaptive design methods were introduced. Six months later I authored a second book, *Adaptive Design Theory and Implementation Using SAS and R* (Chang, 2007a), which provided in-depth and unified theory regarding adaptive designs and implementations, with many trial examples. These two books require a strong statistical background and clinical trial experience.

However, based on feedback from recent adaptive design workshops and conferences, I realize that there are many practitioners who are very good at strategic thinking and solution of practical problems but little interested in or lacking time to study the theory. Although I have kept the SAS and R program units as small as possible, with a clear logic flow from my previous books, there are still minimal requirements for knowledge of SAS or R. Also, many statisticians who are familiar with SAS would prefer to have software with a graphic user interface that can provide user-friendly tools for both classical and adaptive designs and monitoring. Among other options, I believe that ExpDesign Studio® fits the practical needs and provides a one-stop-shopping experience (CTriSoft, www.CTriSoft.net). This book, which avoids dealing with theory, is complementary to the two books mentioned earlier. Readers can jump-start to adaptive design without difficulty if they have one or two years of clinical trial design experience. However, for readers interested in the mathematical details, the mathematical notes at the end of each chapter will provide the key formulations for each method, or they can review *Adaptive Design Theory and Implementation Using SAS and R* (Chang, 2007a) for an in-depth understanding of the theory and algorithms for computer implementation.

ExpDesign is commercial software used by major pharmaceutical companies, universities, and research institutes worldwide. With ExpDesign you can design a classical or adaptive design literately in two minutes if you have the parameters ready. The ExpDesign enterprise version can also generate SAS and R code for an adaptive design.

The book has been written with practitioners in mind. It is not intended to teach adaptive design theory nor to function as a simple software user manual. The objective of the book is to demonstrate the use of ExpDesign in trial design, to assist strategic decision making, and to help solve issues related to classical and adaptive trials. It is written as a tutorial, a self-learning textbook (see the Self-Study and Practice Guide following the preface). Readers are expected to master the basic adaptive trial techniques in about one week. The book, together with the software, makes learning easy and fun. The accompanying software is a fully professional version of ExpDesign Studio 5.0, not a typical trial version. The book and the software, covering both classical and adaptive designs, can be used to leverage drug development in such a way that statisticians and other parties have more freedom and time to focus on the real issues, not the calculation or theory. The book is organized as follows:

In Chapter 1 we present an overview of the software ExpDesign Studio, provide a feeling for what it can do in trial designs, demonstrate simple design examples from classical, group sequential, adaptive, and other trials with ExpDesign Studio, and explain the basic operation of the software.

Chapter 2 provides an overview of a variety of clinical trial designs, their advantages and disadvantages, and when different classical and adaptive designs can be used.

Chapter 3 focuses on classical designs. After a discussion as to how sample size should be determined and on the variety of factors that affect the decision as to what sample size to use in a trial, examples are given on how to utilize ExpDesign to calculate sample size. Among nearly 150 sample-size calculation methods available in ExpDesign, the examples are carefully chosen to include a variety of designs, types of endpoints, and phases of clinical trials.

In Chapter 4 we discuss group sequential design (GSD), a commonly used and probably the simplest adaptive design. Starting with an overview of group sequential design, how to design and monitor a GSD trial using ExpDesign Studio is discussed. Finally, the key mathematic formulations for GSD are summarized for those interested in the mathematical details.

In Chapter 5 we discuss adaptive trial designs and introduce the stagewise test statistic and stopping rules. Interim analysis and trial monitor tools such as conditional power are described. We also discuss how to use ExpDesign Studio to design sample-size reestimation, drop-loser, biomarker-adaptive, response-adaptive randomization, and adaptive dose-finding trials. The mathematic formulations are summarized in the final section.

In Chapter 6 we discuss the specific design of early-phase oncology trials, because of its uniqueness. It includes multiple-stage single-arm design and dose-escalation design for maximum tolerated dose and show how to use ExpDesign to design oncology trials and how to compare and evaluate different designs based on their operating characteristics.

In Chapter 7 we focus on adaptive trial monitoring. The importance of trial monitoring and mathematic tools for monitoring is discussed, and how to use the trial monitor in ExpDesign to monitor an adaptive trial is described in detail using real-world examples.

In Chapter 8 we present a computer simulation approach in which the test statistic is the same as the classical design. The simulation module in ExpDesign allows for any combinations of the following adaptations: early futility and/or efficacy stopping, sample-size reestimation, drop-loser, and response-adaptive randomization based on the dose–response relationship. Step-by-step instructions are presented with trial examples.

In Chapter 9 we discuss how to get further assistance from ExpDesign. ExpDesign provides many toolkits for design, monitoring, and analysis of trials: the graphical calculator, which allows you to plot complicated mathematical expressions, the probability calculator for probability and percentile calculations, and the confidence interval calculator for exact confidence interval calculations. For advanced users, we also discuss how to use ExpDesign to generate univariate and multivariate data that can be used for various purposes of trial design, monitoring, and risk assessment.

In Chapter 10 we present notes on technique for nearly 100 methods for sample-size calculation, grouped by the number of arms, the trial endpoint, and the analysis basis. We describe the purpose of each method, information about the methods, such as when and how to use each one, the formula and/or references, and the assumptions or limitations of the methods.

Appendix A is about validation of ExpDesign. Several reviewers have indicated the importance of software validation and suggested including the validation information in the book. The validation document is also meant to support pharmaceutical end users to meet FDA 21 CFR part 11 requirements.

Installation instructions for the software CD and the license agreement appear at the end of the pages.

Mark Chang

Lexington, Massachusetts
Winter 2007
www.Statisticians.org

SELF-STUDY AND PRACTICE GUIDE

Day 1

- ExpDesign Studio 5.0 Installation (10 minutes)
- Chapter 1: ExpDesign Studio (30 minutes of reading and practice)
- Chapter 2: Clinical Trial Design (3 hours of reading)
- Chapter 3: Classical Trial Design (4 hours of reading and practice)
- Chapter 10: Classical Design Method Reference (15 minutes of reading)
- Appendix A: Validation of ExpDesign Studio (15 minutes of reading)

Day 2

- Chapter 4: Group Sequential Trial Design (8 hours of reading and practice) The classical group sequential design and simplest adaptive design are discussed. Make sure you understand the basic concepts of group sequential design, such as the notion of early stopping, error inflation due to multiple looks, different types of stopping boundaries, and different scales for stopping boundaries. Go through all the trial examples using ExpDesign; it helps you get "hands-on" experience. Trial monitoring requires your effort, which will give you the feeling of running an actual group sequential trial.

Days 3

- Chapter 5: Adaptive Trial Design (8 hours of reading and practice)
- You will learn various adaptive designs. Make sure that you understand the three commonly used statistical methods. Again, go through the trial practice using ExpDesign for hands-on experiences. The practices are straightforward and should take no more than 20 minutes each.

Day 4

- Chapter 6: Adaptive Trial Monitoring (8 hours of reading and practice) Adaptive trial monitoring can be considered as the most challenging part of this book. It is about how you make actual adaptations for an ongoing trial based on the design without undermining the validity and integrity of the trial. Play around with the trial examples using ExpDesign, and spend extra time if needed.

Day 5

- Chapter 7: Oncology Adaptive Trial Design (5 hours of reading and practice)
- Chapter 8: Adaptive Trial Simulator (2 hours of optional reading and practice)
- Chapter 9: Further Assistance with ExpDesign Studio (1 hour of reading and practice)

The mathematical notes in Chapters 3, 4, and 7 are not meant to be studied in your first reading; rather, they are for future reference. Similarly, Chapter 10 and Appendix A can be read as needed.

1 ExpDesign Studio

1.1 INTRODUCTION

ExpDesign Studio (ExpDesign) is an integrated environment for designing experiments or clinical trials. It is a powerful and user-friendly statistical software product that has seven integrated main components: classical design (CD), sequential design (SD), multistage design (MSD), dose-escalation design (DED), adaptive design (AD), adaptive trial monitoring (ATM), and dose-escalation trial monitoring (DTM) modules. In addition, the ExpDesign randomizor can generate random variates from a variety of distributions. The ExpDesign toolkit provides features for distributional calculation, confidence intervals, and function and data plotting (Figure 1.1).

Classical trials are the most commonly used in practice. ExpDesign provides nearly 150 methods for sample-size calculations in CD for different trial designs. It includes methods for single-, two-, and multiple-group designs, and for superiority, noninferiority, and equivalence designs with various endpoints. See the list of classical design methods in Appendix B.

Group sequential trials are advanced designs with multiple analyses. A group sequential trial is usually a cost-effective design compared to a classical design. SD covers a broad range of sequential trials with different endpoints and different types of stopping boundaries.

A multistage design is an exact method for group sequential trials with a binary response, whereas group sequential design uses an asymptotic approach. MSD provides three optimal designs among others: MinMax, MinExp, and MaxUtility, which minimize the maximum sample size, minimize the expected sample size, and maximize the utility index, respectively.

A dose-escalation trial in aggressive disease areas such as oncology has unique characteristics. Due to the toxicity of the testing drug, researchers are allowed to use fewer patients to obtain as much information as possible about the toxicity profile or maximum tolerable dose. By means of computer simulations, DED provides researchers with an efficient way to search for an optimal design for dose-escalation trials with a variety of criteria. It includes traditional escalation rules, restricted escalation rules, two-stage

Classical and Adaptive Clinical Trial Designs Using ExpDesign Studio™,
By Mark Chang

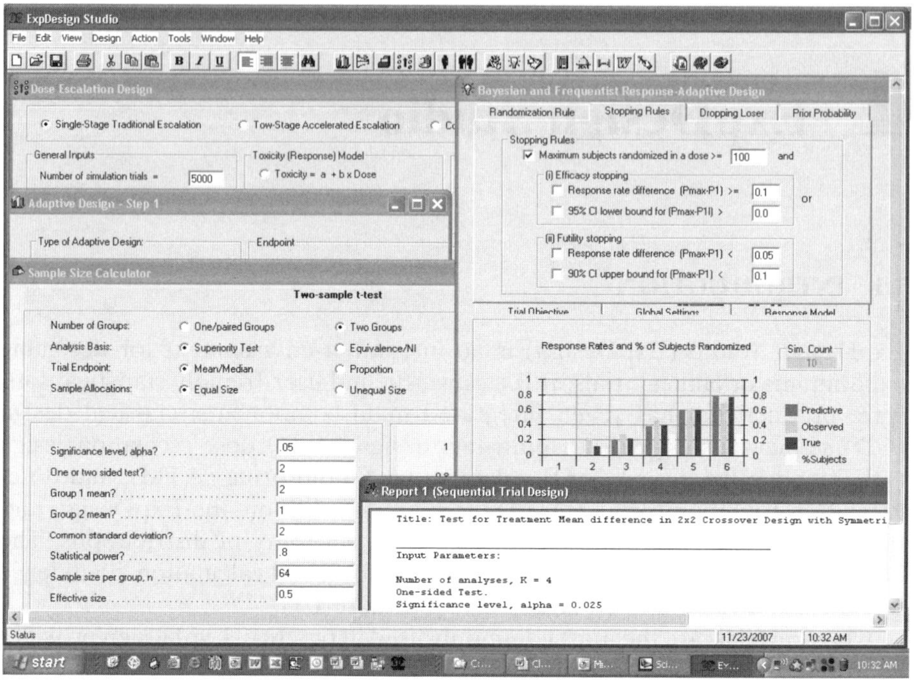

Figure 1.1 ExpDesign integrated environment.

escalation algorithms, and the Bayesian continual reassessment method (CRM).

AD in ExpDesign Studio allows you to design and simulate various adaptive trial, such as sample-size reestimation, dropping a loser, response-adaptive randomization, and biomarker-adaptive designs. You can use response-adaptive randomization to assign more patients to superior treatment groups or to drop a "loser" or inferior group. You may stop a trial prematurely to claim efficacy or futility based on the data observed. You may modify the sample size based on the treatment difference observed. All design reports are generated through an automation procedure that has built-in knowledge of statistical experts in a clinical trial.

ATM and DTM assist in monitoring an ongoing trial. They inform the user if the stopping boundary has been crossed and will also generate interim results such as conditional power, new sample size required, and dynamic randomization to instruct the user to make appropriate adaptations.

Indeed, ExpDesign Studio covers broad statistical tools needed to design a trial. To try ExpDesign, the user simply needs to know the functions of the icons on the toolbar. The black–white icons on the left-hand side of the toolbar are standard for all word processors. The first five icons of the second group of seven icons are used to launch five different types of designs: classical trial

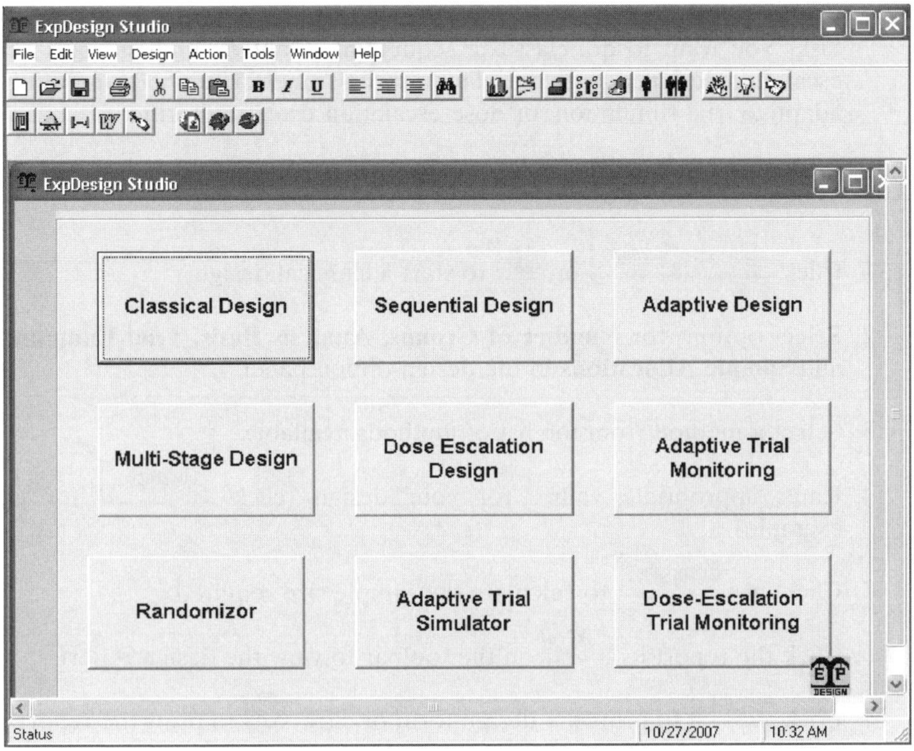

Figure 1.2 ExpDesign Studio startup window.

design, sequential trial design, multistage trial design, dose-escalation trial design, and adaptive design (see Figure 1.2). Alternatively, the user can click one of the nine buttons in the ExpDesign start window to start the corresponding design. The next set of three icons is for launching a design example, computing design parameters, and generating a design report. Following these are five color icons for the toolkits, including a graphic calculator, a distribution calculator, a confidence interval calculator, a word splitter, and TipDay. The mouse can be moved over any icon on the toolbar to see the Tiptext, which describes what the icon is for. We are now ready to design a trial.

1.2 HOW TO DESIGN A TRIAL USING EXPDESIGN STUDIO

1. Double-click on the ExpDesign Studio icon or click Start, the **Start** button. A menu will appear. Click on **Programs** in the **Start** button. The list of available programs will appear. Then click , ExpDesign Studio.

2. On the ExpDesign **Start** window (Figure 1.2), select one of the following tasks you want to do: classical, sequential, adaptive, multistage, dose-escalation design, adaptive trial monitoring, random number generation, adaptive trial simulation, or dose-escalation trial monitoring.

1.2.1 How to Design a Classical Trial

1. Click Classical Design or  to start a classical design.

2. Select options for **Number of Groups, Analysis Basis, Trial Endpoint**, and **Sample Allocations** in the design option panel.

3. Select a method from the list of methods available.

4. Enter appropriate values for your design (click Example for an example).

5. Click on Compute to calculate the sample size required.

6. Click the report icon  on the toolbar to view the design report.

7. Click Print to print the design form or click  to print the report.

8. You can click Copy Graph to copy the graph for the stopping boundaries and use **Paste-Special** to paste it to other applications.

9. Click 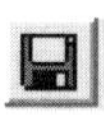 to save the design specification or report (see Figure 1.3).

1.2.2 How to Design a Group Sequential Trial

1. Click Sequential Design or 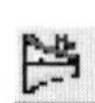 on the toolbar to start a group sequential design.

2. Select options for **Number of Groups, Analysis Basis, Trial Endpoint**, and **Potential Interim Claim** in the design option panel.

3. Select a method from the list of methods available.

4. Enter appropriate values for your design or click Example.

5. Click Compute to generate the design.

6. Click the report icon 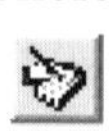 on the toolbar to view the design report.

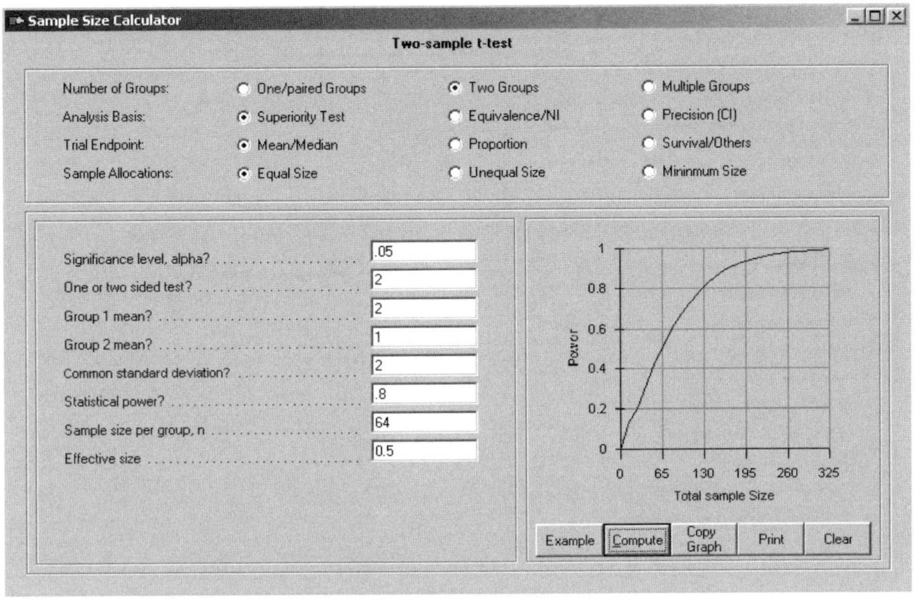

Figure 1.3 Classical design window.

7. Click Print to print the design form or click  to print the report.

8. You can click Copy Graph to copy the graph for the stopping boundaries and use **Paste-Special** to paste it to other applications.

9. Click Save to save the design specification or report (see Figure 1.4).

1.2.3 How to Design an Adaptive Trial

1. Click Adaptive Design or 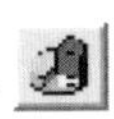 on the toolbar; the **Adaptive Design–Step 1** window will appear (see Figure 1.5).

2. Select the **Sample-Size Reestimation** option in the **Type of Adaptive Design** panel.

3. Select the **Proportion** option in the **Endpoint** panel.

4. Enter appropriate values for the **Response Under Ha** in the **Hypotheses** panel, the noninferiority margin for the noninferiority trial, **One-Sided Alpha,** and **Power**.

5. Click Next; the **Adaptive Design–Step 2** window will appear.

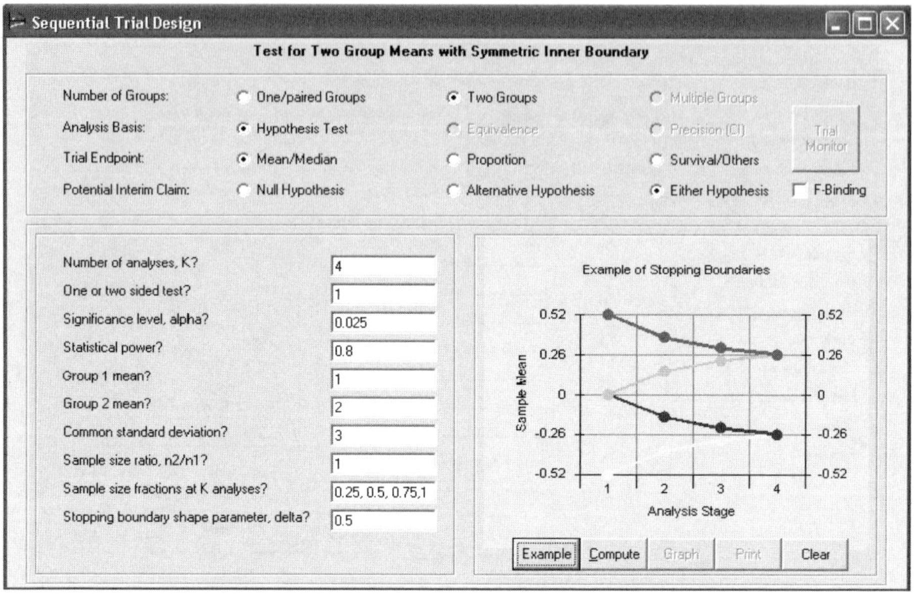

Figure 1.4 Group sequential design window.

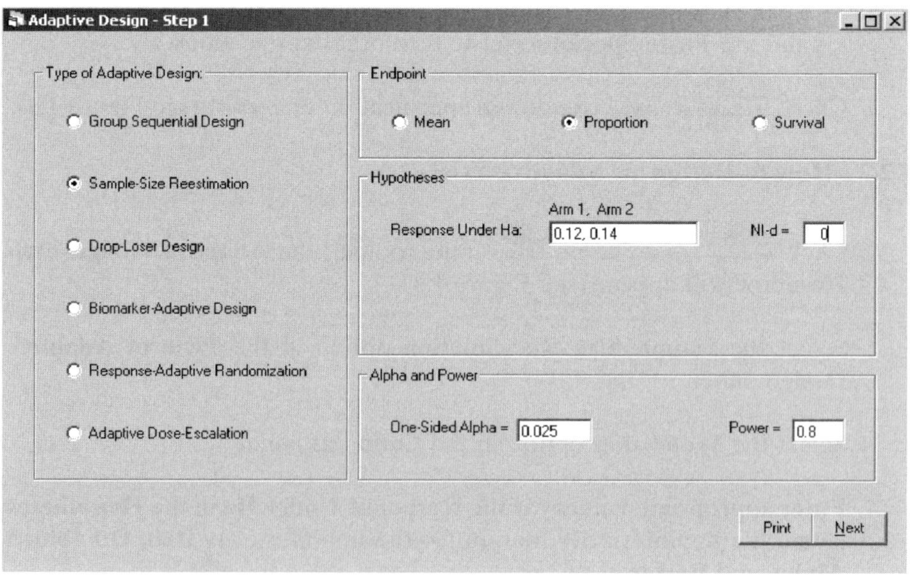

Figure 1.5 Sample size reestimation step 1 window.

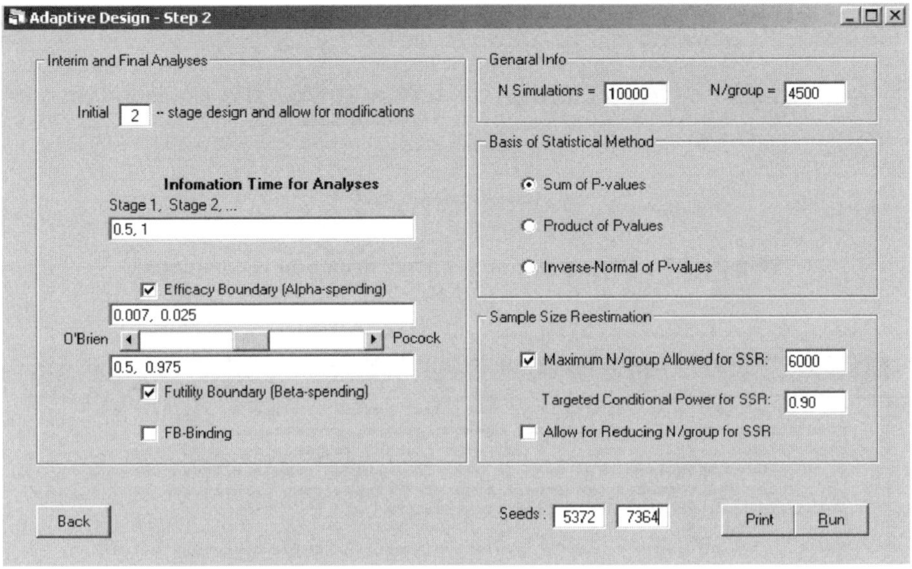

Figure 1.6 Sample size reestimation step 2 window.

In the **Adaptive Design–Step 2** window, do the following (Figure 1.6):

1. Enter values for the initial number of stages and **Information Time for Analyses**.
2. Choose stopping boundaries using the arrow near **O'Brien** or **Pocock**.
3. Enter values for **N Simulations** and **N/group**.
4. Select a statistical method in the panel.
5. Enter values for **Maximum N/group Allowed for SSR** and **Targeted Conditional Power for SSR**.
6. Click Run to start the simulation.

After the simulation is completed, the window in Figure 1.7 will pop up to remind you to click the report icon on the toolbar to view the report that is generated automatically for the adaptive design. Figure 1.8 is an example of the report for the adaptive design.

1.2.4 How to Run Adaptive Trial Simulations

1. Click Adaptive Trial Simulator to set up adaptive trial simulations.
2. Follow the steps specified in the **Simulation Setup** panel.

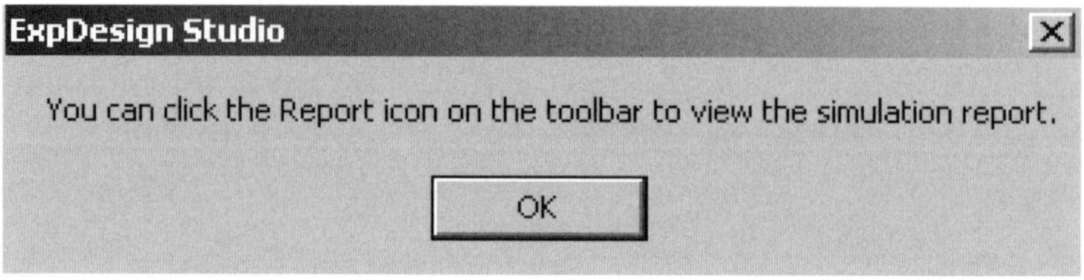

Figure 1.7 Pop-up message when calculation is completed.

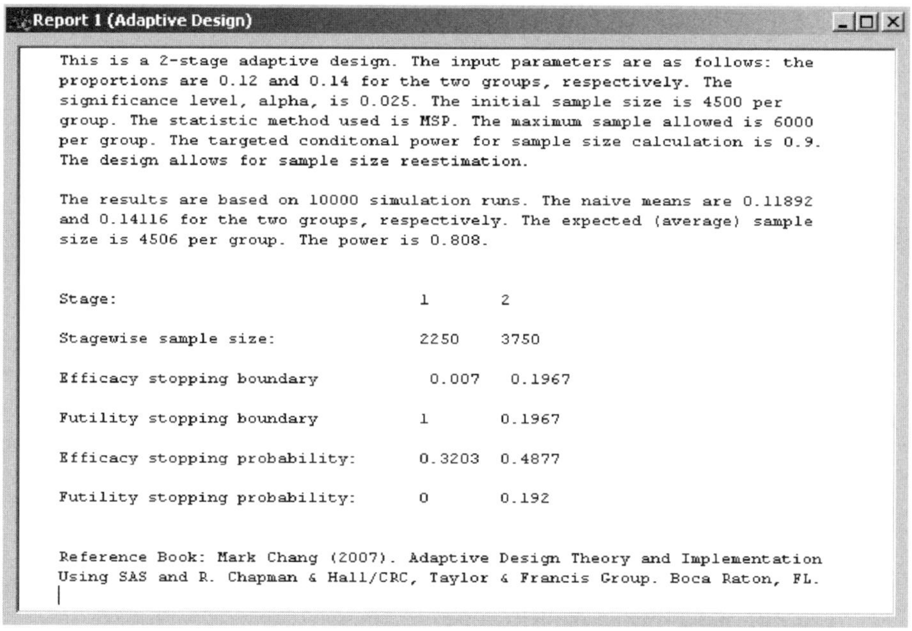

This is a 2-stage adaptive design. The input parameters are as follows: the proportions are 0.12 and 0.14 for the two groups, respectively. The significance level, alpha, is 0.025. The initial sample size is 4500 per group. The statistic method used is MSP. The maximum sample allowed is 6000 per group. The targeted conditonal power for sample size calculation is 0.9. The design allows for sample size reestimation.

The results are based on 10000 simulation runs. The naive means are 0.11892 and 0.14116 for the two groups, respectively. The expected (average) sample size is 4506 per group. The power is 0.808.

Stage:	1	2
Stagewise sample size:	2250	3750
Efficacy stopping boundary	0.007	0.1967
Futility stopping boundary	1	0.1967
Efficacy stopping probability:	0.3203	0.4877
Futility stopping probability:	0	0.192

Reference Book: Mark Chang (2007). Adaptive Design Theory and Implementation Using SAS and R. Chapman & Hall/CRC, Taylor & Francis Group. Boca Raton, FL.

Figure 1.8 Report generated automatically by ExpDesign.

3. Specify parameters in each of the steps or click **Example**.
4. Click **Run** to generate the simulation results.
5. Click the report icon  to view the design report.
6. Click **Print** to print the design form or click 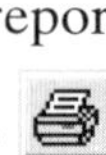 to print the report.
7. Click **Save** to save the design specification or report, whichever is highlighted (see Figure 1.9).

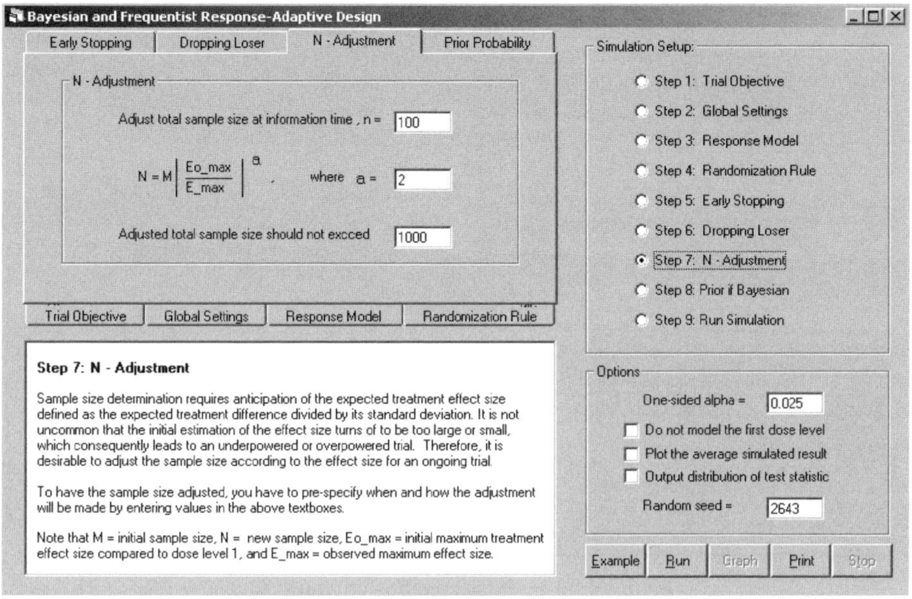

Figure 1.9 Trial simulation window.

1.2.5 How to Design a Multistage Trial

1. Click Multistage Design or 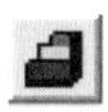 on the toolbar to start a multistage design.
2. Select **2-Stage Design** or **3-Stage Design** in the Multistage design window or open an existing design by clicking  on the toolbar.
3. Enter appropriate values for your design in the textboxes. You may click Example to see an input example.
4. Click Compute to generate the valid designs.
5. Click  on the toolbar to view the design report.
6. Click Print to print the design form or  to print a report.
7. Click 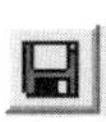 to save the design specification or report (see Figure 1.10).

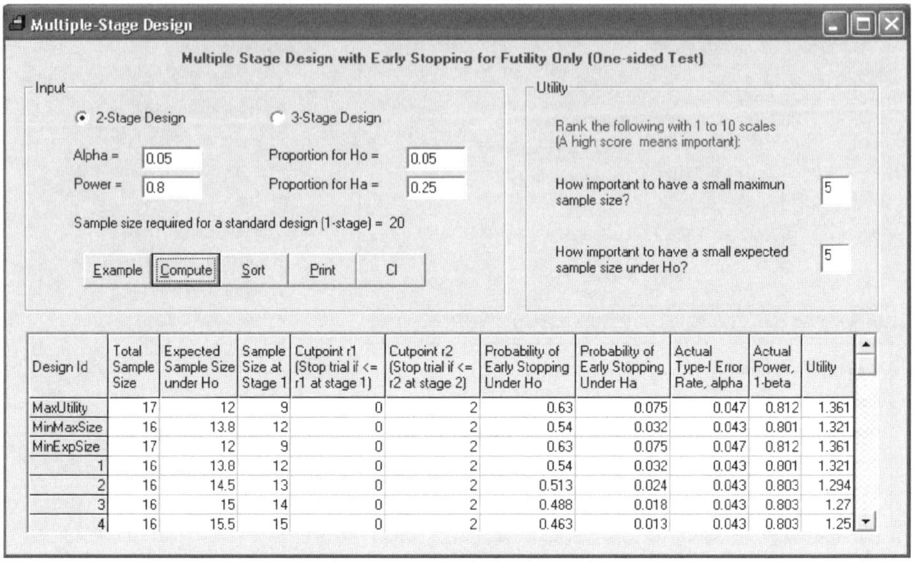

Figure 1.10 Multistage design window.

1.2.6 How to Design a Dose-Escalation Trial

1. Click 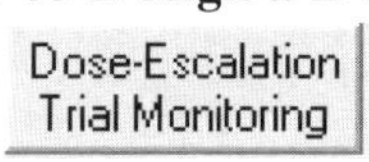

or  on the toolbar to start a dose-escalation design.

2. Enter appropriate values for your design on the *Basic Spec.* panel. You may click 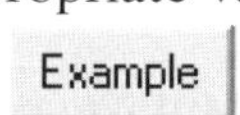

to see an input example.

3. Select *Dose-Response Model, Escalation Scheme*, and *Dose Interval Spec*. or open an existing design by clicking .

4. Click 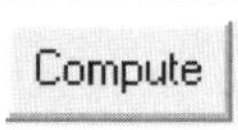

to generate the simulation results.

5. Click 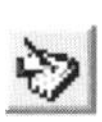 to view the design report.

6. Click 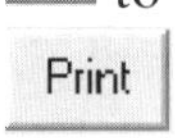

to print the design form or  to print a report.

7. Click 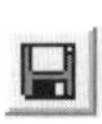 to save the design specification or report, whichever is highlighted (see Figure 1.11).

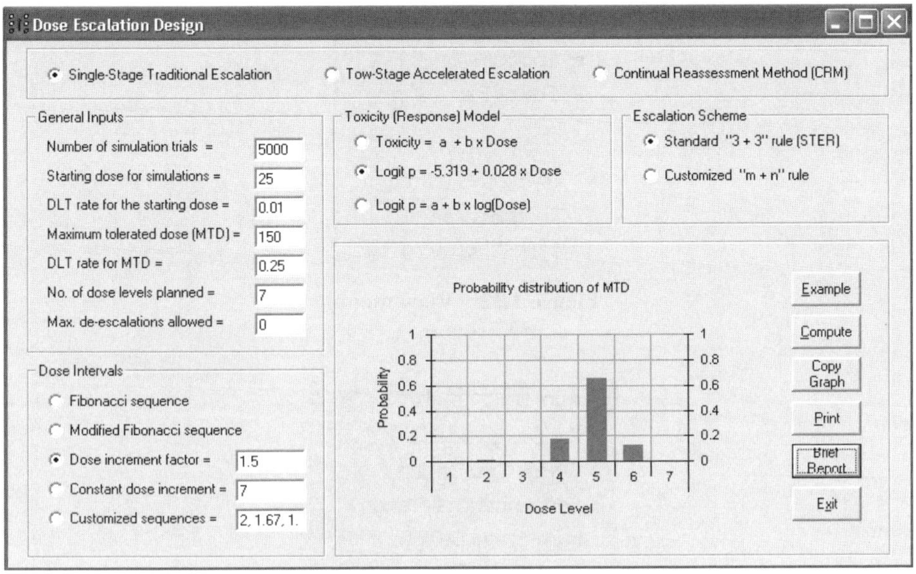

Figure 1.11 Traditional dose-escalation design window.

1.3 EXPDESIGN MENUS

File Menu The ExpDesign file menu is a standard menu similar to that in MS Word. The **Save** option can be used to save a report generated by ExpDesign or design specifications. The **Print** option can be used to print a report generated by ExpDesign.

Edit Menu The edit menu is a standard menu just like the one in MS Word. The hotkey combinations for **cut, copy**, and **paste** are <Ctrl>-X, <Ctrl>-C, and <Ctrl>-V, respectively.

View Menu The view menu is shown in Figure 1.12. The **Toolbar** option toggles between displaying and hiding the toolbar. If the option has a check mark beside it, the toolbar is on and displayed in the ExpDesign window. When you select **Toolbar**, the toolbar will disappear from the ExpDesign window. If the **Toolbar** option has no check mark beside it, the toolbar is off and is not displayed in the ExpDesign window. The **Status Bar** option toggles between displaying and hiding the status bar. It lies at the bottom of your ExpDesign window. The bar displays useful information during the design.

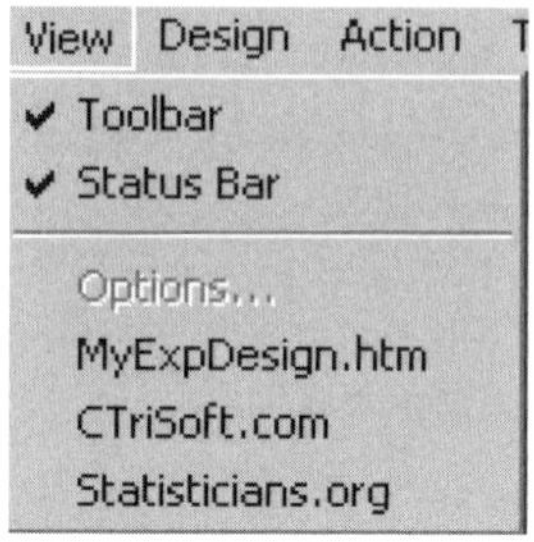

Figure 1.12 View menu.

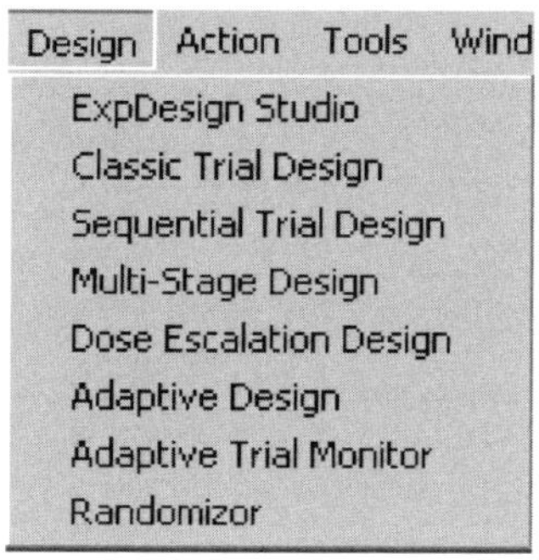

Figure 1.13 Design menu.

The **MyExpDesign Studio.htm** option can be used to access the local Web page, which you can change as you like. To edit the page, you can use MS Word by right-clicking on **MyExpDesignStudio.htm** and selecting the **Edit** item from the pop-up menu. The **CTriSoft.com** option can be used to access the ExpDesign Web site, www.CTriSoft.net, where users can get technical support and product information. The **Statisticians.org** option can be used to access the relevant information to trial design and statistics.

Design Menu The design menu is shown in Figure 1.13. The option **ExpDesign Studio** can be used to display the start window for classical, sequential, multistage, dose-escalation trial, and adaptive designs; and for adaptive trial monitoring, dose-escalation monitoring, the randomizor, and the adaptive trial simulator. The options **Classic Trial Design, Sequential Trial Design, Multi-Stage Design, Dose Escalation Design, Adaptive Design, Adaptive Trial Monitor**, and **Randomizor** can be used for the corresponding task.

Action Menu The action menu has three items: **Example, Compute**, and **Report** (Figure 1.14). The **Example** option can be used to launch an example of a design. The **Compute** option can be used to generate a design after the appropriate inputs. The **Report** option can be used to view a design report.

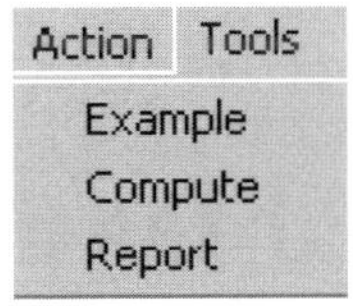

Figure 1.14 Action menu.

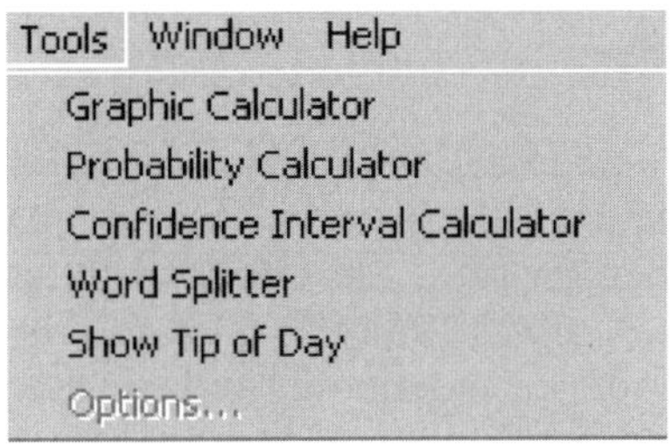

Figure 1.15 Tools menu.

Tools Menu In the tools menu (Figure 1.15) the **Graphic Calculator** option can be used to access the calculator to perform simple arithmetic and complex function calculations, and to plot curves. The **Probability Calculator** option can be used to obtain probabilities and percentiles for various continuous and discrete distributions. The **Confidence Interval Calculator** option can be used to obtain various confidence intervals.

Window and Help Menus The window and help menus are standard, just like those in MS Word.

2 Clinical Trial Design

2.1 INTRODUCTION

As indicated by Chow and Liu (1998), the process of drug research and development is a lengthy and costly process. An adequate and well-controlled study is necessary to demonstrate the efficacy and safety of a drug product under investigation. Section 314.126 of 21 CFR (*Code of Federal Regulations*) provides a definition of an adequate and well-controlled study, which requires:

- *Objectives*: clear statement of an investigation's purpose
- *Methods of analysis*: summary of proposed or actual methods of analysis
- *Design*: valid comparison with a control to provide a quantitative assessment of a drug effect
- *Selection of subjects*: adequate assurance of the disease or conditions under study
- *Assignment of subjects*: minimization of bias and assurance of comparability of groups
- *Participants of studies*: minimization of bias on the part of subjects, observers, and analysis
- *Assessment of responses*: well defined and reliable responses
- *Assessment of the effect*: requirement of appropriate statistical methods

2.2 CLASSICAL CLINICAL TRIAL DESIGN

We review briefly some of the basic concepts of clinical trials. Definitions of the various trials are based on the ICH guidelines (1998) for statistical principles for clinical trials, and the FDA guidelines (2001) for bioequivalence trials (www.fda.gov/cder/guidance/index.htm).

Classical and Adaptive Clinical Trial Designs Using ExpDesign Studio™,
By Mark Chang

2.2.1 Substantial Evidence

For a drug approval, the FDA requires substantial evidence of efficacy and safety. As indicated in the Kefauver–Harris amendments to the Food, Drug and Cosmetics Act of 1962, the term *substantial evidence*, means evidence consisting of adequate and well-controlled investigations, including clinical investigations, by experts qualified by scientific training and experience to evaluate the effectiveness of the drug involved, on the basis of which it could fairly and responsibly be concluded by such experts that the drug will have the effect it purports to have, or is represented to have, under the conditions of use prescribed, recommended, or suggested in the labeling or proposed labeling thereof.

2.2.2 Clinical Trial Endpoint

Clinical trial endpoints can be classified as primary or secondary. *Primary endpoints* measure outcomes that will answer the most important question being asked by a trial, such as whether a new treatment will reduce the incidence of heart attack or mortality, or prolong survival. *Secondary endpoints* ask other important relevant questions in the same study, so they may potentially be included in the drug labeling. It is important to consider a reasonable number of secondary endpoints, because every endpoint added will usually have to pay the multiplicity penalty statistically. An endpoint may be based on a binary, continuous, or time-to-event clinical outcome, indicating whether an event such as death from any cause has occurred.

In choosing endpoints, it is important to ensure that they:

- Are clinically meaningful and related to the "intend-to-treat" disease
- Answer the important question to be answered by the trial
- Are practical so that they can be assessed in all subjects in the same way
- Are easily assessed with reasonable precision such that the study will have adequate statistical power or the size of the trial is feasible

2.2.3 Confirmatory Trials

A *confirmatory trial* is an adequately controlled trial in which the hypotheses are stated in advance and evaluated. As a rule, confirmatory trials are necessary to provide firm evidence of efficacy or safety. In such trials the key hypothesis of interest follows directly from the trial's primary objective, is always predefined, and is the hypothesis that is subsequently tested when the trial is complete. In a confirmatory trial it is equally important to estimate with due precision the size of the effects attributable to the treatment of interest and to relate these effects to their clinical significance. ExpDesign provides designs, including sample-size calculation methods, for both confirmatory and exploratory trials (see below).

2.2.4 Exploratory Trials

The rationale and design of confirmatory trials nearly always rests on earlier clinical work carried out in a series of *exploratory studies*. Like all clinical trials, exploratory studies should have clear and precise objectives. However, in contrast to confirmatory trials, their objectives may not always lead to simple tests of predefined hypotheses. In addition, exploratory trials may sometimes require a more flexible approach to design so that changes can be made in response to accumulating results. Their analysis may entail data exploration; tests of hypothesis may be carried out, but the choice of hypothesis may be data dependent. Such trials cannot be the basis of the formal proof of efficacy, although they may contribute to the total body of relevant evidence. Any individual trial may have both confirmatory and exploratory aspects.

2.2.5 Multicenter Trials

Multicenter trials are carried out for two main reasons. First, a multicenter trial is an accepted way of evaluating a new medication more efficiently; under some circumstances, it may present the only practical means of accruing sufficient subjects to satisfy the trial objective within a reasonable time frame. Second, a trial may be designed as a multicenter (and multi-investigator) trial primarily to provide a better basis for the subsequent generalization of its findings. ExpDesign features various sample-size calculation methods for trials with or without a center effect.

2.2.6 Trials to Show Superiority

Scientifically, efficacy is established most convincingly by demonstrating superiority to a placebo in a placebo-controlled trial, by showing superiority to an active control treatment, or by demonstrating a dose–response relationship. This type of trial is referred to as a *superiority trial*. For serious illnesses, when a therapeutic treatment that has been shown to be efficacious by superiority trial(s) exists, a placebo-controlled trial may be considered unethical. In that case, the scientifically sound use of an active treatment as a control should be considered. The appropriateness of placebo control versus active control should be considered on a trial-by-trial basis. A large portion of the methodologies in ExpDesign are for trials showing superiority.

2.2.7 Trials to Show Equivalence or Noninferiority

In some cases, an investigational product is compared to a reference treatment without the objective of showing superiority. This type of trial is divided into two major categories according to its objective; one is an *equivalence trial* and the other is a *noninferiority trial*. *Bioequivalence trials* fall into the former category. In some situations, clinical equivalence trials are also undertaken for other regulatory reasons, such as demonstrating the clinical equivalence of a generic product to a marketed product when the compound is not absorbed and therefore is not present in the bloodstream. Many active control trials are designed to show that the efficacy of an investigational product is no worse than that of the active comparator, and hence fall into the latter category. Another possibility is a trial in which multiple doses of the investigational drug are compared with the recommended dose or multiple doses of the standard drug. The purpose of this design is to show simultaneously a dose–response relationship for the investigational product and a comparison of the investigational product with the active control. ExpDesign has implemented a list of methods or designs for equivalence, noninferiority, and bioequivalence trials.

2.2.8 Trials to Show a Dose–Response Relationship

How response is related to the dose of a new investigational product is a question to which answers may be obtained in all phases of development and by a variety of approaches. Dose–response trials may serve a number of objectives, among which the following are of particular importance: confirmation of efficacy, investigation of the shape and location of the dose–response curve, estimation of an appropriate starting dose, identification of optimal strategies for individual dose adjustments, and determination of a maximal dose beyond which additional benefits would be unlikely to occur. These objectives should be addressed using the data collected at a number of doses under investigation, including a placebo (zero dose) wherever appropriate. Various sample-size calculation methods are available for a dose–response trial with different endpoints.

2.2.9 Parallel Design

A *parallel design* is a design in which each patient receives one and only one treatment, usually in a random fashion. A parallel design can be two or more treatment groups with one or more control groups. Parallel designs are commonly used in clinical trials because they are simple, universally accepted, and applicable to acute conditions. ExpDesign provides comprehensive tools for the parallel designs, including classical sequential designs.

2.2.10 Crossover Design

A common and generally satisfactory use of the 2 × 2 *crossover design* is to demonstrate the bioequivalence of two formulations of the same medication. In this particular application in healthy volunteers, carryover effects on the relevant pharmacokinetic variable are most unlikely to occur if the washout time between the two periods is sufficiently long. However, it is still important to check this assumption during analysis on the basis of the data obtained: for example, by demonstrating that no drug is detectable at the start of each period. ExpDesign provides sample calculation methods for crossover designs.

2.2.11 Factorial Design

In a *factorial design*, two or more treatments are evaluated simultaneously through the use of varying combinations of treatments. The simplest example is the 2×2 factorial design, in which subjects are randomly allocated to one of the four possible combinations of two treatments: A and B, say. These are A alone, B alone, both A and B, neither A nor B. In many cases the design is used for the specific purpose of examining the interaction of A and B. The statistical test of interaction may lack power to detect an interaction if the sample size was calculated based on the test for main effects. This consideration is important when the design is used for examining the joint effects of A and B: in particular, if the treatments are likely to be used together. Another important use of a factorial design is to establish the dose–response characteristics of the simultaneous use of treatments C and D, especially when the efficacy of each monotherapy has been established at some dose in prior trials. A number m of doses of C is selected, usually including a zero dose (placebo), and a similar number n of doses of D. The full design then consists of $m \times n$ treatment groups, each receiving a different combination of doses of C and D. The resulting estimate of the response surface may then be used to help identify an appropriate combination of doses of C and D for clinical use. ExpDesign provides users with a variety of sample-size calculation methods for trials with interaction terms presented in the model.

2.3 SELECTION OF A TRIAL DESIGN

2.3.1 Balanced Versus Unbalanced Designs

Balanced designs are commonly used in clinical trials, but unbalanced designs have several advantages and can be used in the following situations.

1. When recruiting one group is easier than recruiting other groups, allocating more patients in one group could be cost-effective.
2. When the treatment variability or incidence rate is different among experimental groups, allocating more subjects in the group with the greatest variability could reduce the total sample size.
3. In a placebo-controlled trial, when there is a requirement for the minimum number of exposures to a test drug but a balanced design is overpowered, allocating more subjects in the active group could reduce the total sample size.
4. For ethical considerations regarding the control (e.g., the placebo), one can allocate more patients to receive the active treatment.

2.3.2 Crossover Versus Parallel Designs

Parallel Design As mentioned earlier, parallel designs are commonly used in clinical trials because they are simple, universally accepted, and applicable to acute conditions. However, a parallel design usually requires more patients than do comparative designs. A parallel design can be stratified using prognostic characteristics, which can be accomplished using a stratified randomization scheme. The *matched-pairs parallel design* is a design in which each patient is *matched* with another patient of similar prognostic characteristics for the disease under investigation. One patient in each pair is assigned the treatment, and the other receives the control. A matched-pairs parallel design can reduce the sample size, but matched-pairs designs make patient recruitment difficult and slow and therefore are uncommon in clinical trials. Although at the planning stage it is almost impossible to identify all of the covariates that may have an impact on a disease, an unbiased estimate of the treatment effect can still be obtained by adjusting these covariates, regardless of whether or not they are used for stratification.

For a parallel design, each patient receiving one treatment, the variability observed for any comparisons between groups contains both interpatient and intrapatient variabilities, which cannot be separated and estimated, due to the nature of the parallel design. As a result, a parallel design does not provide independent estimates of interpatient and intrapatient variabilities. In practice, a parallel-group design is an appropriate design for comparative clinical trials if the interpatient variability is relatively small compared to the intrapatient variability. This is because a valid and efficient comparison between treatments is often assessed based on the intrapatient variability.

Crossover Design A crossover trial is a special type of repeated-measurements experiment. The main feature that distinguishes a crossover trial from the traditional repeated-measures trial is that a sequence of two or more treatments is applied to each subject. A crossover design can be viewed as a modified randomized block design in which each block receives more than one treatment in different dosing periods. A block can be a patient or a group of patients. Patients in each block receive different sequences of treatments. A crossover design is called a *complete crossover design* if each sequence contains all treatments under investigation. For a crossover design it is not necessary that the number of treatments in each sequence be greater than or equal to the number of treatments to be compared. We refer to a crossover design as a *$p \times q$ crossover design* if there are p sequences of treatments administered at q different time periods (Ratkowsky et al., 1993).

A crossover design has the following advantages: (1) it allows a within-patient comparison between treatments, since each patient serves as his or her own control; (2) it removes the interpatient variability from the comparison between treatments; and (3) with proper randomization of patients to the treatment sequences, it provides the best unbiased estimates for the differences between treatments.

An important feature of crossover designs is the presence of, and the ability to measure, *carryover effects*. Carryover effects are commonly viewed as a manifestation of treatment at a future time and may result from a "late response" to treatment in a clinical trial, as may happen with human subjects in a psychological experiment. Sometimes, steps are taken by the experimenter to prevent or mitigate the occurrence of carryover effects by use of a *washout period* between applications of drugs or treatments. However, in other experiments, such as psychological tests and certain clinical trials, the ability to estimate carryover may be the main focus of interest in the experiment (Ratkowsky et al., 1993).

The separability of treatment and carryover effects is an important characteristic of a crossover design. There are two major reasons for concern about one's ability to separate direct treatment effects from carryover effects and both concern the interpretability of the results of the analysis of variance of a crossover design. The first reason relates to circumstances where the investigator will not know whether a treatment effect is truly a direct treatment effect or rather, a residual effect of some other treatment. The second reason for wishing to separate direct and carryover effects relates to a phenomenon akin to multicollinearity in multiple regression applications with continuous variables. There, the presence of two multicollinear explanatory (regressor) variables in the model may lead to the erroneous interpretation that there are neither significant direct treatment effects nor carryover effects (Ratkowsky et al., 1993). This is illustrated further in the following example.

A 2×2 crossover design (two-treatment, two-period, two-sequence) yields only four cell means (the responses for each of two sequences in each of two periods), which cannot be used to estimate more than four parameters. If a carryover parameter is present in the model, the 2×2 design is not analyzable without making some strong assumptions. This is because one of these parameters is the overall grand mean, another represents differences between periods, and a third, differences between treatments. One can get an estimate of differential carryover effects as the fourth parameter only by making a strong assumption, such as that there is no sequence effect, or there is no period-by-treatment interaction.

When more than two treatments are to be compared, complete crossover becomes much more complicated and may not be of practical interest because (1) potential residual effects make the assessment of efficacy and/or safety almost impossible; (2) it takes longer to complete the study; and (3) patients are likely to drop out if they are required to return frequently for tests.

Note that crossover designs may be used in clinical trials in the following situations, where (1) objective measures and interpretable data are obtained for both efficacy and safety; (2) chronic (relatively stable) diseases are under study; (3) prophylactic drugs with a relatively short half-life are being investigated; (4) relatively short treatment periods are considered; (5) baseline and washout periods are feasible and (6) an adequate number of patients for detection of the carryover effect with sufficient power that accounts for expected dropouts is feasible, or extra study information is available to rule on the carryover effect (Ratkowsky et al., 1993; Chow and Liu, 1998).

2.3.3 Dose Escalation Versus Titration Designs

Dose-escalation design is used for early phases of clinical trials. The primary goal of a dose-escalation trial is to identify the *maximum tolerated dose* (MTD). The participants are usually healthy volunteers. The first group (usually about 8 to 12 subjects) is treated with the lowest dose level. If there is no or low toxicity, the second group of patients will be enrolled and treated at a higher dose level. The procedure continues until the highest tolerated dose is identified. Sometimes different doses are applied to the same group of subjects to determine, for example, the maximum efficacy dose. In this case, the dose-escalation trial is called *titration design*. One of the advantages of using different groups for different doses is that it can avoid drug accumulation in the body. Otherwise, a washout period is required between dosages, thus prolonging the trial duration.

For aggressive disease treatment, such as oncology, the use of healthy volunteers is considered nonethical, due to the fact that oncology drugs for testing are usually highly toxic. In addition, the patient population is usually rather heterogeneous, with some medical complications. A limited number of patients are available for trials and there is a high chance of withdrawals, which may or may not be related to the toxicity of the study drug. For these reasons, there are usually three to six patients at each dose level in oncology trials. To identify the MTD, a special dose-escalation algorithm has to be used. The most popular one is the *3 + 3 traditional escalation rule.*

2.3.4 Bioavailability Versus Bioequivalence Designs

The *bioavailability* of a drug is defined as the rate and extent to which the active drug ingredient or therapeutic moiety is absorbed and becomes available at the site of drug action. A *comparative bioavailability study* involves a comparison of bioavailabilities of different formulations of the same drug or different drug products. When two formulations of the same drug or two drug products are claimed to be *bioequivalent*, it is assumed that they will provide the same therapeutic effect or that they are therapeutically equivalent. Two drug products are considered *pharmaceutical equivalents* if they contain identical amounts of the same active ingredient. Two drugs are identified as *pharmaceutical alternatives* to each other if both contain an identical therapeutic moiety but not necessarily in the same amount or dosage form or as the same salt or ester. Two drug products are said to be bioequivalent if they are pharmaceutical equivalents (i.e., similar dosage forms made, perhaps, by different manufacturers) or pharmaceutical alternatives (i.e., different dosage forms) and if their rates and extents of absorption do not show a significant difference when administered at the same molar dose of the therapeutic moiety under similar experimental conditions. For more on the bioequivalence test, see the book by Chow and Liu (2003).

2.3.5 Equivalence Versus Bioequivalence

The criteria for equivalence or, more often, noninferiority are usually dependent on the particular disease targeted by the drugs. However, for a bioequivalance study, there are some strict rules. In the July 1992 FDA guidelines on statistical procedures for bioequivalence studies using a standard two-treatment crossover design, the Center for Drug Evaluation and Research (CDER) recommended that a standard in vivo bioequivalence study design be based on the administration of either single or multiple doses of the treatment and response (T and R) products to healthy subjects on separate occasions, with random assignment to the two possible sequences of drug product administration. The 1992 guidance further recommended that statistical analysis for pharmacokinetic measures, such as area under the curve (AUC) and peak concentration ($C_{\max}$), be based on the *two one-sided test procedure* to determine whether the average values for the pharmacokinetic measures determined after administration of the T and R products were comparable. This approach, termed *average bioequivalence*, involves calculation of a 90% confidence interval for the ratio of the averages (population geometric means) of the measures for the T and R products. To establish bioequivalence, the confidence interval calculated should fall within a bioequivalence (BE) limit, usually 80 to 125% for the ratio of the product averages. In addition to this general approach, the 1992 guidance provided specific recommendations for (1) logarithmic transformation of pharmacokinetic data, (2) methods to evaluate sequence effects, and (3) methods to evaluate outlier data. In practice, people also use parallel designs and a 90% confidence interval for nontransformed data. To establish bioequivalence, the confidence interval calculated should fall within a BE limit, usually 80 to 120% for the difference of the product averages (Ratkowsky et al., 1993; Chow and Liu, 2003).

Although average bioequivalence is recommended for a comparison of BE measures in most studies, the FDA 2001 guidance describes two new approaches, *population* and *individual bioequivalence*. These new approaches may be useful, in some instances, for analyzing in vitro and in vivo BE studies. The average BE approach focuses on a comparison of population averages of a BE measure of interest and not on the variances of the measure for the T and R products. The average BE method does not assess a subject-by-formulation interaction variance, that is, variation in the average T and R difference among individuals. In contrast, population and individual BE approaches include comparisons of averages and variances of the measure. The population BE approach assesses the total variability of the measure in the population. The individual BE approach assesses within-subject variability for T and R products as well as subject-by-formulation interaction. For population and individual bioequivalences, 95% confidence intervals are recommended, with the same BE limits as those for average bioequivalence (Ratkowsky et al., 1993; Chow and Liu, 2003).

2.3.6 Sample-Size Determination

The number of subjects in a clinical trial should always be large enough to provide a reliable answer to the questions addressed. This number is usually determined by the primary objective of the trial. If the sample size is determined on some other basis, this should be made clear and justified. For example, a trial sized on the basis of safety questions or requirements, or important secondary objectives, may require larger numbers of subjects than those required for a trial sized on the basis of the primary efficacy question. Using the most common method for determining the appropriate sample size, the following items should be specified: a primary variable, the test statistic, the null hypothesis, the alternative hypothesis at the dose(s) chosen, the probability of erroneously rejecting the null hypothesis (type I error), and the probability of erroneously failing to reject the null hypothesis (type II error), as well as the approach to dealing with treatment withdrawal and protocol violations. Sample-size calculations should refer to the number of subjects required (sometimes the number of events for a survival endpoint) for the primary analysis. Assumptions about variability may also need to be revised. The sample size of an equivalence or noninferiority trial should normally be based on the objective of obtaining a confidence interval for the treatment difference which shows that the treatments differ at most by a clinically acceptable difference. When the power of an equivalence trial is assessed at a true difference of zero, the sample size necessary to achieve this power is underestimated if the true difference is not zero. When the power of a noninferiority trial is assessed at a zero difference, the sample size needed to achieve that power will be underestimated if the effect of the investigational product is less than that of the active control. The choice of a clinically acceptable difference needs justification with respect to its meaning for future patients and may be smaller than the clinically relevant difference referred to above in the context of superiority trials designed to establish that a difference exists.

2.4 ADAPTIVE CLINICAL TRIAL DESIGN

As indicated by a white paper by the PhRMA Adaptive Design Group (Gallo et al., 2006), an adaptive design is a clinical study design that uses accumulating data to decide how to modify aspects of the study as it continues, without undermining the validity and integrity of the trial (see Figure 2.1). As indicated further by a white paper by the BIO Adaptive Design Working Group (M. Chang et al., 2007), an adaptive design usually consists of two or more stages; at each stage, data analyses are conducted and adaptations are made based on updated information to maximize the chance of success. Various aspects of a

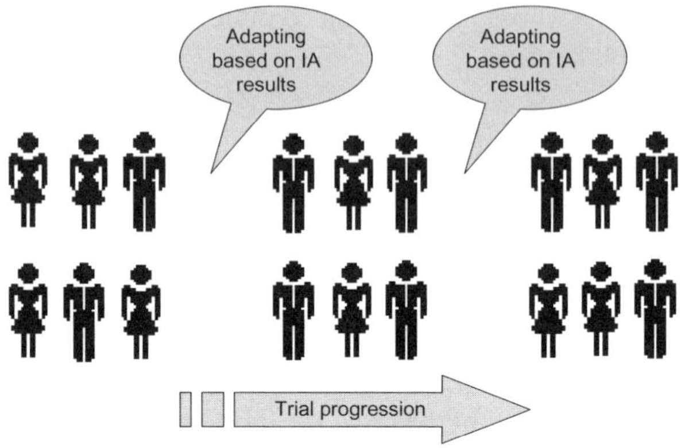

Figure 2.1 Adaptive design.

trial design can be modified or adapted. The adaptations may include, but are not limited to, (1) adjusting sample size, (2) stopping early due to efficacy or futility, (3) changing the timing and the number of analyses, (4) dropping inferior treatment groups, (5) adding new treatment groups, (6) response-adaptive randomization, (7) modifying the target population, (8) changing study endpoints, (9) treatment switch (crossover), and (10) any combination of the foregoing adaptations.

An adaptive design has to preserve the validity and integrity of a trial. The validity includes internal and external validities. *Internal validity* is the degree to which we are successful in eliminating confounding variables and establishing a cause–effect relationship (treatment effect) within the study itself. A study that readily allows its findings to generalize to the population at large has high *external validity*. *Integrity* involves minimizing operational bias (M. Chang, 2007a).

2.4.1 Group Sequential Design

A *group sequential design*, the most commonly used adaptive design, consists of multiple stages. An *interim analysis* (IA) is planned at each stage. Based on results from an IA, a decision can be made either to stop to reject the null hypothesis of no treatment effect, or to accept the null hypothesis, or to continue on to the next stage. For a trial with a positive result, early stopping ensures that a new drug product can be exploited sooner. If a negative result is indicated, early stopping avoids wasting resources. Sequential methods typically lead to savings in sample size, time, and cost compared with a classical design with a fixed sample size.

There are three different types of group sequential designs: early efficacy stopping design if permitting only early claiming efficacy, early futility stopping design if permitting only claiming futility, and early efficacy or a futility stopping design if permitting either efficacy or a futility claim. If we believe (based on prior knowledge) that the test treatment is very promising, an early efficacy stopping design should be used. If we are very concerned that the test treatment may not work, an early futility stopping design should be employed. If we are not certain about the magnitude of the effect size, a group sequential design permitting early stopping for both efficacy and futility should be considered. In practice, if we have good knowledge regarding the effect size, a classical design with a fixed sample size may be more efficient.

2.4.2 Sample-Size Reestimation Design

A *sample-size reestimation* (SSR) *design* is an adaptive design that allows for sample-size adjustment or reestimation based on unblinded interim analysis results. The sample-size requirement for a trial is sensitive to the treatment effect and its variability. An inaccurate estimation of the effect size and its variability could lead to an underpowered or overpowered design, neither of which is desirable. If a trial is underpowered, it will not be able to detect a clinically meaningful difference, and consequently, could prevent a potentially effective drug from being delivered to patients. On the other hand, if a trial is overpowered, it could lead to the unnecessary exposure of many patients to a potentially harmful compound when the drug is, in fact, not effective. In practice, it is often difficult to estimate effect size and variability because of many uncertainties during protocol development. Thus, it is desirable to have the flexibility to reestimate the sample size in the middle of a trial.

2.4.3 Drop-Loser Design

A *drop-loser design* (DLD) is an adaptive design consisting of multiple groups. At each stage, interim analyses are performed and the losers (i.e., inferior treatment groups) are dropped based on certain criteria. Ultimately, the best group and the control group are retained. This type of design can be used in a combination of phase I–II and phase II–III trials. A typical phase II clinical trial is often a dose–response study, where the goal is to assess whether there is a treatment effect. If there is, the goal becomes finding the appropriate dose level (or treatment groups) for the phase III trials. This type of traditional design is not efficient with respect to time and resources because the phase II efficacy data are not pooled with data from phase III trials. Therefore, it is desirable to combine phases II and III so that the data can be used efficiently. This type of drop-loser design is often called *seamless design*.

2.4.4 Response-Adaptive Randomization Design

In a *response-adaptive randomization design* (RARD), the allocation probability is based on the responses of previous patients. If a positive response is observed in a treatment group, the probability of allocating future patients to this group will be increased. The well-known response-adaptive models include the randomized *play-the-winner* (RPW) *model*, an optimal model that minimizes the number of failures.

2.4.5 Adaptive Dose-Escalation Design

In early phases of clinical development, dose escalation is often considered to identify the maximum tolerated dose (MTD) and is commonly used for oncology trials. In an *adaptive dose-escalation design*, the dose level used to treat the next-entered patient is dependent on the toxicity of previous patients. The *continual reassessment method* (CRM) (O'Quigley et al., 1990; M. Chang and Chow, 2005) is a popular escalation algorithm. CRM can reduce the sample size and overall toxicity in a trial and improve the accuracy and precision of estimation of the MTD. The main difference between the common RARD and the CRM is that the former usually has a fixed number of arms (e.g., two arms), whereas the latter does not have a fixed number of arms or dose levels and the escalation starts from the lowest dose level and then gradually proceeds to higher dose levels if the data show that there is a limit safety concern.

2.4.6 Biomarker-Adaptive Design

Biomarker-adaptive design refers to a design in which adaptations are made based on biomarker response at interim analyses and the final analysis is based on the primary endpoint that differs from the *biomarker*. A *biomarker* is a characteristic that is measured and evaluated objectively as an indicator of normal biological or pathogenical processes or as a pharmacological response to a therapeutic intervention (Chakravarty, 2005). A biomarker can be a classifier or a prognostic or predictive marker. It is often the case that a pharmaceutical company has to make a decision as to whether to target a very selective population for whom the test drug probably works well or to target a broader population for whom the test drug is less likely to work well. However, the size of the selective population may be too small to justify the overall benefit to the patient population. In this case, a biomarker-adaptive design may be used, where the biomarker response at interim analysis points can be used to determine on which target populations the trial should be focused (M. Chang, 2007a).

2.4.7 Multistage Design of Single-Arm Trials

Single-arm trial multistage design is a special type of sequential design with a single experiment group which permits early futility stopping. It is often used in oncology trials. The response variable is a binary type and the statistical methods used are exact without the normality assumption because of the small size of the trial.

3 Classical Trial Design

3.1 INTRODUCTION

3.1.1 Hypothesis Test

In clinical trials a *hypothesis* is usually referred to as a *postulation, assumption*, or *statement* that is made about a population regarding the effectiveness and safety of a drug under investigation. For example, the statement that there is a direct drug effect is a hypothesis regarding the treatment effect. For testing hypotheses of interest, a random sample is usually drawn from the targeted population to evaluate hypotheses about the drug product. A statistical test is then performed to determine whether the null hypothesis would be rejected at a prespecified significance level (Chow et al., 2003). Based on the test result, conclusion(s) can be drawn regarding the hypotheses. Selection of a hypothesis depends on the study objectives. In clinical research, hypotheses commonly considered include tests for equality, equivalence, noninferiority, and superiority.

When testing a null hypothesis H_0: $\varepsilon < 0$ against an alternative hypothesis H_a: $\varepsilon > 0$, where ε is the treatment effect (difference in response), the *type I error rate* is defined as

$$\alpha(\varepsilon) = \Pr(\text{reject } H_0 \text{ when } H_0 \text{ is true}). \tag{3.1}$$

Note that the type I error rate is a function of the true treatment difference. More often, the type I error rate can be defined (implicitly) as $\sup\{\alpha(\varepsilon)\}$. Similarly, the type II error rate function β is defined as

$$\alpha(\varepsilon) = \Pr(\text{fail to reject } H_0 \text{ when } H_a \text{ is true}). \tag{3.2}$$

For hypothesis testing, knowledge of the distribution of the test statistic under H_0 is required. For sample-size calculation, knowledge of the distribution of the test statistic under a particular H_a value ais also required. To control the overall type I error rate at level α under any point of the H_0 domain, the condition $\alpha(\varepsilon) < \alpha^*$ for all $\varepsilon \le 0$ must be satisfied, where α^* is a threshold that

---

Classical and Adaptive Clinical Trial Designs Using ExpDesign Studio™,
By Mark Chang

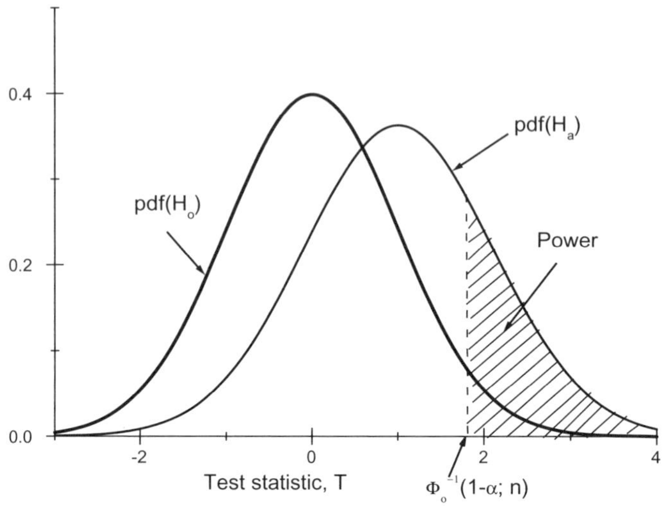

Figure 3.1 Power function.

is usually larger than 0.025 unless it is a phase III trial. If $\alpha(\varepsilon)$ is a monotonic function of ε, the maximum type I error rate occurs when $\varepsilon = 0$. The rejection region should be constructed under this condition. Under normal conditions the power can be derived as follows (M. Chang, 2007a, pp. 21–22):

$$\text{power}(\varepsilon) = 1 - \beta = \Phi\left(\frac{\sqrt{n}\varepsilon}{2\sigma} - z_{1-\alpha}\right), \tag{3.3}$$

where Φ is the cumulative distribution function (c.d.f.) of the standard normal distribution, ε is the treatment difference, and $z_{1-\beta}$ and $z_{1-\alpha}$ are the percentiles of the standard normal distribution. Figure 3.1 illustrates the power function of the type I error rate α and the sample size n. From (3.3), the total sample size can be obtained:

$$n = \frac{4(z_{1-\alpha} + z_{1-\beta})^2\sigma^2}{\varepsilon^2}. \tag{3.4}$$

3.1.2 Importance of Sample-Size Calculation

The importance of power in the determination of sample size has been well recognized. One should take steps to ensure that the power of an experiment is sufficient to justify the effort involved. On the other hand, if the power in detecting a specified practical difference is sufficiently high, failure to achieve significant results may properly be interpreted as probably indicating negligible relevant difference between the comparison groups. Thus, the proper interpretation of a negative result is based largely on a consideration of the power of the experiment.

3.1.3 Factors Affecting Sample Size

Many factors can affect the sample size for conducting a study: for example, the estimated difference between (i.e., variability in) two populations, the statistical power for detecting the difference, and the significance level. An increase in power, decrease in significant level, or increase in variability will result in an increase in sample size. The difference between two groups, or the effective size, could increase or decrease the sample size required. In hypothesis testing for a difference, the larger the difference, the smaller the sample size. For an equivalent test, the smaller the difference, the smaller the sample size. Other factors, such as the type of experimental design (e.g., parallel or crossover), the type of parameter (e.g., continuous or discrete), and the statistical methods used for the analysis will also affect the sample size.

3.1.4 Avoiding Under- or Overpowered Designs

To avoid an under- or overpowered design, we have to understand the meaning of power. *Power* is the probability of showing statistical significance (i.e., p-value $\leq \alpha$). When the sample size is calculated based on a particular power (e.g., 80%), the power is assured if the parameters for the populations are estimated accurately. For example, in a placebo-controlled two-parallel-arm clinical trial, the null hypothesis H_0: mean difference $\Delta = 0$ between the two groups and the alternative hypothesis H_a: mean difference $\Delta \neq 0$. Assuming that the true difference $\Delta = 5$ and the common standard deviation $\sigma = 10$, with level of significance $\alpha = 0.05$ (two-sided) and power = 0.8, the sample size required will be 64 per group based on a two-sample t-test. The question is: If we design the study with 64 per group, does the design have 80% probability (conditional probability) to detect the true difference $\Delta = 5$ when true $\sigma = 10$? The answer is "yes." Does the design have the 80% probability (unconditional probability) to show the statistical significance? The answer is "no," because practically, we don't know the true Δ and σ. Instead, we estimate these two parameters. When the true Δ is larger than the estimate or the true σ is smaller than the estimate, the actual power is greater than 80%; in contrast, if the true Δ is smaller than the estimate or the true σ is larger than the estimate, the power will be below 80%.

Suppose that the trial described above is designed with 90% power. When the trial has been completed, the mean difference observed and pooled standard deviation based on the trial data are identical to the estimates: $\hat{\Delta} = 5$ and $\hat{\sigma} = 10$, respectively. Then the p-value from a two-sample t-test will be 0.0055, which is much less than the prespecified $\alpha = 0.05$. If the sample mean difference $\hat{\Delta} = 3.5$, much less than the true (population) difference $\hat{\Delta} = 5$, but the sample standard deviation $\hat{\sigma} = 10$, the p-value will be 0.05.

Practically, investigators would only be interested in the effective size beyond a particular threshold, Δ_{min}, which could be a minimal clinically and commercially meaningful difference. For example, in a clinical trial on patients with asthma, the minimal clinically meaningful difference is identified to be $\Delta_{min} = 5\%$ difference in % FEV1 (percent forced expiration volume in the first second) change from baseline, but that difference will not be commercially meaningful because a better drug is available on the market. Therefore, the clinical trial design team sets a minimal difference to be $\Delta_{min} = 10\%$, which is considered as both a clinically and commercially meaningful cut point. Now the question is: Should we use 80% or 90% power to design the trial such that we can show a statistically significant difference even when Δ is much less than 10%? The suggestion is to use a lower power when the standard deviation estimation is accurate. If not, sample-size reestimation technology can be used to reestimate the standard deviation during the study.

3.2 HOW TO CALCULATE SAMPLE SIZE USING EXPDESIGN

For confirmary clinical trials, it is common practice to use $\alpha = 0.05$ and power = 0.8 to 0.9, as indicated in most of the examples in this book.

3.2.1 Testing the Mean Difference Between Two Groups

Suppose that we are planning a clinical trial to test a new drug called ABC for treatment of patients with mild to moderate asthma. A double-blind randomized parallel design with two treatment groups (placebo vs. ABC) is chosen for this phase II trial. The primary efficacy parameter is percentage change from baseline in FEV1. The mean difference in % change in FEV1 between placebo and ABC is estimated to be 9% with a standard deviation of 18%.

Based on this information, we can specify the options in ExpDesign as follows: two groups, hypothesis test, mean/median, and equal size. In the list of methods, choose the two-sample *t*-test. Enter "0.05" for the level of significance, "2" for a two-sided test, "3" for the group 1 mean, "12" for the group 2 mean, "18" for the standard deviation, and "0.8" for the power (Figure 3.2). Clicking Compute, we obtain a sample size of 64 per group for the trial. The power curve shows that the sample size required increases when the power increases. (*Note*: Double-click to see the finest grids.)

3.2.2 Testing the Proportion Difference Between Two Groups

Suppose that we want to design a phase III clinical trial to evaluate the efficacy of a new compound, ABC, in patients with a dermatological disease. Qualified patients will be randomized to receive either of the treatments: ABC or

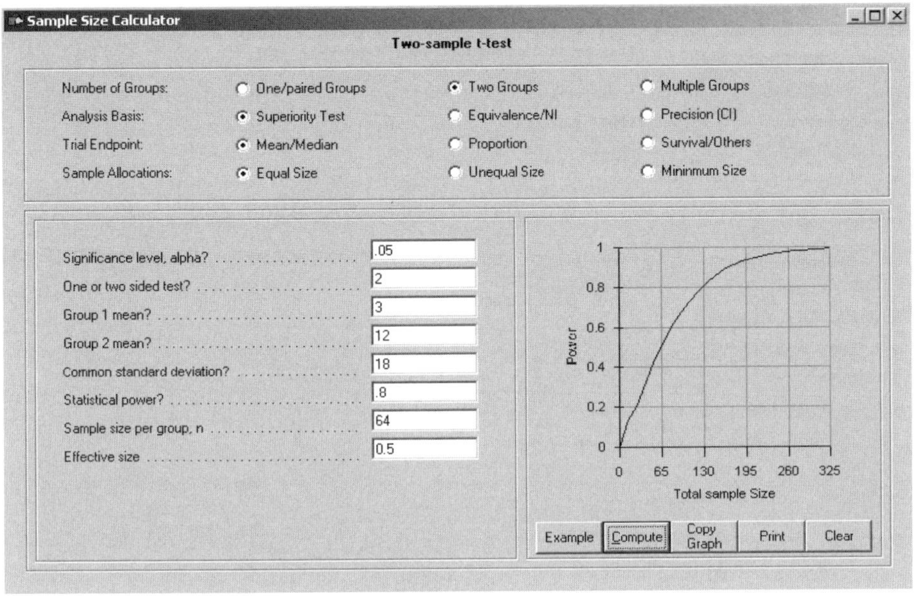

Figure 3.2 Two-sample *t*-test for an asthma trial.

placebo. After a year's treatment, the clinical outcome will be evaluated as cured or not cured. It was estimated that the response rates (cured) is 1% in placebo and 12% in the active treatment group.

Based on this information, we specify the options in ExpDesign as follows: two groups, hypothesis test, proportion, and equal size. In the list of methods, choose Pearson's chi-square test. Enter "0.05" for the level of significance α, a two-sided test, "0.01" for the proportion in group 1, "0.12" for the proportion in group 2, and "0.90" for the power. Clicking 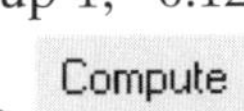

, we obtain a sample size of 121 per group for the trial. The power curve shows the relationship between the power and the required sample size (Figure 3.3).

3.2.3 Testing the Survival Difference Between Two Groups

Suppose that we are designing a phase III clinical trial for a potential oncology drug, ABC. The study drug, ABC, will be combined with an approved drug, XYZ, as second-line therapy in patients with multiple myeloma. The combined treatment will be compared with XYZ alone for effectiveness in prolonging survival time. It is estimated that the proportion of deaths is 50% in the XYZ group and 40% in the combined group a year after the randomization.

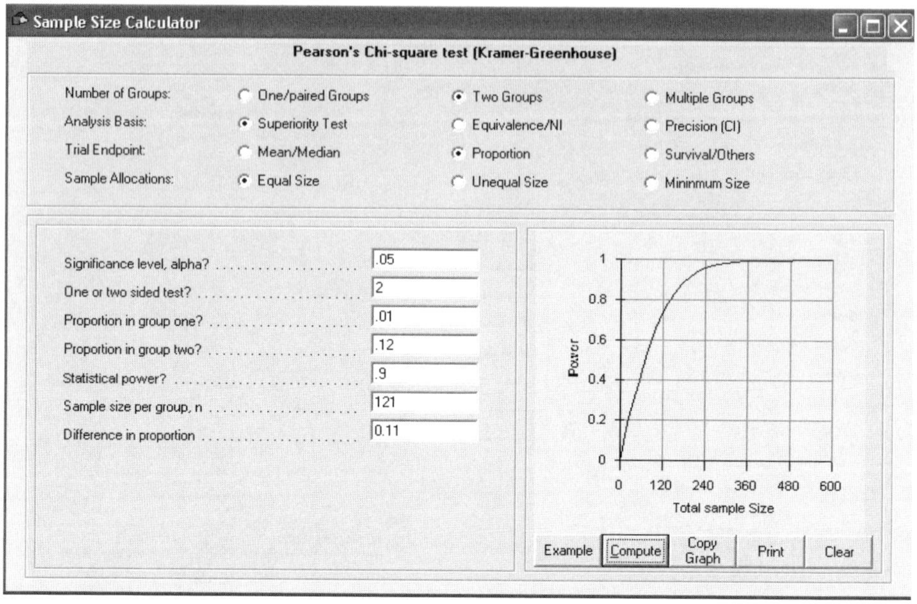

Figure 3.3 Pearson's chi-square test for a dermatological disease trial.

Based on this information, we specify the options in ExpDesign as follows: two groups, hypothesis test, survival/others, and equal size. In the list of methods, choose the log-rank test for survival analysis. Enter "0.05" for the level of significance, "2" for a two-sided test, "0.50" for the proportion in group 1, "0.40" for the proportion in group 2, and "0.8" for the power (Figure 3.4). Clicking 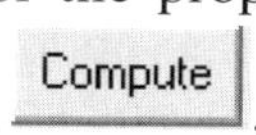

, we obtain a sample size of 371 per group and or 408 for the total number of events. The hazard ratio, 1.322, was calculated by using $\ln p_1/\ln p_2$.

3.2.4 Testing the Survival Difference with a Follow-up Period

Suppose that we want to design a phase III clinical trial for a potential oncology drug, ABC. The study drug, ABC, will be combined with an approved drug, XYZ, as second-line therapy in patients with multiple myeloma. The combined treatment will be compared with XYZ alone for effectiveness in prolonging patients' survival time. It is estimated that the median survival time is 8 months for XYZ alone and 10.5 months for the combined treatment group. The duration of patient enrollment is anticipated to be 9 months with a maximum follow-up period or total study duration of 23 months.

Based on this information, we specify the options in ExpDesign as follows: two groups, hypothesis test, survival/others, and equal size. In the list of methods, choose the exponential survival distribution method with uniform

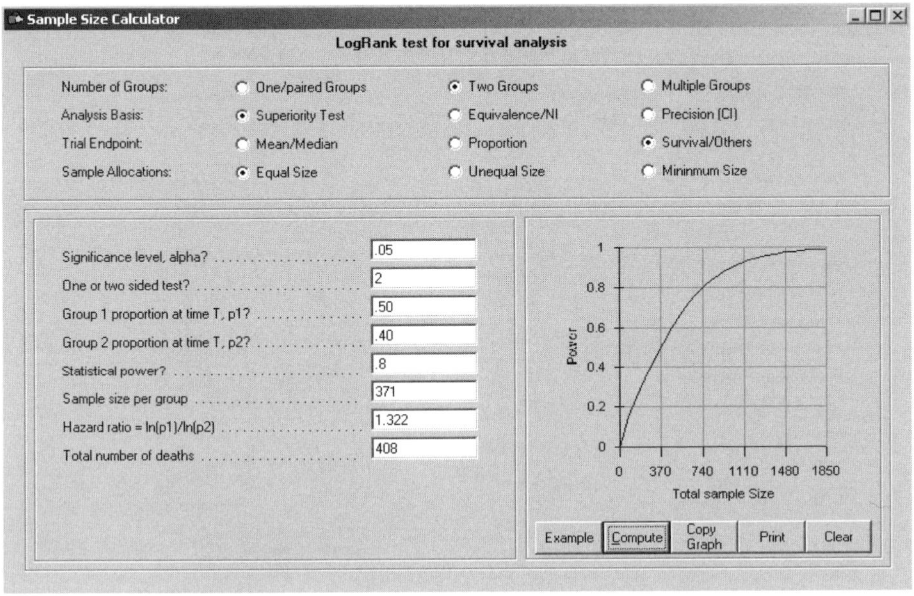

Figure 3.4 Log-rank test for an oncology trial.

enrollment and a follow-up. Enter "0.05" for the level of significance, "2" for a two-sided test, "0.066" (= ln 2/8) for the hazard rate in group 1, "0.0866" (= ln 2/10.5) for the hazard rate in group 2, "9" for the duration of enrollment, "23" for the total trial duration, and "0.8" for the power. Clicking Compute, we obtain a sample size of 288 per group (Figure 3.5).

3.2.5 Exact Test for a One-Sample Proportion

In designing a phase II single-arm oncology trial, suppose that the investigator is interested in the response rate of the test drug. If the response rate is greater than 20%, the drug will be considered very promising and will be pursued further in the next-phase study. If the response rate is less than 5%, it will not be pursued further.

Based on this information, we specify the options in ExpDesign as follows: one group, hypothesis test, proportion, and equal size. In the list of methods, choose the one-sample exact test for proportion using binomial distribution. Enter "0.05" for the level of significance, "1" for a one-sided test, "0.05" for the H_0 proportion, "0.2" for the H_a proportion, and "0.8" for the power. Clicking Compute, we obtain a sample size of 21 (Figure 3.6).

Note that the power does not increase monotonically with sample size based on binomial distribution. ExpDesign adoptes a conservative approach;

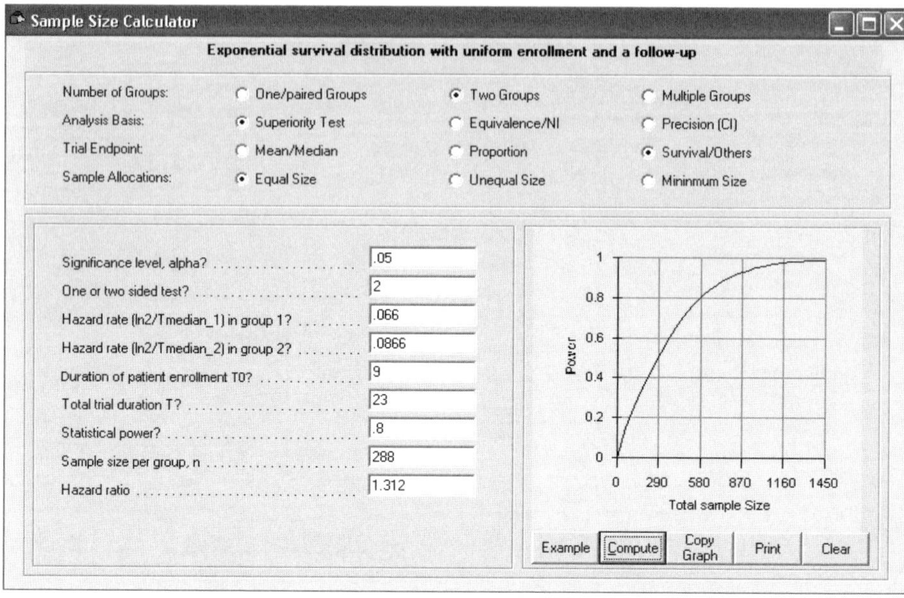

Figure 3.5 Oncology trial with uniform enrollment.

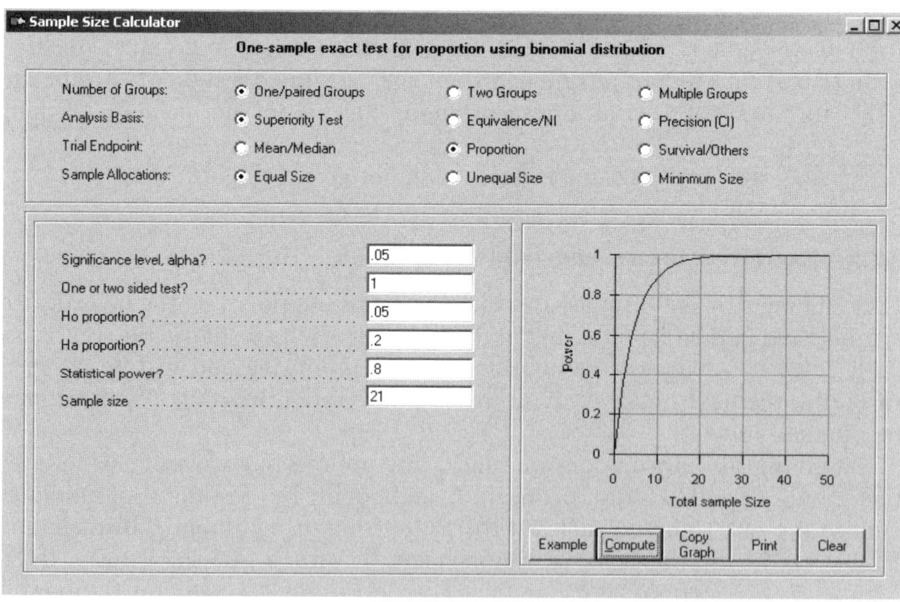

Figure 3.6 Exact test for a single-group oncology trial.

that is, with the required sample size n it will ensure that the power will be larger than or equal to the power specified for all sample sizes $\geq n$.

3.2.6 McNemar's Test for Paired Data

A researcher is investigating the effect of an experimental drug on bilirubin abnormalities. Pre- and postdose clinical laboratory results will be collected and compared using McNemar's test for the paired data. The estimated difference between pre- and postdose in proportions of abnormalities is 20%, and the estimated sum of proportions of shifts from the normal to the abnormal and the abnormal to the normal is 30%.

Based on the information, we specify the options in ExpDesign as follows: one/paired groups, hypothesis test, proportion, and equal size. In the list of methods, choose McNemar's test for a paired sample. Enter "0.05" for the level of significance, "2" for a two-sided test, "0.2" for the difference in proportion, "0.3" for the proportion of discordant pairs, and "0.8" for the power. Clicking Compute, we obtain a sample of 52 subjects per group for the trial (Figure 3.7).

3.2.7 Noninferiority Test for Two Means

Suppose that in an asthma study, the objective is to prove that the test drug is noninferior to the active control. It is estimated that both the control and

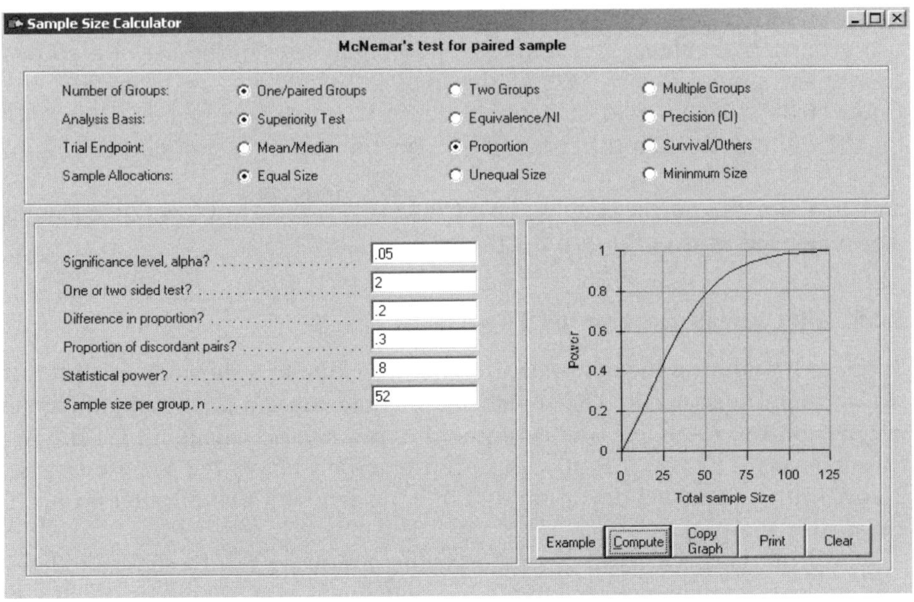

Figure 3.7 McNemar's test for a bilirubin abnormality study.

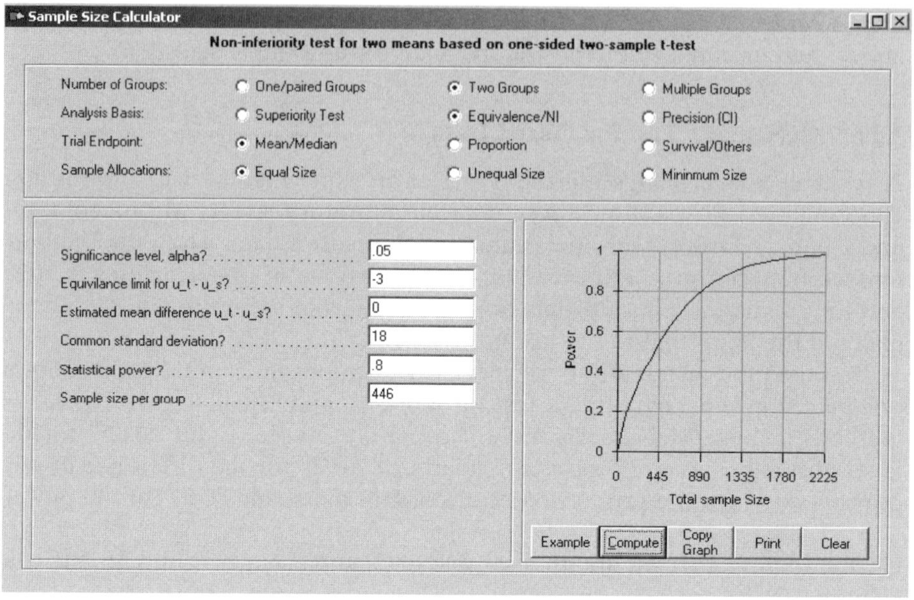

Figure 3.8 Noninferiority asthma trial in mean FEV1 changes.

the test drug have 10% improvement in FEV1. The criterion for noninferiority is –3% in FEV1 improvement. The common standard deviation is estimated to be 18%.

Based on this information, we specify the options in ExpDesign as follows: two groups, equivalence, mean/media, and equal size. In the list of methods, choose the noninferiority test of two means based on a two-sample *t*-test. Enter "0.05" for the level of significance, "–3" for the equivalence limit, "0" for the estimated mean difference, "18" for the common standard deviation, and "0.8" for the power (Figure 3.8). Clicking 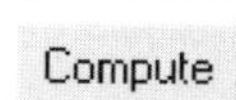

, we obtain a sample size of 446 subjects per group for the trial.

3.2.8 Bioequivalence Test for Two Means

Suppose that during the manufacture of a drug, due to a shortage of material, replacement must occur. The replacement could cause a potentially different polymorphism. A clinical trial is required to prove bioequivalence for the two formulations. The two formulations are expected to have the same response: 2 units with a standard deviation of 1.0. A design with two parallel groups is chosen for the trial.

Based on this information, we specify the options in ExpDesign as follows: two groups, equivalence, mean/media, and equal size. Then in the list of methods, choose the two one-sided *t*-tests for equivalence based on difference

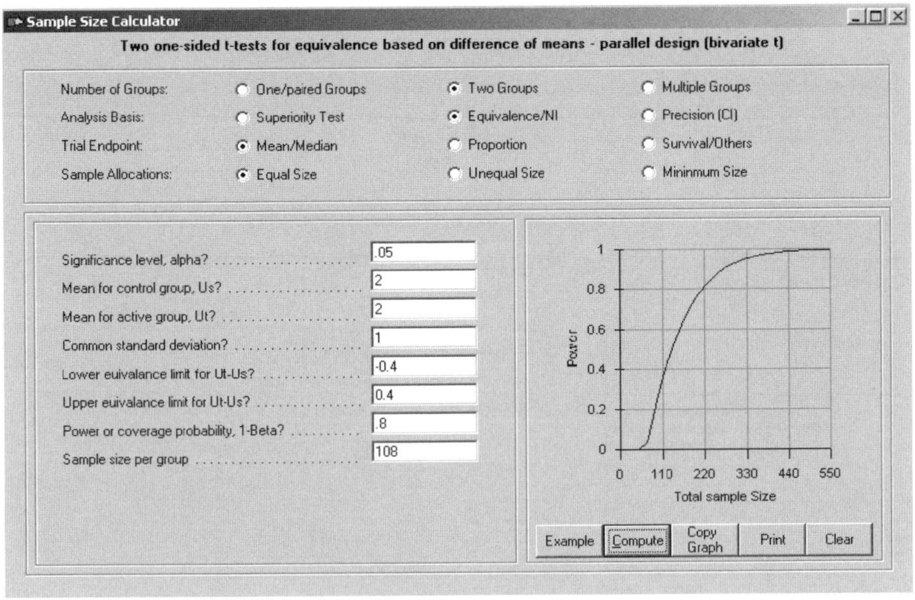

Figure 3.9 Bioequivalence trial for two means.

of means for parallel design (using bivariate t). Enter "0.05" for the level of significance, "2" for means in both groups, "–0.4" for the lower limit and "0.4" for the higher limit, "1.0" for the standard deviation, and "0.8" for the power. Clicking 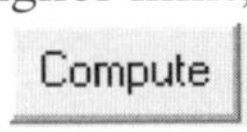

, we obtain a sample size of 108 per group (Figure 3.9). [*Note*: The equivalence limits 0.4 are based on the 20% rule: 2(20%) = 0.4.]

3.2.9 Bioequivalence Test for Two Means of Lognormal Data

Suppose that due to safety concerns, a drug formulation is modified for asthma patients. A clinical trial is required to prove bioequivalence between the new and earlier formulations. The two are expected to have the same response of 2 on the original scale or 0.693 on the log scale. The standard deviation is 0.55 on the log scale. A design with two parallel groups is chosen for the trial.

Based on this information, we can specify the options in ExpDesign as follows: two groups, equivalence, mean/media, and equal size. In the list of methods, choose two one-sided t-tests for equivalence based on difference of means for parallel design (bivariate t). Enter "0.05" for the level of significance, "0.693" for the means of both groups, "–0.223" for the lower limit and "0.223" for the higher limit, "0.55" for the standard deviation, and "0.8" for the power. Clicking 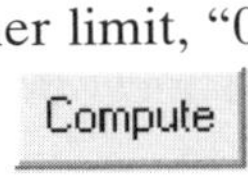

, we obtain a sample size of 104 per group

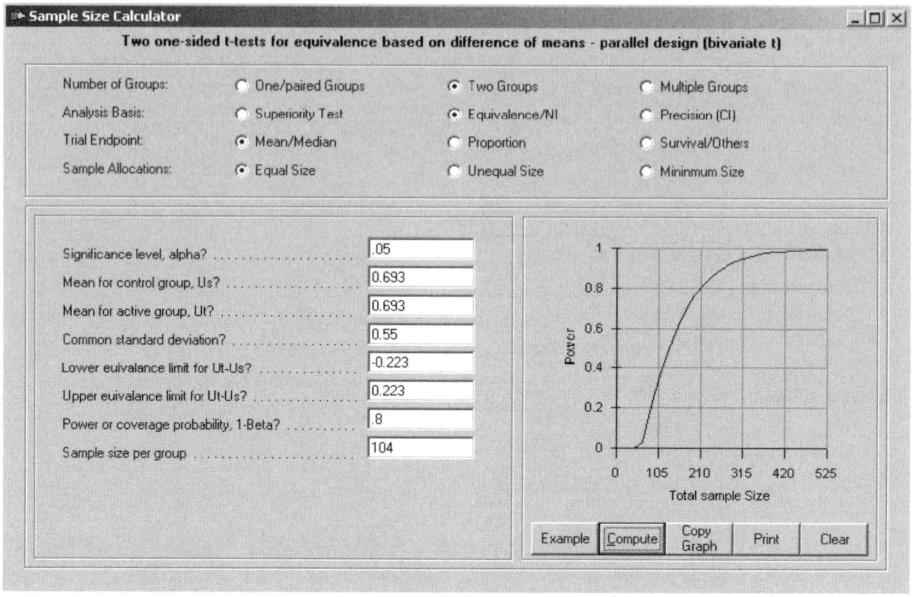

Figure 3.10 Bioequivalence trial with lognormal data.

(Figure 3.10). (*Note*: The equivalence limits, 0.223, are based on an FDA guideline.)

3.2.10 Equivalence Test Based on the Ratio of Two Means

Suppose that a bioequivalence trial is designed based on the area under the concentration curve (AUC). The pharmacokinetic parameter (AUC) is believed to be lognormally distributed with a mean of 2.5 mg/m$^3 \cdot$h for both formulations. The coefficient of variation between subjects is 0.2, and the coefficient of variation within subjects is 0.5 on the original scale. A 2 × 2 crossover design is chosen for the trial.

Based on the information, we can specify the options in ExpDesign as follows: two groups, equivalence, mean/media, and equal size. In the list of methods, choose the two one-sided *t*-tests for equivalence based on the ratio of two means for crossover design (bivariate *t*). Enter "0.05" for the level of significance, "2.5" for the means in both groups, "0.2" for the coefficient of variation between subjects, "0.5" for the coefficient of variation within subjects, "0.8" for the lower limit and "1.25" for the higher limit, and "0.8" for the power (Figure 3.11). Clicking 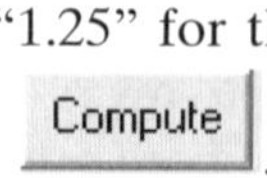

, we obtain 44 subjects per sequence for the trial. (*Note*: If more than one parameter is concerned, calculate the sample size for each parameter and pick the largest one, to be conservative.)

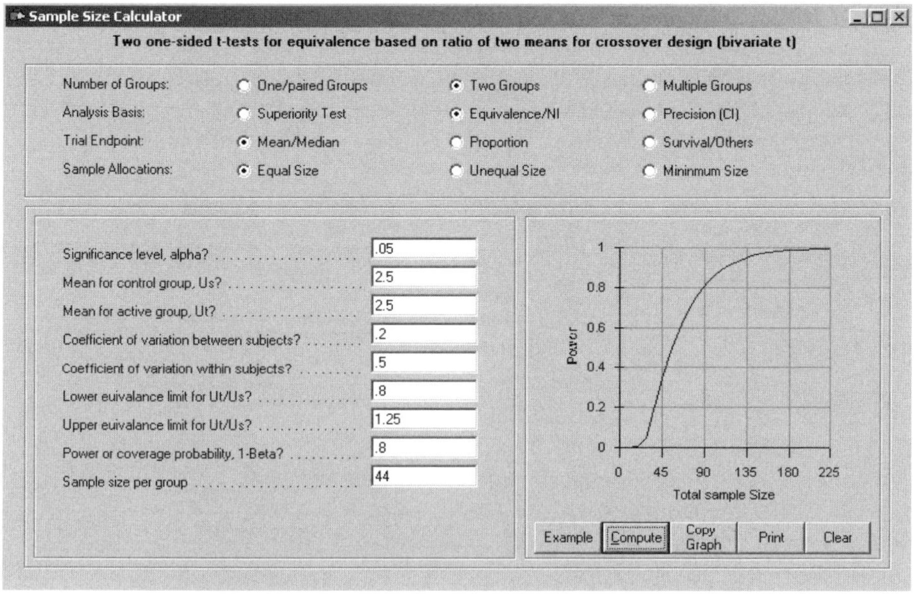

Figure 3.11 Bioequivalence trial on the ratio of means.

3.2.11 Precision Method for the Mean Difference for a Paired Sample

Suppose that a biotech company is developing a new appetite-suppressing compound, ABC, for weight reduction. The mean weight reduction after 10 weeks-treatment with ABC is estimated to be 33.5 pounds with a standard deviation of 6.3 pounds. The researchers want to know if ABC is effective in weight reduction by investigating the confidence interval for the difference. It is believed that a confidence interval with a precision (distance between the limit and the mean difference) of 1 pound would be adequate.

Based on the information, we specify the options in ExpDesign as follows: one/paired groups, precision(CI), mean/median, and equal size. In the list of methods, choose the paired sample confidence interval using a t-distribution. Enter "0.05" for the level of significance, "2" for the two-sided confidence interval, "1" for precision, and "6.3" for the standard deviation of the difference. Clicking 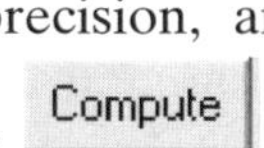

, we obtain a sample size of 152 pairs for the trial (Figure 3.12).

3.2.12 Mantel–Haenszel Test for an Odds Ratio with Two Strata

Suppose that we are designing a trial to investigate the effectiveness of a new drug, ABC, in treating patients with acute myelogenous leukemia (AML). Patients will be randomized into one of two groups, 10-day infusion with ABC

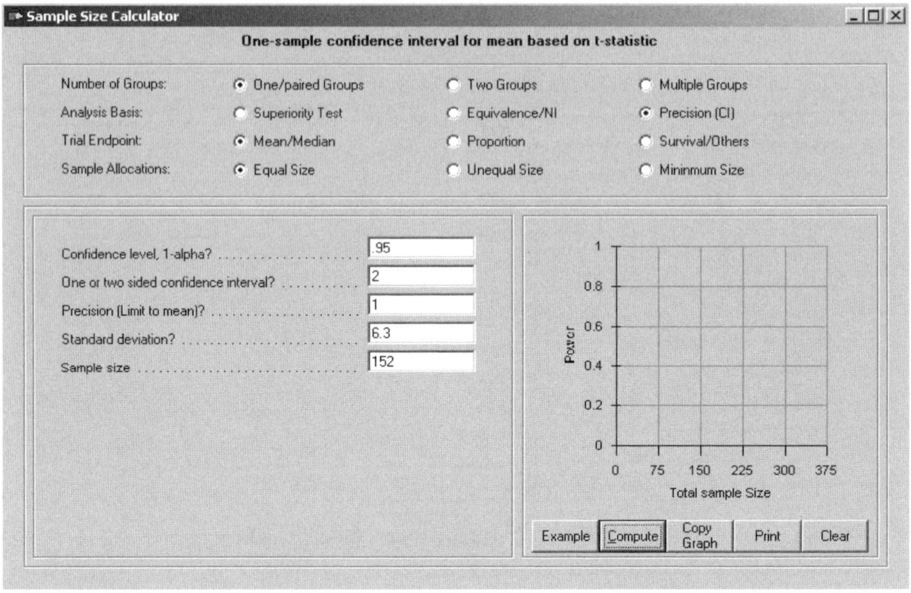

Figure 3.12 Precision method for paired means in a weight reduction study.

or control, and will be followed for 90 days. The time of remission from diagnosis or prior relapse at study is considered an important covariate in predicting the response, which is defined as relapse, death, or major intervention (e.g., bone marrow transplant before day 90). The investigator wants to know if there is any evidence that administration of ABC is associated with a decreased relapse rate. To design this study, patients are stratified by their time to remission: 60% of patients are in stratum 1, with a remission time of less than 10 months, and 40% of patients are in stratum 2, with a remission time greater than or equal to 10 months. The responses in the control group are estimated to be 0.55 and 0.75 for the two strata. The common odds ratio (control vs. ABC) is estimated to be 0.33.

Based on the information, we can specify the options in ExpDesign as follows: two groups, hypothesis test, proportion, and equal size. In the list of methods, choose the Mantel–Haenszel test for an odds ratio with k strata. Enter "0.05" for the level of significance, "2" for a two-sided test, "2" for the number of strata, "0.33" for the common odds ratio, " 0.55" and "0.75" for rates in the control group, "0.6" and "0.4" for fractions of observations, and "0.8" for the power. Clicking 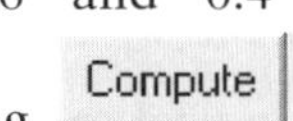

, we obtain a sample size of 55 subjects per group, calculated with 33 in stratum 1 and 22 in stratum 2 (Figure 3.13).

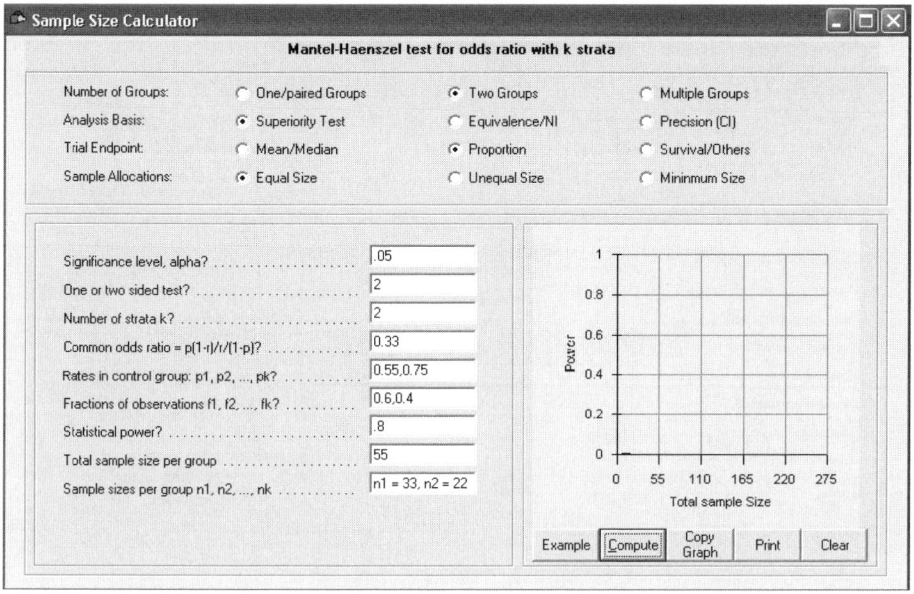

Figure 3.13 Mantel–Haenszel test for the odds ratio in an AML trial.

3.2.13 Pearson's Chi-Square Test for Rate Difference

Let's use the preceding example but without stratification. The response rate for the control is about 0.63, and the common odds ratio (OR) is 0.33. Since the proportion $p_2 = p_1 \cdot \mathrm{OR}/[1 - p_1(1 - \mathrm{OR})]$, we can use a method for proportions to calculate the sample size for odds ratio problems. For the current case, $p_1 = 0.3$ and OR = 0.33. We calculate $p_2 = (0.63 \times 0.33)/[1 - 0.63 \times (1 - 0.33)] = 0.36$.

Based on the information, we can specify the options in ExpDesign as follows: two groups, hypothesis test, proportion, and equal size. In the list of methods, choose Pearson's chi-square test (Kramer–Greenhouse) for a large sample. Enter "0.05" for the level of significance, "2" for a two-sided test, "0.63" for the proportion in group 1, "0.36" for the proportion in group 2, and "0.8" for the power. Clicking 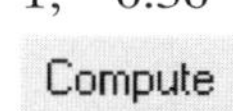

, a sample size of 60 subjects per group is calculated (Figure 3.14).

3.2.14 One-Way Analysis of Variance for Parallel Groups

Suppose that a phase II trial is to be designed to investigate the efficacy of a new serotonin-uptake inhibiting agent, ABC, in subjects with a general anxiety disorder (GAD). Subjects diagnosed with a GAD value of moderate or greater severity will be randomized into one of three treatment groups: placebo, 25 mg of ABC, and 100 mg of ABC. After 12 weeks of once-daily dosing in a double-

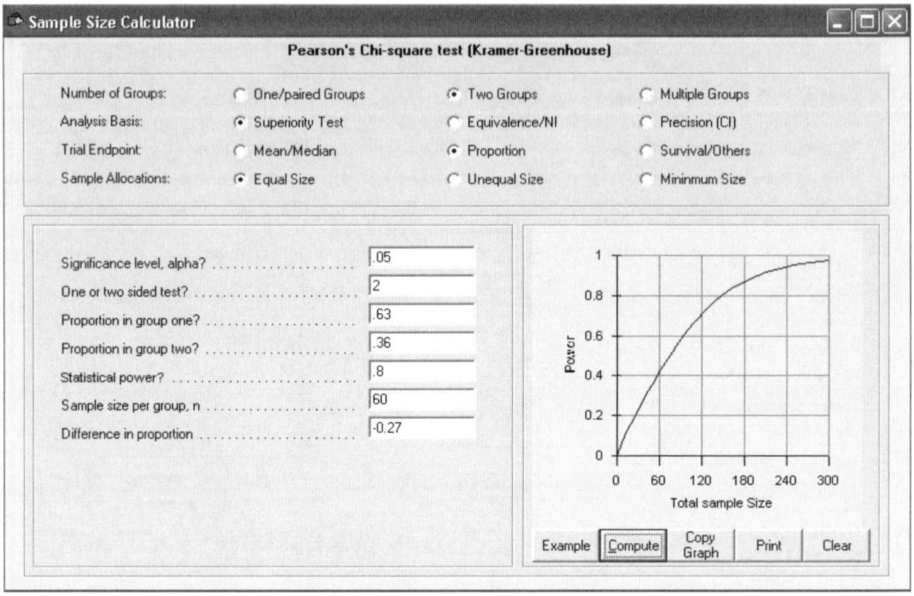

Figure 3.14 Chi-square test for the rate difference in an AML trial.

blind fashion, a test based on the Hamilton rating scale for anxiety (HAM-A) will be administrated. This test consists of 14 anxiety-related items. The HAM-A test scores are the sums of the code values over all 14 items. It is estimated that the mean HAM-A scores are 28, 25, and 24 for the placebo, 25 mg of ABC, and 100 mg of ABC groups, respectively, with a common standard deviation of 6. We want to know if there is any difference in mean HAM-A test scores among the three groups.

Based on the information, we specify the options in ExpDesign as follows: multiple group, hypothesis test, mean/media, and equal size. In the list of methods, choose the one-way ANOVA for parallel groups. Enter "0.05" for the level of significance; "3" for the number of treatment groups; "28, 26, 24" for the treatment means; "6" for the common standard deviation; and "0.9" for the power (Figure 3.15). Clicking 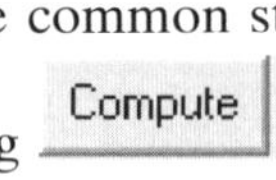

, we obtain a sample size of 58 subjects per group for the trial.

3.2.15 Dose–Response Trial for a Myocardial Infarction

Suppose that a trial is to be designed for patients with acute ischemic stroke of recent onset. The composite endpoint (death and myocardial infarction) is the primary endpoint. Four dose levels are planned, with event rates of 14%, 12%, 11%, and 10%, respectively. The first group is the active control group (the 14% event rate). Comparisons are made between the active control and

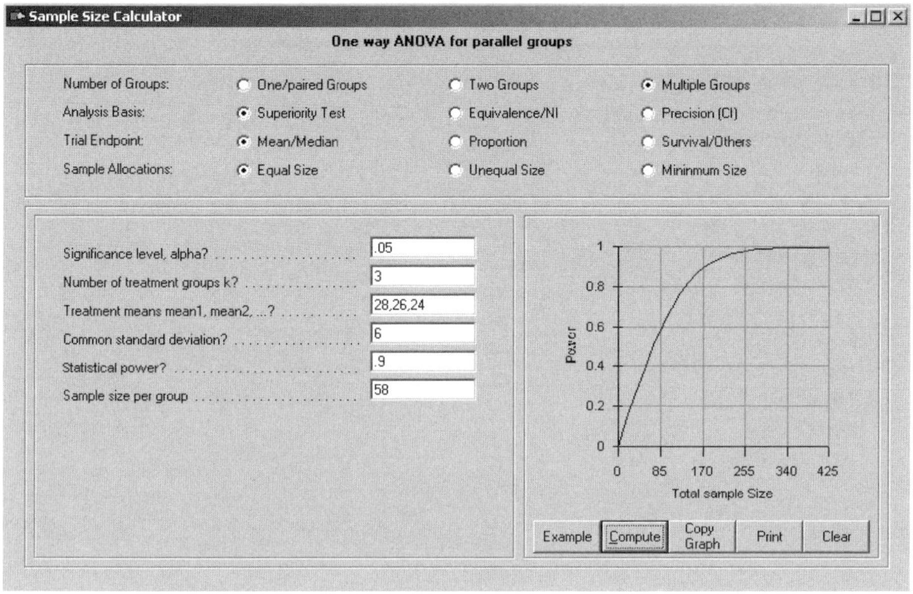

Figure 3.15 ANOVA for a parallel general anxiety disorder trial.

the test groups; therefore, the contrast for the active control should have a different sign than the contrasts for the test groups. Let $c_1 = -6$, $c_2 = 1$, $c_3 = 2$, and $c_4 = 3$. It is assumed that the event rate is $p_0 = 0.14$ under the null hypothesis.

Based on the information, we can specify the options in ExpDesign as follows: multiple groups, hypothesis test, proportion, and equal size. In the list of methods, choose the Cochran–Armitage test for linear/monotonic trend (dose–response). Enter "0.1" for the level of significance, "1" for a one-sided test; "4" for the number of groups; "–6, 1, 2, 3" for the (virtual) dose levels; "0.15, 0.12, 0.11, 0.10" for the proportions in k groups, and "0.8" for the power. Clicking 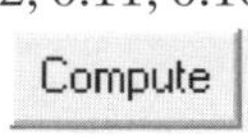

, we obtain a total sample size of 1473 for the trial (Figure 3.16).

3.3 MATHEMATICAL NOTES ON CLASSICAL DESIGN

3.3.1 Large-Sample-Size Calculation for Classical Design

Testing a single mean:

$$N = \left[\left(\Phi^{-1}\left(1 - \frac{\alpha}{s}\right) + \Phi^{-1}(1-\beta) \right) \frac{\sigma}{\theta} \right]^2, \tag{3.5}$$

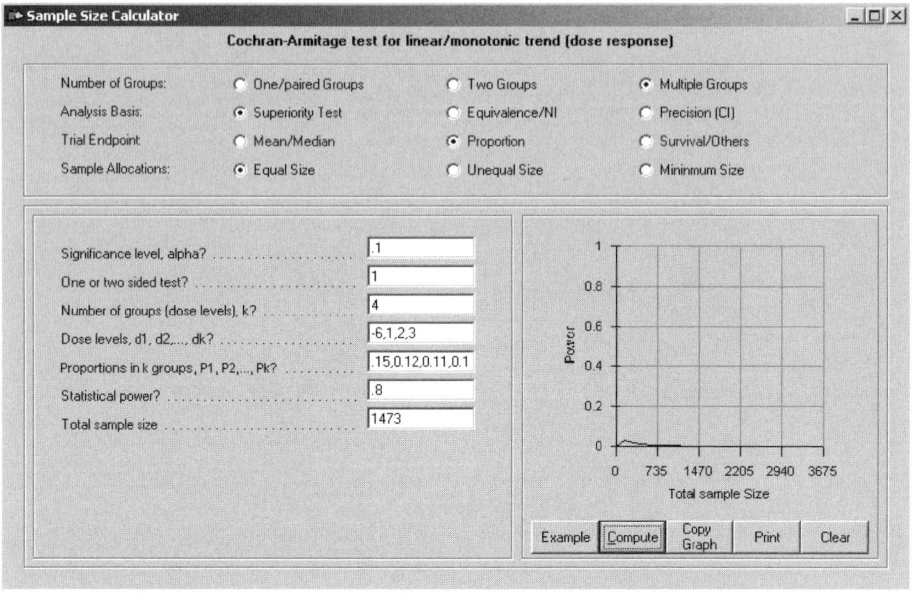

Figure 3.16 Dose–response design for a myocardial infarction trial.

where θ is the parameter difference between the null and alternative conditions; $s = 1$ for a one-sided test and 2 for a two-sided test.

Testing paired means:

$$N = \left[\left(\Phi^{-1}\left(1 - \frac{\alpha}{s}\right) + \Phi^{-1}(1-\beta) \right) \frac{\sigma}{\theta} \right]^2. \tag{3.6}$$

Testing two independent means:

$$N = 4\left[\left(\Phi^{-1}\left(1 - \frac{\alpha}{s}\right) + \Phi^{-1}(1-\beta) \right) \frac{\sigma}{\theta} \right]^2. \tag{3.7}$$

Testing one proportion:

$$N = \left[\left(\Phi^{-1}\left(1 - \frac{\alpha}{s}\right) + \Phi^{-1}(1-\beta) \right) \frac{\sigma}{\theta} \right]^2, \tag{3.8}$$

where $\sigma = \sqrt{P_0(1-P_0)}$.

Testing two independent proportions:

$$N = 4\left[\left(\Phi^{-1}\left(1 - \frac{\alpha}{s}\right) + \Phi^{-1}(1-\beta) \right) \frac{\sigma}{\theta} \right]^2, \tag{3.9}$$

where

$$\sigma = \sqrt{\bar{p}(1-\bar{p})}, \qquad \bar{p} = \frac{p_{\mathrm{A}} + p_{\mathrm{B}}}{2}. \tag{3.10}$$

Log-rank test for two survival distributions:

$$N = \frac{1}{(\lambda_2 - \lambda_1)^2}\left[\left(\Phi^{-1}\left(1-\frac{\alpha}{s}\right)\sqrt{\phi\left(\frac{1}{Q_1}+\frac{1}{Q_2}\right)} + \Phi^{-1}(1-\beta)\right)\sqrt{\frac{\phi_1}{Q_1}+\frac{\phi_2}{Q_2}}\right]^2, \tag{3.11}$$

where

$$Q_1 = \frac{1}{1+r}, \qquad Q_2 = \frac{r}{1+r},$$

$$\lambda = Q_1\lambda_1 + Q_2\lambda_2, \qquad r = \frac{n_2}{n_1},$$

$$\phi_i = \lambda_i^2\left(1 - \frac{e^{-\lambda_i(T_{\max}-T_0)} - e^{-\lambda_i T_{\max}}}{\lambda_i T_0}\right)^{-1}, \qquad i = 1, 2 \tag{3.12}$$

$$\phi = \lambda^2\left(1 - \frac{e^{-\lambda(T_{\max}-T_0)} - e^{-\lambda T_{\max}}}{\lambda T_0}\right)^{-1}. \tag{3.13}$$

3.3.2 Commonly Used Terms and Their Mathematical Expressions

Relative risk:

$$\mathrm{RR} = \frac{P(\text{response} \mid \text{drug A})}{P(\text{response} \mid \text{drug B})}. \tag{3.14}$$

Odds given drug A:

$$\text{odds}_{\mathrm{A}} = \frac{P(\text{response} \mid \text{drug A})}{P(\text{nonresponse} \mid \text{drug A})}. \tag{3.15}$$

Odds ratio:

$$\mathrm{OR} = \frac{\text{odds}_{\mathrm{A}}}{\text{odds}_{\mathrm{B}}} \frac{p_{11}p_{22}}{p_{12}p_{21}}. \tag{3.16}$$

Proportions versus odds ratio: Because of the relationships between the odds ratio and proportions: $\mathrm{OR} = p_{\mathrm{B}}(1 - p_{\mathrm{A}})/p_{\mathrm{A}}(1 - p_{\mathrm{B}})$ and $p_{\mathrm{B}} = p_{\mathrm{A}}\mathrm{OR}/[1 - p_{\mathrm{A}}(1 - \mathrm{OR})]$, all sample-size formulas for proportion difference can be used to calculation the sample size for an odds ratio.

Standard deviation of ln x:

$$\sigma_{\ln x} = \sqrt{\ln(1+\text{CV}^2)}, \tag{3.17}$$

where CV is the coefficient of variation.

Confidence interval for ln OR:

$$\ln \hat{\text{OR}} \pm \sqrt{\frac{1}{n_{11}} + \frac{1}{n_{12}} + \frac{1}{n_{21}} + \frac{1}{n_{22}}}, \tag{3.18}$$

where n_{ij} is the number of patients in cell (i, j) of a 2×2 table.

Exponential survival distribution:

$$S(t) = e^{-\lambda t}, \tag{3.19}$$

where λ is the hazard rate.

Hazard ratio: The hazard ratio is defined as HR = λ_1/λ_2. For two exponential survival curves, HR can be expressed as

$$\text{HR} = \frac{\lambda_1}{\lambda_2} = \frac{t_{\text{median}2}}{t_{\text{median}1}} = \frac{t_{\text{mean}2}}{t_{\text{mean}1}} = \frac{\ln S_1(t)}{\ln S_2(t)} \approx \frac{\ln p_1}{\ln p_2}, \tag{3.20}$$

where S_i is a survivorship function.

Median survival time versus hazard rate:

$$S(t_{\text{median}}) = 0.5 \Rightarrow e^{-\lambda t_{\text{median}}} = 0.5 \Rightarrow t_{\text{median}} = \frac{\ln 2}{\lambda}. \tag{3.21}$$

Mean survival time versus hazard rate:

$$t_{\text{mean}} = \int_0^{+\infty} S(t)dt = \int_0^{+\infty} e^{-\lambda t} dt = \frac{1}{\lambda}. \tag{3.22}$$

Confidence interval for mean survival time: Suppose that the trial is terminated after d of n patients have died. Denote the survival times as

$$t_1 \le t_2 \le \ldots \le t_d = t_1^+ = t_2^+ = \ldots = t_{n-d}^+, \tag{3.23}$$

where t_i^+ represents a censored observation. Under an assumption of exponential survival distribution, the maximum likelihood estimates lead to the following results (E. T. Lee, 1992):

$$\hat{\mu} = \frac{1}{d}\left(\sum_{i=1}^{d} t_i + \sum_{i=1}^{n-d} t_i^+\right) \tag{3.24}$$

and

$$\frac{2d\hat{\mu}}{\chi^2_{2d,\alpha/2}} < \mu < \frac{2d\hat{\mu}}{\chi^2_{2d,1-\alpha/2}}. \tag{3.25}$$

Confidence interval for hazard rate for large sample size:

$$\hat{\lambda} = \frac{1}{\hat{\mu}} \quad \text{and} \quad \frac{\hat{\lambda}\chi^2_{2d,1-\alpha/2}}{2d} < \lambda < \frac{\hat{\lambda}\chi^2_{2d,\alpha/2}}{2d} \tag{3.26}$$

or

$$\hat{\lambda} - \frac{\hat{\lambda} Z_{\alpha/2}}{\sqrt{d-1}} < \lambda < \hat{\lambda} + \frac{\hat{\lambda} Z_{\alpha/2}}{\sqrt{d-1}}, \tag{3.27}$$

where d is the number of deaths and n is the number of patients.

Two-sided confidence interval for log-hazard ratio, θ:

$$\mathrm{CI}_\theta = \hat{\theta} \pm \frac{1+r}{\sqrt{r}} \frac{z_{1-\alpha/2}}{\sqrt{d}}, \tag{3.28}$$

where r is the sample-size ratio between the two treatment groups and d is the total number of deaths.

Assume that there are a total of d deaths in the study. Under the condition of no ties, we denote the survival times of these subjects by $\tau_1 < \tau_2 < \ldots < \tau_d$, where the τ_i represent elapsed times between entry in the study and failure. Let the numbers known to have survived up to time τ_i after treatment be r_{i1} and r_{i2} for treatments A and B, respectively. The log-rank score statistic is given as (Jennison and Turnbull, 2000)

$$\hat{\theta} = \frac{(1+r)^2}{rd} \sum_{i=1}^{d} \left(\delta_{i2} - \frac{r_{i1}}{r_{i1} + r_{i2}}\right), \tag{3.29}$$

where $\delta_{i2} = 1$ is the failure at τ_i for treatment B, and $\delta_{i2} = 0$, otherwise.

Two-sided confidence interval for hazard ratio:

$$\mathrm{CI}_{\mathrm{HR}} = \exp\left(\hat{\theta} \pm \frac{1+r}{\sqrt{r}} \frac{z_{1-\alpha/2}}{\sqrt{d}}\right) \tag{3.30}$$

Two-sided confidence interval for difference in hazard rates:

$$\mathrm{CI}_{\lambda_1-\lambda_2} = \left(\hat{\lambda}_1 - \hat{\lambda}_2\right) \pm \frac{1}{\sqrt{N}} z_{1-\alpha/2} \hat{\sigma}_{\lambda_1-\lambda_2}, \tag{3.31}$$

where

$$\hat{\sigma}_{\lambda_1-\lambda_2} = \sqrt{\frac{\phi_1}{f_1} + \frac{\phi_2}{f_2}} \tag{3.32}$$

and

$$\phi_i = \lambda_i^2 \left(1 - \frac{e^{-\lambda_i(T-T_0)} - e^{-\lambda_i T}}{\lambda_i T_0}\right)^{-1}, \qquad i = 1, 2, \tag{3.33}$$

where f_i is the sample-size fraction n_i/N, T_0 the patient accrual time, and T the follow-up time (Lachin, 1981).

3.3.3 Relationship Between Enrollment Rate and Number of Events

A common question to be answered by a statistician during a protocol design for a clinical trial involving the time to an events as the primary efficacy end-point is: What would be the number of events at a particular time, or when would a particular number of events occur? The information is particularly useful when the design involves interim analyses.

Notation:

$S(t)$	survival function: the probability of a patient surviving longer than age t
$F(t) = 1 - S(t)$	probability of a patient dying before age t
$f(t) = dF(t)/dt$	density function
$R(t)$	enrollment rate; usually a step function
D	number of events
T_0	enrollment duration

Exponential Distribution Without Censoring Before T Assume no censoring before time T (i.e., no early dropouts):

$$D = \int_0^T \int_0^t R(\tau) d\tau f(t-\tau) dt. \tag{3.34}$$

Given $S(t) = \exp(-\lambda t)$, $f(t) = \lambda \exp(-\lambda t)$, and

$$R(t) = \begin{cases} R & t \le T_0 \\ 0 & t > T_0, \end{cases} \tag{3.35}$$

$$D = \begin{cases} R\lambda \int_0^T \int_0^t e^{-\lambda(t-\tau)} d\tau dt, & T \leq T_0 \\ R\lambda \int_0^T \int_0^{T_0} e^{-\lambda(t-\tau)} d\tau dt, & T > T_0, \end{cases} \tag{3.36}$$

$$D = \begin{cases} R\left(T - \frac{1}{\lambda} + \frac{1}{\lambda} e^{-\lambda T}\right), & T \leq T_0 \\ R\left[T_0 - \frac{1}{\lambda}(e^{\lambda T_0} - 1)e^{-\lambda T}\right], & T > T_0. \end{cases} \tag{3.37}$$

(*Note*: The number of events is proportional to the constant enrollment rate R.)

$$T = \begin{cases} -\frac{1}{\lambda} \ln\left(\frac{\lambda D}{R} - T\lambda + 1\right), & T \leq T_0 \\ -\frac{1}{\lambda} \ln\left[\lambda\left(T_0 - \frac{D}{R}\right)(e^{\lambda T_0} - 1)^{-1}\right], & T > T_0. \end{cases} \tag{3.38}$$

Illustrative Example Suppose that a trial requires $N = 300$ patients to be enrolled in 9 months; the median survival time for the test drug, $t_{\text{median}} = 7.91$ months; and the total study duration = 23 months. Therefore, $T_0 = 9$ months, $R = 300/9 = 33.333$, and $\lambda = \ln 2/t_{\text{median}} = 0.0876$. The predictions for the number of events at 9, 11, and 12 months are 92, 126, and 140, respectively.

Exponential Distribution with Censoring Let $R(t)$ be the enrollment rate at time t (the clock starts when the first patient is enrolled in the trial), and $E(\tau, t)$ is the probability of early withdrawal (censoring) before time t for a patient enrolled at time τ. Let $f(t)$ be the probability density function for dying at time t. The number of patients enrolled during the time interval $(\tau, \tau + d\tau)$ is approximately equal to $R(\tau)\, d\tau$, where $d\tau$ is small. The probability of censoring before time t for these patients is $E(\tau, t)$. In other words, the probability of staying in the trial at time t for these patients is $1 - E(\tau, t)$. Furthermore, the patient who stays in the trial at time t has a probability of dying at the time interval $(t, t + dt)$ of $f(t)\, dt$, where dt is a small interval such that $f(t)$ is constant within the interval $(t, t + dt)$. Therefore, the number of deaths at time T will be

$$D = \int_0^T \int_0^t R(\tau)[1 - E(\tau, t)] d\tau f(t - \tau) dt. \tag{3.39}$$

For an exponential survival model we have $S(t) = \exp(-\lambda t)$ and $f(t) = \lambda \exp(-\lambda t)$. If $E(\tau, t)$ does not depend on how long a patient has stayed in the trial, $E(\tau, t) = E(t)$. If $E(\tau, t)$ does not depend on how long it has been since the trial started (i.e., it does not depend on seasons), then $E(\tau, t) = E(\tau)$. The simplest case is $E(\tau, t) =$ constant. In the following we consider only the exponential survival model with $E(\tau, t) = E(t)$ and use a discrete form to approximate the integration above, which is very practical:

$$D = \sum_{i=1}^{N_T} \sum_{j=1}^{i} R(\tau_j)[1 - E(t_i)]\lambda \exp[-\lambda(t_i - \tau_j)] \tag{3.40}$$

or

$$D = \sum_{i=1}^{N_T} \sum_{j=1}^{i} R_j(1 - E_i)\lambda \exp[-\lambda(i - j)]. \tag{3.41}$$

If we use a monthly rate for R and E, then N_T will be equal to the number of months from time zero to the time of interest. To calculate the number of deaths in each month, one needs to know (or make assumptions regarding) the R and E values in each month to the time of interest, and the hazard rate λ.

4 Group Sequential Trial Design

4.1 INTRODUCTION

A group sequential design involves multiple stages. At each stage an interim analysis is performed. An interim analysis is intended to compare treatment arms with respect to efficacy or safety at any time prior to formal completion of a trial. Because the number and methods of these comparisons will affect the interpretation of the trial, all interim analyses should be planned carefully in advance and described in the protocol, including the timing of the analyses and stopping rules. (Later we will see that these requirements may be eased in adaptive designs.) An interim analysis planned with the intention of deciding whether or not to terminate a trial is usually accomplished through the use of a group sequential design that employs statistical monitoring schemes or a data monitoring committee charter as guidelines. The goal of such an interim analysis is to stop the trial early if the superiority of the treatment under study is clearly established, if the demonstration of a relevant treatment difference has become unlikely, or if unacceptable adverse effects are apparent. When the trial design and monitoring objective involve multiple endpoints, another layer of multiplicity (in addition to the multiplicity due to multiple looks over time) may also need to be taken into account. In some circumstances, an unplanned interim analysis may be necessary. In these cases, a protocol amendment describing the interim analysis should be completed prior to "unblinding" the data.

4.2 BASICS OF GROUP SEQUENTIAL DESIGN

Group Sequential Test The key feature of a group sequential test, as contrasted with a fully sequential test, is that the accumulating data are analyzed at intervals rather than after each new observation.

Error Inflation For a classical single-stage trial with $\alpha = 0.05$, H_0 will be rejected if the statistic $z > 1.96$. For a sequential trial with K analyses, if at the kth analysis ($k = 1, 2, \ldots, K$) the absolute value of Z_k is sufficiently large, the

Classical and Adaptive Clinical Trial Designs Using ExpDesign Studio™,
By Mark Chang

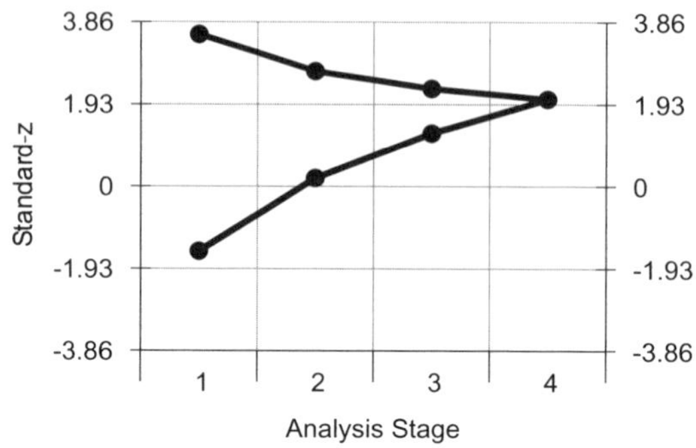

Figure 4.1 Efficacy and futility stopping boundaries.

study stops with rejection of H_0. It is not appropriate simply to apply a level α two-sided test at each analysis since the multiple tests at the data would lead to a type I error well in excess of α. In fact, for $K = 5$, the actual α level is 0.142, nearly three times the 0.05 significance level applied at each individual analysis.

Stopping Boundary Stopping boundaries consist of a set of critical values that are compared against the statistics calculated from actual data to determine whether to continue or terminate a trial. A typical set of stopping boundaries with early stopping for efficacy or futility is presented in Figure 4.1.The stopping rules for a group sequential design with early stopping for H_a can be specified as follows: At the kth stage ($k = 1, \ldots, K - 1$), if $p_k \leq \alpha_k$, stop and reject H_0; otherwise, continue the trial. At the final stage, K, if $p_K \leq \alpha_K$, stop and reject H_0; otherwise, accept H_0.

The stopping rules for a group sequential design with early stopping for either H_0 or H_a can be specified as follows: At the kth stage ($k = 1, \ldots, K - 1$), if $p_k \leq \alpha_k$, stop and reject H_0; if $p_k \geq \beta_k$, stop and accept H_0; otherwise, continue the trial. At the final stage K, if $p_K \leq \alpha_K$, stop and reject H_0; otherwise, accept H_0. The stopping rules for a group sequential design with early stopping for H_0 can be specified as follows: At the kth stage ($k = 1, \ldots, K - 1$), if $p_k \geq \beta_k$, stop and accept H_0; otherwise, continue the trial. At the final stage, K, if $p_K \leq \alpha_K$, stop and reject H_0; otherwise, accept H_0.

Boundary Scales Different scales can be used to construct the stopping boundaries. The two commonly used scales are the standardized z-statistic and the p-scale. The scale definitions can be given as follows:

Standardized z-statistic:

$$Z_k = \theta_k \sqrt{I_k}, \tag{4.1}$$

where the information level is defined as $I_k = n_k/2\sigma^2$, and θ_k is the treatment difference.

p-Value scale or p-scale:

$$p_k = 1 - \Phi(Z_k). \tag{4.2}$$

If the z-scale is used, the usual z test statistic is calculated at each stage and compared with the stopping boundary on the z-scale. When the p-scale is used, the p-value is calculated at each stage and compared with the stopping boundary on the p-scale.

ExpDesign Studio allows users to select different shapes for the stopping boundaries. All these boundaries are determined to control the overall type I error, α. The difference between the types of boundaries is that some (e.g., Pocock's) may spend more α in the early stages, and others (e.g., O'Brien and Fleming's) may spend more α in later stages. ExpDesign has implemented a more generalized boundary type (Wang and Tsiatis) to meet different boundary requirements. The Wang–Tsiatis boundary was originally defined on the standardized z-scale, but can equivalently be defined as $\alpha_k = 1 - \Phi(ct_k^{\Delta-0.5})$ on the p-scale, where $t_k = k/K$; c is a constant determined by the significance level α. The inner futility boundary type can be symmetrical (on the sample mean scale): $\beta_k = 2c\sqrt{t_k} - ct_k^{\Delta-0.5}$ or trianglular: $\beta_k = c(k - k_0)/(K - k_0)$, where $k_0 = (K/2) + 1 = \text{Int}(K/2) + 1$. When the parameter $\Delta = 0$, 0.5, and 0.688, the Wang–Tsiatis boundary degenerates to the O'Brien–Fleming, linear, and Pocock boundaries, respectively.

Futility Binding In futility binding the futility rules have to be followed (i.e., if the futility boundary is crossed, the trial must stop). With no futility binding, the futility boundary does not have to be followed. In current practice, not every company follows the futility rules specified in the protocols, and regulatory agencies usually apply a nonbinding rule, which means that a futility boundary in the earlier part of a trial cannot be used for the construction of efficacy boundaries in the later part of the trial.

4.3 HOW TO DESIGN SEQUENTIAL TRIALS USING EXPDESIGN

There are many factors that can be used to characterize a group sequential design, such as the expected sample size under the hypotheses and the maximum sample size in selecting a group sequential design. If you wish to reduce the expected cost, you might want to choose a design with a minimum expected sample size; if you wish to reduce the maximum possible cost, you might want to consider a design with a minimum total sample size. In any case, you should compare all the stopping probabilities between designs carefully before determinating an appropriate design. O'Brien–Fleming boundaries, with the corresponding $\Delta = 0$, are very conservative in early rejection of the null hypothesis. Pocock's method, with the corresponding $\Delta = 0.5$, uses a constant stopping boundary (on the z-scale) over time. Generally speaking, a large value of Δ (e.g., 0.8) will lead to a design that spends type I error more at earlier stages than at later stages. To increase the probability of accepting the null hypothesis at earlier stages, you can use the triangular inner boundaries. If you don't want to accept the null hypothesis at all at interim analyses, you should choose a design with rejection of the null hypothesis only. If you don't want to reject the null hypothesis at interim analyses, you should choose a design with acceptance of the null hypothesis only. Adjusting the size fractions is also an effective way to achieve a desired design. Although balanced designs are commonly used, one can, if desired, use an unbalanced design with a difference size for each experimental group.

The basic steps in designing a group sequential trial with ExpDesign are presented in Section 1.2.2. You will be shown below, through examples, how to design various sequential trials using ExpDesign Studio. However, before we discuss these, it will be helpful to explain some of the input parameters. The potential early claim can be "the null hypothesis is true" (i.e., the futility design), "the alternative hypothesis is true" (i.e., the efficacy design), or "either of the hypotheses is true." The sample-size fractions at K analyses should be a sequence of numbers between 0 and 1, separated by commas. When you enter the number of stages, the fractions are filled into the textbox automatically based on an equal-sample-size design (an equal-information-interval design). You can change them anytime afterward. The stopping boundary shape parameter, delta, is the Δ in the Wang–Tsiatis boundary family, in which a low value will lead to a low probability of rejecting the alternative hypothesis. The allowable range for Δ is (–0.5, 1). You can move the mouse over each input box and wait for a second to see the hint. You can always click the example button 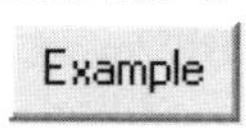

to see the input example.

4.3.1 Design Featuring Early Efficacy Stopping for Two Means

Consider a trial to test the effectiveness of a new drug, ABC, in treating patients with mild to moderate asthma. A parallel design with two treatment groups (placebo vs. ABC) is chosen for the design. The primary efficacy parameter is percentage change from baseline in FEV1. The mean difference in percent change in FEV1 between placebo and ABC is estimated to be 6% (5% vs. 11%), with a standard deviation of 18%.

A single-stage design with a fixed sample of 282 will allow us to have 80% power to detect the difference at a one-sided significance level $\alpha = 0.025$. The sponsors believe that there is a good chance that the test drug will be superior to the placebo and want to stop the trial early if the superiority becomes evident.

Based on the information, we specify the options in ExpDesign as follows: two groups, hypothesis test, mean/median, and alternative hypothesis. Enter "2" for the number of analyses, "1" for a one-sided analysis, "0.025" for α, "0.05" for the group 1 mean, "0.11" for the group 2 mean, "0.18" for the

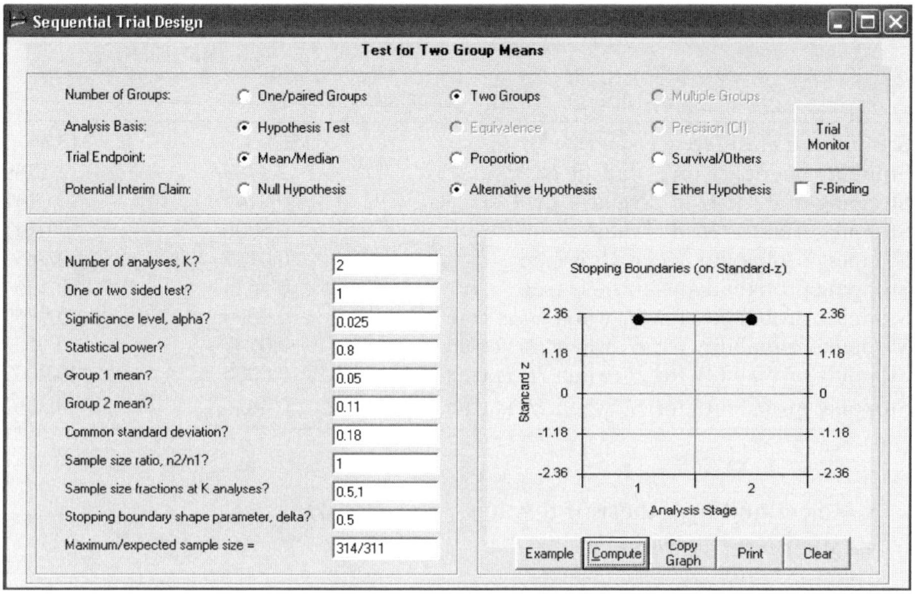

Figure 4.2 Two-stage group sequential design for two means.

common standard deviation, "1" for the sample-size ratio, "0.5, 1" for the sample-size fractions, "0.5" for the stopping boundary shape parameter Δ, and "0.8" for the power (Figure 4.2). Click 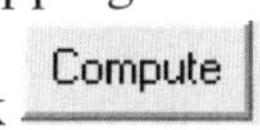

to run the simulation. When it is finished, click  on the toolbar; the outputs reported below will be generated.

Design Outputs See Table 4.1. Sample size for the single-stage design = 282; maximum sample size (combined total) = 314; sample size expected under H_0 = 311; sample size expected under H_a = 241.

Report This experimental design has one interim analysis and a final analysis. The sample sizes for the two analyses are 157 and 314, respectively. The sample-size ratio between the two groups is 1. The maximum sample size for the design is 314, and the expected sample size is 311 under the null hypothesis and 241 under the alternative hypothesis. The calculation is based on a level of significance $\alpha = 0.025$, power = 0.8, mean difference = 0.06, and standard deviation = 0.18.

The decision rules are specified as follows:

At stage 1:

- Accept null hypothesis if p-value > 0.5.

TABLE 4.1

	Analysis Stage	
	1	2
Sample size at difference stages	156.90	313.80
Stopping boundary on z-statistic scale	2.1789	2.1789
Stopping trial for H_a if p-value < or =	0.0147	0.0147
Stopping trial for H_0 if p-value >	0.5000	0.0147
Stopping probability when H_0 is true	0.0147	0.9853
Stopping probability when H_a is true	0.4636	0.5364
Stopping probability for H_0 when H_0 is true	0.0000	0.9750
Stopping probability for H_a when H_0 is true	0.0147	0.0103
Stopping probability for H_0 when H_a is true	0.0000	0.2002
Stopping probability for H_a when H_a is true	0.4636	0.3362

- Reject null hypothesis if p-value < or = 0.0147.
- Otherwise, continue.

At stage 2:

- Accept null hypothesis if p-value > 0.0147.
- Reject null hypothesis if p-value < or = 0.0147.

It is important to know that the sponsors are more interested in the expected sample size (241) under the alternative hypothesis than the sample size (309) under the null hypothesis. The maximum sample size is 314, whereas it is 284 for the classical single-stage design. The sponsors believe that there is a good chance to stop the trial early, which means that only 157 patients are required. This will lead not only to a reduction in the number of patients but also a savings in time.

4.3.2 Design Featuring Early Futility Stopping for a Proportion

A phase III trial is to be designed for patients with acute ischemic stroke of recent onset. The composite endpoint (death and MI) is the primary endpoint, and the event rate is 14% for the control group and 12% for the test group. For classical design, a sample size of 5937 per group will provide 90% power to detect the difference at a one-sided α of 0.025.

To design the trial, we specify the options in ExpDesign as follows: two groups, hypothesis test, proportion, and null hypothesis. Enter "3" for the number of analyses, "1" for a one-sided test; "0.025" for the significance level; "0.9" for the statistical power; "0.12" for the proportion for group 1; "0.14" for the proportion for group 2; "1" for the sample size ratio; "0.333, 0.667, 1" for the sample-size fractions; and "0" for the stopping boundary

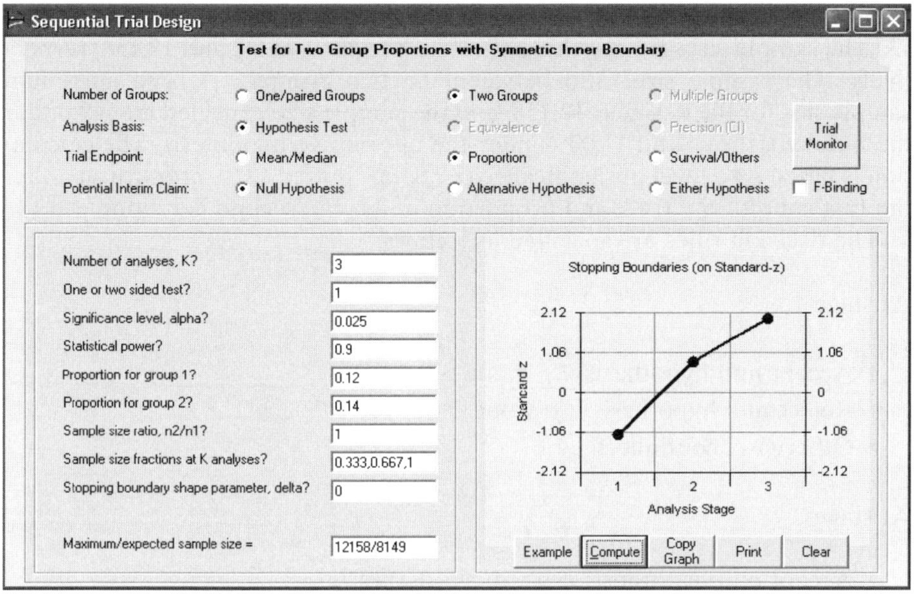

Figure 4.3 One-sided futility group sequential design.

shape parameter Δ (Figure 4.3). After clicking 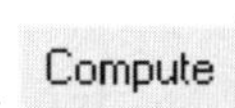 and then 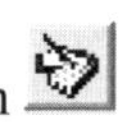 on the toolbar, the outputs reported below will be generated.

Design Outputs See Table 4.2. Sample size for the single-stage design = 11,884; maximum sample size (combined total) = 12,158; sample size expected under H_0 = 8149; sample size expected under H_a = 12,029.

TABLE 4.2

	Analysis Stage		
	1	2	3
Sample size at difference stages	4,048.6	8,109.3	12,158
Stopping boundary on z-statistic scale	−1.1344	0.8015	1.9599
Stopping trial for H_a if p-value < or =	0.0000	0.0000	0.0250
Stopping trial for H_0 if p-value >	0.8717	0.2114	0.0250
Stopping probability when H_0 is true	0.1283	0.6609	0.1867
Stopping probability when H_a is true	0.0012	0.0294	0.9694
Stopping probability for H_0 when H_0 is true	0.1283	0.6609	0.1867
Stopping probability for H_a when H_0 is true	0.0000	0.0000	0.0000
Stopping probability for H_0 when H_a is true	0.0012	0.0294	0.0694
Stopping probability for H_a when H_a is true	0.0000	0.0000	0.9000

Report This experimental design has two interim analyses and a final analysis. The sample sizes for the three analyses are 4049, 8109, and 12,158, respectively. The sample size ratio between the two groups is 1. The maximum sample size for the design is 12,158, and the sample size expected is 8149 under the null hypothesis and 12,029 under the alternative hypothesis. The calculation is based on a level of significance $\alpha = 0.025$, power = 0.9, proportion under the first condition = 0.12, and proportion under the second condition = 0.14.

The decision rules are specified as follows:

At stage 1:

- Accept null hypothesis if p-value > 0.8717.
- Reject null hypothesis if p-value < or = 0.
- Otherwise, continue.

At stage 2:

- Accept null hypothesis if p-value > 0.2114.
- Reject null hypothesis if p-value < or = 0.
- Otherwise, continue.

At stage 3:

- Accept null hypothesis if p-value > 0.025.
- Reject null hypothesis if p-value < or = 0.025.

4.3.3 Design Featuring Early Stopping for a Survival Endpoint

An oncology trial is to be conducted to investigate the efficacy of the test drug ABC. A two-arm unbalanced design is chosen for the trial with a sample size ratio of 1.2 (ABC vs. control). The median survival time is 7.8 months for the control and 10 months for the ABC group. The accrual time is estimated to be 8 months, and the total trial duration, 23 months. The calculation indicates that 667 patients are required for a classical single-stage design. There is great interest in determining if a sequential trial will save time and money.

To design this trial, we specify the following options in ExpDesign: two groups, hypothesis, survival, and either hypothesis. Enter "4" for the number of analyses; "1" for a one-sided test; "0.025" for α; "0.8" for the statistical power; "7.8" for the median time for group 1; "10" for the median time for group 2; "8" for the patient accrual time; "23" for the total follow-up time; "1.2" for the sample-size ratio; "0.25, 0.5, 0.75, 1" for the sample-size fractions at K analyses; and "0.25" for the stopping boundary shape parameter δ

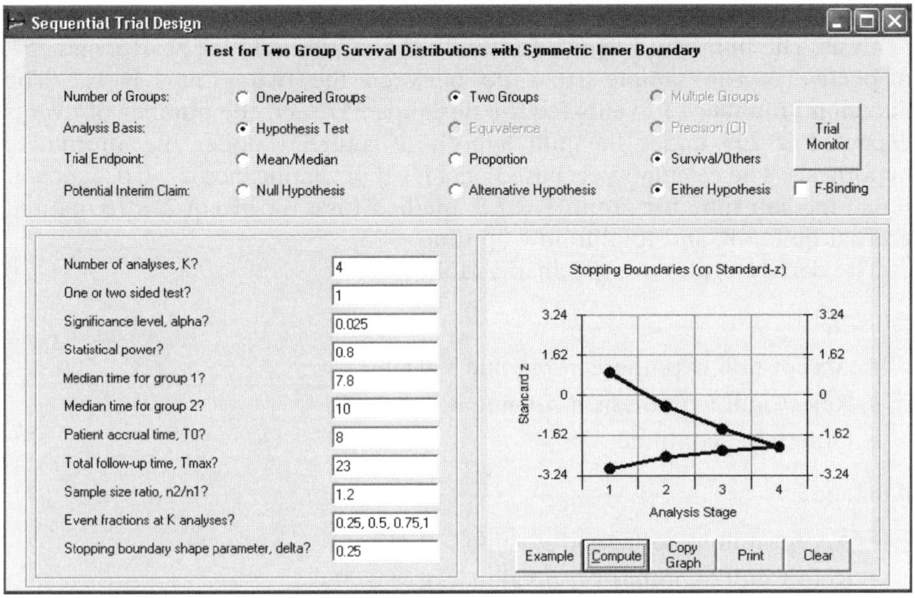

Figure 4.4 Group sequential design with efficacy or futility stopping.

(Figure 4.4). After Clicking 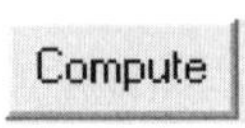

and then 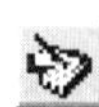 on the toolbar, the outputs reported below will be generated.

Design Outputs See Table 4.3. Sample size for the single-stage design = 667; maximum sample size (combined total) = 838; maximum number of events required = 586; number of events expected under H_0 = 319; number of events expected under H_a = 403.

TABLE 4.3

	Analysis Stage			
	1	2	3	4
Sample size at difference stages	146.60	293.20	439.80	586.40
Stopping boundary on z-statistic scale	0.8753	−0.4755	−1.3893	−2.1131
	−2.9883	−2.5129	−2.2706	−2.1131
Stopping trial for H_a if p-value < or =	0.0014	0.0060	0.0116	0.0173
Stopping trial for H_0 if p-value >	0.8093	0.3172	0.0824	0.0173
Stopping probability when H_0 is true	0.1921	0.5025	0.2425	0.0630
Stopping probability when H_a is true	0.0769	0.3298	0.3626	0.2308
Stopping probability for H_0 when H_0 is true	0.1907	0.4970	0.2342	0.0551
Stopping probability for H_a when H_0 is true	0.0014	0.0054	0.0083	0.0079
Stopping probability for H_0 when H_a is true	0.0088	0.0445	0.0740	0.0728
Stopping probability for H_a when H_a is true	0.0681	0.2853	0.2886	0.1581

Report This experimental design has three interim analyses and a final analysis. The number of events for the four analyses is 139, 279, 418, and 557, respectively. The sample-size ratio between the two groups is 1.2. The maximum number of events for the design is 557, and the number of events expected is 295 under the null hypothesis and 531 under the alternative hypothesis. The calculation is based on a level of significance $\alpha = 0.025$, power = 0.8, median time for group 1 = 7.8, median time for group 2 = 10, patient accrual time = 8, and total follow-up time = 23.

The decision rules are specified as follows:

At stage 1:

- Accept null hypothesis if *p*-value > 0.8093.
- Reject null hypothesis if *p*-value < or = 0.0014.
- Otherwise, continue.

At stage 2:

- Accept null hypothesis if *p*-value > 0.3172.
- Reject null hypothesis if *p*-value < or = 0.006.
- Otherwise, continue.

At stage 3:

- Accept null hypothesis if *p*-value > 0.0824.
- Reject null hypothesis if *p*-value < or = 0.0116.
- Otherwise, continue.

At stage 4:

- Accept null hypothesis if *p*-value > 0.0173.
- Reject null hypothesis if *p*-value < or = 0.0173.

It is obvious that a four-stage sequential design could save a great deal. However, it is important to examine the practical issues. Can we suspend enrollment while waiting for the interim analysis results? If four analyses are impractical, can we use a sequential design with two or three analyses?

4.3.4 Design Featuring Early Stopping for Paired Proportions

Proliferative diabetic retinopathy is a chronic complication of diabetes that after a long asymptomatic period can progress to severe visual loss. It is a leading cause of blindness in the United States. The diabetic retinopathy study, a randomized, controlled clinical trial, was sponsored by the National Eye Institute in the early 1970s to assess the ability of photocoagulation to treat retinopathy. One eye was randomly selected for photocoagulation while the other eye remained untreated. A five-year follow-up was planned for each

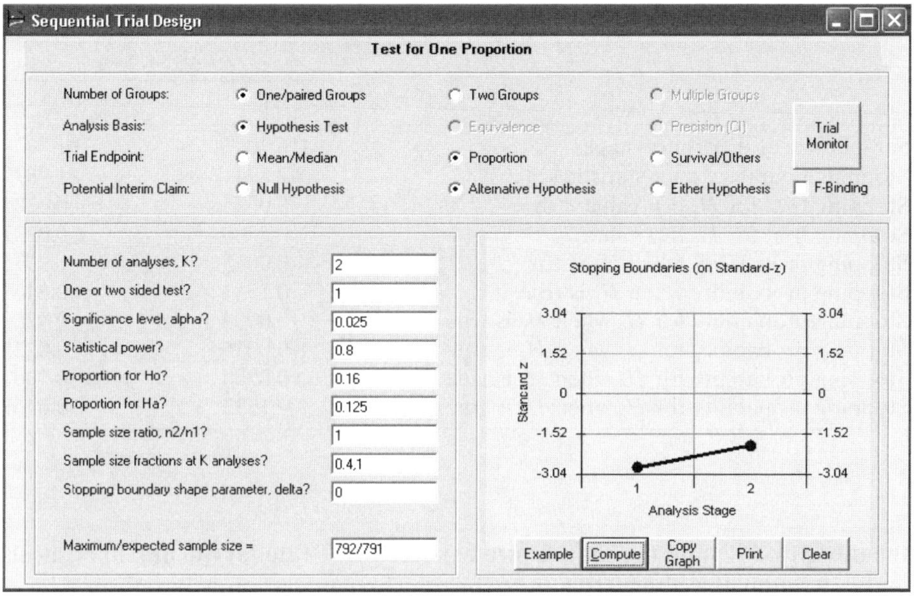

Figure 4.5 GSD for a proliferative diabetic retinopathy trail (paired means).

patient, and the principal response for gauging the efficacy of the treatment was the occurrence of severe visual loss (blindness). This was defined as visual acuity of less than 5/200 at two or more consecutive follow-up visits scheduled at 4-month intervals (DeMets et al., 2006, p. 56).

Suppose that we use group sequential design (GSD) with one interim analysis (Pocock boundary) for the trial. The estimated event rates for the two groups are 16% and 12.5% for the control and treated groups, respectively. To design a group sequential trial, we specify options in ExpDesign as follows: two groups, hypothesis, proportion, and alternative hypotheses. Enter "2" for the number of analyses, "1" for a one-sided test; "0.025" for α, "0.8" for the power, "0.16" for the proportion for H_0, "0.125" for the proportion for H_a, "1" for the sample-size ratio, "0.4, 1" for the sample-size fractions, and "0" for δ (Figure 4.5). After clicking 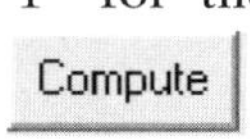

and then 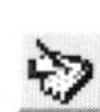 on the toolbar, the outputs reported below will be generated.

Design Outputs See Table 4.4. Sample size for the single-stage design = 783; maximum sample size (combined total) = 792; sample size expected under H_0 = 791; sample size expected under H_a = 719.

Report This experiment design has one interim analysis and a final analysis. The sample sizes for the two analyses are 317 and 792, respectively. The sample-size ratio between the two groups is 1. The maximum sample size for

TABLE 4.4

	Analysis Stage	
	1	2
Sample size at difference stages	316.70	791.70
Stopping boundary on z-statistic scale	−2.8043	−1.9829
Stopping trial for H_a if p-value < or =	0.0025	0.0237
Stopping trial for H_0 if p-value >	0.5000	0.0237
Stopping probability when H_0 is true	0.0025	0.9975
Stopping probability when H_a is true	0.1533	0.8467
Stopping probability for H_0 when H_0 is true	0.0000	0.9750
Stopping probability for H_a when H_0 is true	0.0025	0.0225
Stopping probability for H_0 when H_a is true	0.0000	0.2000
Stopping probability for H_a when H_a is true	0.1533	0.6467

the design is 792, and the sample size expected is 791 under the null hypothesis and 719 under the alternative hypothesis. The calculation is based on a level of significance $\alpha = 0.025$, power = 0.8, proportion under $H_0 = 0.16$, and proportion under $H_a = 0.125$.

The decision rules are specified as follows:

At stage 1:

- Accept null hypothesis if p-value > 0.5.
- Reject null hypothesis if p-value < or = 0.0025.
- Otherwise, continue.

At stage 2:

- Accept null hypothesis if p-value > 0.0237.
- Reject null hypothesis if p-value < = 0.0237.

4.4 HOW TO MONITOR A GROUP SEQUENTIAL TRIAL USING EXPDESIGN

4.4.1 Need for Trial Monitoring

The stopping rule chosen in the design phase serves as a guideline to a data monitoring committee (DMC) (Ellenberg et al., 2002) as it makes a decision recommending continuing or stopping a clinical trial. If all aspects of the conduct of a clinical trial adhere exactly to the conditions stipulated during the design phase, the stopping rule obtained during the design phase could be used directly. However, there are usually complicating factors that must be dealt with during the conduct of a trial.

Deviation in Analysis Schedule DMC meetings are typically based on the availability of the members, which may differ from the schedules set at the design phase. The enrollment may be different from the assumption made during the design phase. The deviation in the analysis schedule will affect the stopping boundaries; therefore, the boundaries should be recalculated based on the actual schedules.

Deviation in Efficacy Variable Estimation The true variability of the response variable is never known, but the actual data collected from an interim analysis may show that the initial estimates in the design phase are inaccurate. In this case we may want to know the likelihood of success of a trial based on current data, known as *conditional power* or *predictive power*, and use sample size reestimation technique (Chapter 5).

Safety Factors Efficacy is not the only factor that will affect a DMC's decision. Safety factors are critical for the DMC to make an appropriate recommendation to stop or continue a trial. The benefit–risk ratio is the composite criterion used most commonly to assist in the decision making. In this respect it is desirable to know the likelihood of success of the trial based on current data (i.e., the conditional power or predictive power).

4.4.2 Techniques for Monitoring a Sequential Trial

The sequential stopping boundaries are the simplest tool available to use in determining whether to continue or terminate a trial. The original methodology for group sequential boundaries required that the number and timing of interim analyses be specified in advance. Whitehead (1983) introduced another type of stopping boundary method: Whitehead triangle boundaries. This method permits unlimited analyses as a trial progresses and thus is called a continuous monitoring procedure.

A practical but more complicated method utilizes the operating characteristics desired for the design, which typically include type-I error $[P(H_a|H_0)]$, the power curve $[P(H_a|\theta)$ vs. $\theta]$, the sample-size distribution or information levels (I_k), estimates of the treatment effect that would correspond to early stopping, the naive confidence interval, the repeated confidence interval, curtailment (conditional power or predictive power), and the futility index. The conditional power and predictive power both represent the likelihood of rejecting the alternative hypothesis conditioning on the current data. The difference is that the conditional probability is based on a frequentist approach, whereas the predictive power is a Bayesian approach. The *futility index* is a measure of the likelihood of failing to reject H_0 at the k analysis given that H_a

is true. (Sometimes, the futility index is defined as 1–conditional power.) The defining property of a $(1 - \alpha)$-level sequence of repeated confidence interval (RCI) for θ is

$$\Pr_\theta(\theta \in I_k \text{ for all } k = 1, \ldots, K) = 1 - \alpha \qquad \text{for all } \theta. \tag{4.3}$$

Here each I_k ($k = 1, \ldots, K$) is an interval computed from the information available at analysis k. Calculation of the RCI at analysis k is similar to the naive confidence interval, but $z_{1-\alpha}$ ($z_{1-\alpha/2}$) is replaced by C_k, the stopping boundary on the standard z-statistic (Jennison and Turnbull, 2000). For example, CI = $d \pm z_{1-\alpha/2}\sigma$; RCI = $d \pm C_k\sigma$.

The conditional power method can be used to assess whether an early trend is sufficiently unfavorable that reversal to a significant positive trend is very unlikely or nearly impossible. The futility index can also be used to monitor a trial. Premature termination of a trial with a very small futility index might be inappropriate. The same is true for continuing a trial with a very high futility index (Jennison and Turnbull, 2000).

4.4.3 How to Monitor a Trial Using ExpDesign

A simple example of trial monitoring is to use observed data to check if the stopping boundaries have been crossed. We discuss monitoring of the proliferative diabetic retinopathy trial in Section 4.3.4. The patient enrollment began in 1972 and ended in 1975. Suppose that the group sequential design has one interim analysis with a Pocock stopping boundary at month 15. The efficacy stopping boundaries occur at 0.0142 on the p-scale for both interim and final analyses. Suppose that at a planned interim analysis, the two-year cumulative incidence of blindness was 16.3% in untreated eyes but only 6.4% in treated eyes. Based on a large-sample assumption, the p-value is less than 0.001. Therefore, the efficacy stopping boundary was crossed and the trial met the early efficacy criterion. However, the actual trial was continued due to the uncertainty of long-term safety (see DeMets et al., 2006, for details).

ExpDesign has built-in tools for trial monitoring. To carry out the monitoring, we proceed as follows:

1. Open the file for the design if it has been saved previously, or reenter values for the input parameters (if the analysis schedule or enrollment changed, use the actual sample-size fractions for the input) and click 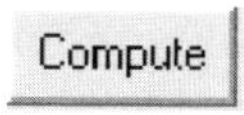

 to create the design.
2. Click 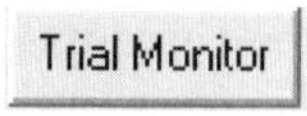

 in the **Group Sequential Design** window. The **Trial Monitor** window will appear.
3. Enter the values for **Observed Stage, Theta**, and **Observed Info**. For the current case with a survival endpoint θ = ln(hazard ratio), the informa-

tion level observed, $I = rd/(1 + r)^2$, where r is the sample size ratio and d is the number of deaths.

4. Click 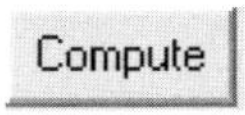

on the **Trial Monitor** window to produce the results.

We now use the oncology trial in Section 4.3.3 to illustrate how to monitor a trial using ExpDesign. First, rerun the oncology trial design as in Section 4.3.3 (Figure 4.4). After the calculation has been made, the **Trial Monitor** button 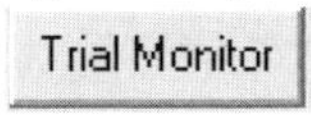

will be enabled. Click the button and enter the information required.

It is helpful to explain the input parameters before discussing the example further. The stage observed is the current stage. The θ value is the treatment difference expected; in practice the difference observed [mean difference, proportion difference, or log(hazard ratio)] is generally used. The information observed at stage k is defined as $I_k = n_k/\hat{\sigma}$ and $I_k = (\hat{\sigma}_A^2/n_{Ak} + \hat{\sigma}_B^2/n_{Bk})^{-1}$ for one- and two-group designs with a continuous endpoint. The same formulations can be used for a proportion endpoint with the variance defined as $\hat{\sigma}_i^2 = p_i(1-p_i)$, where p_i is the proportion in the ith group.

For a survival endpoint, the information level is defined as $I_k = d_k$ and $I_k = rd_k/(1 + r)^2$ for one- and two-group designs, respectively, where d_k is the number of deaths at stage k and r is the sample-size ratio between the two groups. Let's use the oncology trial example in Section 4.3.3 to illustrate the steps for trial monitoring.

Assume at stage 1 that the total deaths = 147, as scheduled; the proportions of deaths are 0.15 and 0.22 for the two groups, respectively. The log hazard ratio is given by

$$\hat{\theta} = \ln(\frac{\ln p_2}{\ln p_1}) = \ln(\frac{\ln 0.22}{\ln 0.15}) = -0.225.$$

The information level is calculated using the formula

$$I_1 = \frac{r}{(1+r)^2} d_1 = \frac{1.2}{(1+1.2)^2} 147 = 36.45.$$

Similarly, suppose that at stage 2, the deaths observed = 293; the proportions of deaths are 0.43 and 0.52 for the two groups, respectively. We then obtain $\hat{\theta} = -0.255$ and $I_2 = 72.64$.

At stage 3, suppose that the deaths observed = 440; the proportions of deaths are 0.61 and 0.68 for the two groups, respectively. We then obtain $\hat{\theta} = -0.248$ and $I_3 = 109.09$.

In practice, we calculate $\hat{\theta}$ and I_k at each stage, then perform the following steps using the ExpDesign trial monitor for decision making.

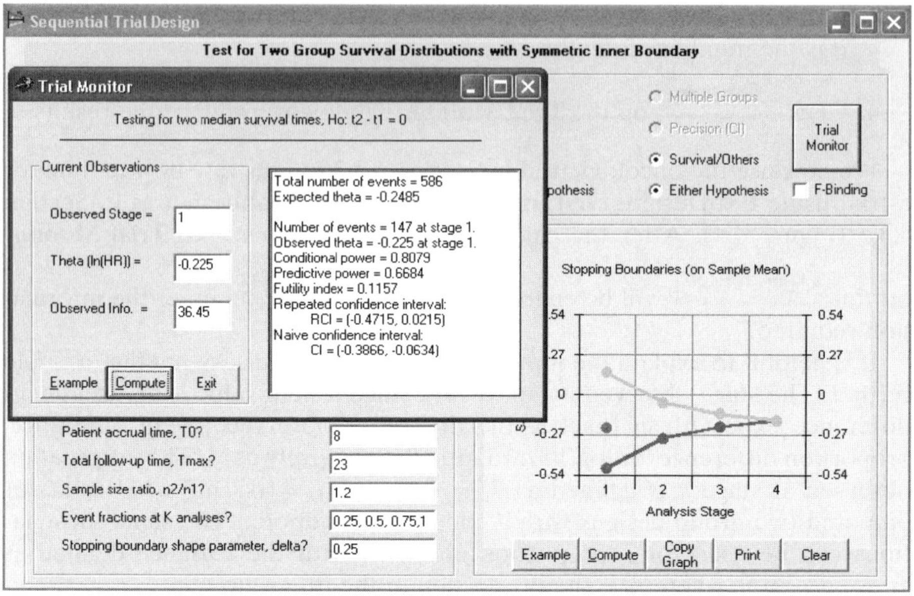

Figure 4.6 Trial monitoring using ExpDesign at stage 1.

1. Regenerate the group sequential design (or open the design if you have saved it) as shown in Figure 4.6. The **Trial Monitor** button 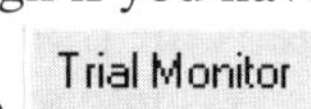

 is enabled.
2. Enter the stagewise observed treatment difference $\hat{\theta}$ and information level I_k into the **Trial Monitor** window; then click 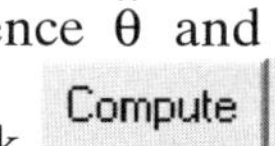

 to calculate the conditional and predictive power, futility index, and the naive and repeated confidence intervals (Figures 4.6 to 4.8). A summary of the trial monitoring is presented in Table 4.5.

At each stage, the p-value is calculated using $p\text{-value} = \Phi^{-1}\left(\hat{\theta}\sqrt{I_k}\right)$. For stage 1 the p-value is 0.0872, which lies within the continuation range between 0.0014 and 0.8093; hence, the trial continues to the next stage. The conditional power is reasonable (81%). At stage 2 the p-value is 0.015 and the conditional power is 0.94, and the trial continues according to the predefined stopping boundary. At stage 3 the p-value is 0.0048, which is smaller than the efficacy stopping boundary 0.0116, so the trial is stopped and the null hypothesis is rejected. For normal and binary endpoints, the calculations are simpler than using the survival endpoint. You may want to try this yourself.

If the information fraction is different from that originally scheduled, the stopping boundaries have to be recalculated based on the actual information fraction. We discuss this in detail in Chapter 6.

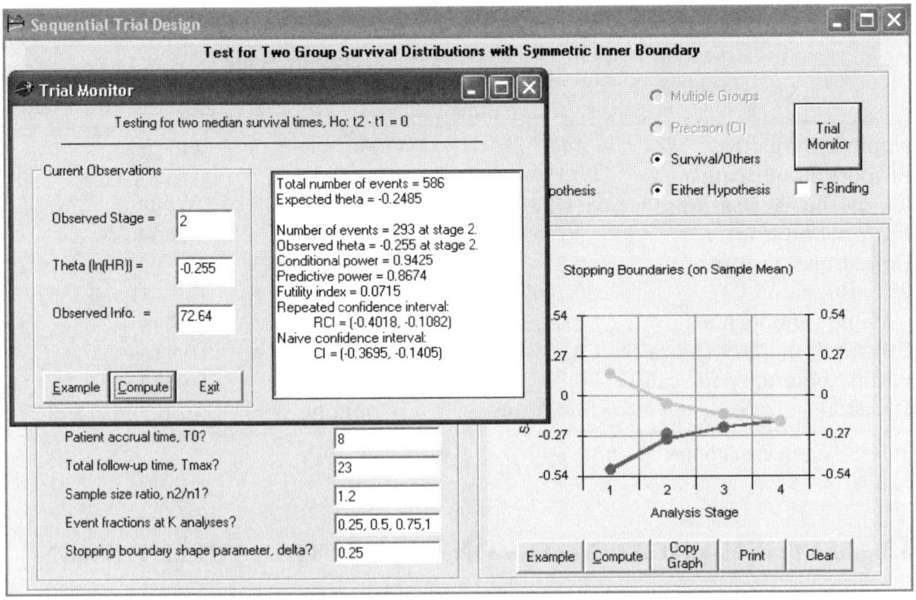

Figure 4.7 Trial monitoring using ExpDesign at stage 2.

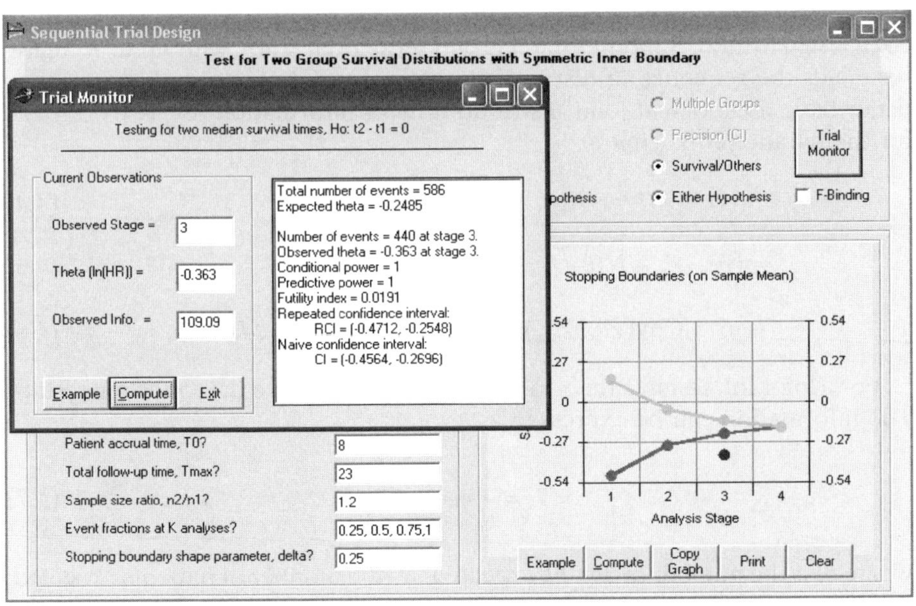

Figure 4.8 Trial monitoring using ExpDesign at stage 3.

TABLE 4.5 Summary of Oncology Trial Monitoring[a]

	Design Stage		
	1	2	3
Number of deaths	147	293	440
Proportion of deaths	0.15 vs. 0. 22	0.43 vs. 0.52	0.61 vs. 0.68
$\hat{\theta}$ = log(ha zard ratio)	–0.225	–0.255	–0.248
Information level, I_k	36.45	72.64	109.09
Conditional power	0.81	0.94	1
95% Repeated CI	(–0.672, 0.022)	(–0.40, –0.108)	(–0.471, –0.255)
p-Value (unadjusted)	0.0872	0.015	0.0048
Efficacy boundary (p-scale)	0.0014	0.0060	0.0116
Futility boundary (p-scale)	0.8093	0.3172	0.0824
Decision	Continue	Continue	Stop and reject H_a

[a]For the survival endpoint, $\hat{\theta} \approx \ln(\ln p_1/\ln p_2)$, p-value $= \Phi^{-1}\left(\hat{\theta}\sqrt{I_k}\right)$.

4.5 MATHEMATICAL NOTES ON SEQUENTIAL TRIAL DESIGN

4.5.1 Unified Formulation for Sequential Trial Design

A unified formulation for sequential trial designs (Lan and DeMets 1983; Lan and Zucker 1993; Jennison and Turnbull, 2000) has been implemented in ExpDesign Studio. Suppose that a group sequential study with up to K analyses yields the sequence of test statistics $\{Z_1, \ldots, Z_K\}$. Assume that these statistics have a canonical joint distribution with information levels $\{I_1, \ldots, I_k\}$ for the parameter θ. That is,

$$\text{(i)}\quad \{Z_1, \ldots, Z_K\}, \tag{4.4}$$

$$\text{(ii)}\quad Z_k \sim N(\theta\sqrt{I_k}, 1), \qquad 1, \ldots, K, \tag{4.5}$$

$$\text{(iii)}\quad \mathrm{Cov}(Z_{k_1}, Z_{k_2}) = \sqrt{I_{k_1}/I_{k_2}}, \qquad 1 \le k_1 \le k_2 \le K. \tag{4.6}$$

For a log-rank test in a time-to-event analysis, we have the following results. The information can be expressed as

$$I_k = \frac{r}{(1+r)^2} d_k, \tag{4.7}$$

where d_k is the number of deaths expected, N_k the number of patients expected, and r the sample-size ratio (this should be consistent with θ as to which treatment is chosen.) Under the conditions of exponential survival distribution, the relationship between an accrual time of T_0 and death can be expressed as

$$d_{ik} = \frac{N_{1i}}{T_0}\left[T_0 - \frac{1}{\lambda_i e^{\lambda_i T_k}}(e^{\lambda_i T_0} - 1)\right], \qquad T > T_0;\ \ i = 1, 2;\ \ k = 1, 2, \ldots, K, \tag{4.8}$$

where d_{ik} is the number of deaths in group i at stage k, T_k the time of first-patient-in to the kth death, and N_{ik} the number of patients in group i at stage k. Therefore, the patient–death ratio is given by

$$\eta = \frac{N_{1k} + N_{2k}}{d_{1k} + d_{2k}} = \frac{1+r}{\xi_1 + r\xi_2}, \tag{4.9}$$

where $\xi_i = 1 - (e^{\lambda_i T_0} - 1)/(T_0 \lambda_i e^{\lambda_i T})$.
From Eq. (4.7) we can obtain the number of deaths required for the sequential design by mimicking a normal endpoint with a treatment difference equal to log(hazard ratio) and a standard deviation of 1. After the number of deaths d is obtained, the number of patients can be obtained by $N = \eta d$.

Testing a Single Mean

Test statistic:

$$Z_k = (\bar{x}_k - \mu_0)\sqrt{I_k}. \tag{4.10}$$

Information level:

$$I_k = \frac{n_k}{\sigma^2}. \tag{4.11}$$

Difference expected:

$$\theta = \mu - \mu_0. \tag{4.12}$$

Testing Paired Means

Test statistic:

$$Z_k = \bar{d}_k \sqrt{I_k}, \tag{4.13}$$

where $\bar{d}_k$ is the mean treatment difference.

Information level:

$$I_k = \frac{n_k}{\tilde{\sigma}^2}, \tag{4.14}$$

where $\tilde{\sigma}$ is the standard deviation of the difference, and

$$\tilde{\sigma}^2 = 2(1-p)\sigma^2, \tag{4.15}$$

where ρ is the correlation coefficient.

Difference expected:

$$\theta = \mu_d. \tag{4.16}$$

Testing Two Independent Means

Test statistic:

$$Z_k = (\bar{x}_{Ak} - \bar{x}_{Bk})\sqrt{I_k}. \tag{4.17}$$

Information level:

$$I_k = \left(\frac{\sigma_A^2}{n_{Ak}} + \frac{\sigma_B^2}{n_{Bk}}\right)^{-1}. \tag{4.18}$$

Difference expected:

$$\theta = \mu_B - \mu_A. \tag{4.19}$$

Testing One Proportion

Test statistic:

$$Z_k = (p_k - p_0)\sqrt{I_k}. \tag{4.20}$$

Information level:

$$I_k = \frac{n_k}{\sigma^2}, \qquad \sigma^2 = \bar{p}(1-\bar{p}), \qquad \bar{p} = 0.5(p_0 + p_a). \tag{4.21}$$

Difference expected:

$$\theta = P - P_0. \tag{4.22}$$

Testing Two Independent Proportions

Test statistic:

$$Z_k = (p_{Bk} - p_{Ak})\sqrt{I_k}. \tag{4.23}$$

Information level:

$$I_k = \frac{1}{\sigma^2}\left(\frac{1}{n_{Ak}} + \frac{1}{n_{Bk}}\right)^{-1}, \qquad \sigma^2 = \bar{p}(1-\bar{p}), \quad \bar{p} = 0.5(p_A + p_B). \tag{4.24}$$

Difference expected:

$$\theta = P_B - P_A. \tag{4.25}$$

Log-rank Test for Two Survival Distributions

Test statistic:

$$Z_k = \frac{S_k}{\sqrt{I_k}}, \tag{4.26}$$

where S_k is the log-rank score statistic.

Information level:

$$I_k = \frac{r}{(1+r)^2} d_k, \tag{4.27}$$

where d_k is the number of deaths expected.

Log(hazard ratio) expected:

$$\theta = \log\left(\frac{\lambda_B}{\lambda_A}\right). \tag{4.28}$$

2 × 2 Crossover Design

Test statistic:

$$Z_k = \frac{1}{2}(\bar{d}_{xk} + \bar{d}_{yk})\sqrt{I_k}, \tag{4.29}$$

where $\bar{d}_{xk}$ and $\bar{d}_{yk}$ are the mean treatment differences in sequences x and y.

$$I_k = 4\left(\frac{\sigma_A^2}{n_{xk}} + \frac{\sigma_B^2}{n_{yk}}\right)^{-1}. \tag{4.30}$$

4.5.2 Calculation of Conditional Probability

Suppose that a group sequential test with a maximum of K analyses is defined in terms of standardized statistics:

$$Z_k\sqrt{I_k} - Z_{k-1}\sqrt{I_{k-1}} \sim N(\theta\Delta_k, \Delta_k), \tag{4.31}$$

where $\Delta_k = I_k - I_{k-1}$, independent of $Z_1, \ldots, Z_{k-1}$. A fundamental quantity to compute for a group sequential test is the probability of exiting by a specific boundary at a particular analysis. For each $k = 1, \ldots, K$, define

$$\psi_k(a_1, b_1, \ldots, a_k, b_k; \theta) = \Pr_\theta(a_1 < Z_1 < b_1, \ldots, a_{k-1} < Z_{k-1} < b_{k-1}, Z_k > b_k), \tag{4.32}$$

$$\xi_k(a_1, b_1, \ldots, a_k, b_k; \theta) = \Pr_\theta(a_1 < Z_1 < b_1, \ldots, a_{k-1} < Z_{k-1} < b_{k-1}, Z_k < a_k). \tag{4.33}$$

These quantities are the two key formulas for a test's error probabilities and expected sample size. They are also used in constructing error-spending boundaries and in computing p-values and confidence intervals on termination.

The two quantities are carried out numerically as follows:

$$\psi_k(a_1, b_1, \ldots, a_k, b_k; \theta) \approx \sum_{i_{k-1}=1}^{m_{k-1}} h_{k-1}(i_{k-1};\theta) e_{k-1}(z_{k-1}(i_{k-1}), b_k; \theta), \tag{4.34}$$

$$h_k(i_k; \theta) = \sum_{i_{k-1}=1}^{m_{k-1}} h_{k-1}(i_{k-1};\theta) w_k(i_k) f_k(z_{k-1}(i_{k-1}), z_k(i_k); \theta), \tag{4.35}$$

$$f_1(z_1; \theta) = \phi(z_1 - \theta\sqrt{I_1}), \qquad f_k(z_{k-1}, z_k; \theta) = \frac{\sqrt{I_k}}{\sqrt{\Delta_k}}\phi\left(\frac{z_k\sqrt{I_k} - z_{k-1}\sqrt{I_{k-1}} - \theta\Delta_k}{\sqrt{\Delta_k}}\right), \tag{4.36}$$

$$e_{k-1}(z_{k-1}, b_k; \theta) = \Phi\left(\frac{z_{k-1}\sqrt{I_{k-1}} + \theta\Delta_k - b_k\sqrt{I_k}}{\sqrt{\Delta_k}}\right), \tag{4.37}$$

where $\phi(x) = \exp(-x^2/2)/\sqrt{2\pi}$ is the standard normal probability density function (p.d.f.) and Φ is the standard normal c.d.f. The weight w_k is defined by numerical integration as follows:

$$\int_l^u q(z)dz \approx \sum_{i=1}^{m} w_k q(z_k). \tag{4.38}$$

The values of $\psi_k(a_1,b_1, \ldots, a_k,b_k;\theta)$ and $\xi_k(a_k,(a_1,b_1, \; , a_k,b_k;\theta)$ for $k = 1, \ldots, K$ determine the distribution of the stopping time and associated decision for a group sequential test. Hence, we can obtain from them the test's error probabilities and expected information on termination for any θ. For example, a two-sided test of H_0: $\theta = 0$ has K analyses at information levels $I_1, \ldots, I_K$ with continuation regions $(a_1, b_1), \ldots, (a_K, b_K)$ for $Z_1, \ldots, Z_K$. Then the test's type I error probability is

$$\Pr_{\theta=0}(\text{reject } H_0) = \sum_{k=1}^{K} [\psi_k(a_1, b_1, \ldots, a_k, b_k; 0) + \xi_k(a_1, b_1, \ldots, a_k, b_k; 0)]. \quad (4.39)$$

If $\delta > 0$ is large enough that we can ignore the probability of crossing the lower boundary, the test's power when $\theta = \delta$ is

$$\sum_{k=1}^{K} \psi_k(a_1, b_1 \ldots, a_k, b_k; \delta). \quad (4.40)$$

For a test defined by error spending,

$$\psi_k(-c_1, c_1, \ldots, -c_k, c_k; 0) = \frac{\pi_k}{2}, \quad (4.41)$$

where π_k is a two-sided type I error probability assigned to analysis k. Equivalently, the problem becomes that of finding the value c_k for which

$$\sum_{i_{k-1}=1}^{m_{k-1}} h_{k-1}(i_{k-1}; 0) e_{k-1}(z_{k-1}(i_{k-1}), c_k; 0) = \frac{\pi_k}{2}. \quad (4.42)$$

4.5.3 Conditional and Predictive Power and RCI for Trial Monitoring

One-sided *conditional power* at analysis k is given by

$$P_k(\theta) = \Phi\left(\frac{Z_k\sqrt{I_k} - z_\alpha\sqrt{I_k} + (I_K - I_k)\theta}{\sqrt{I_K - I_k}}\right), \quad k = 1, \ldots, K, \quad (4.43)$$

where $\Phi(\cdot)$ is the standard normal probability function. The two-sided *conditional power* at analysis k is given by

$$P_k(\theta) = \Phi\left(\frac{Z_k\sqrt{I_k} - z_{\alpha/2}\sqrt{I_k} + (I_K - I_k)\theta}{\sqrt{I_K - I_k}}\right) + \Phi\left(\frac{-Z_k\sqrt{I_k} - z_{\alpha/2}\sqrt{I_k} - (I_K - I_k)\theta}{\sqrt{I_K - I_k}}\right), \quad k = 1, \ldots, K. \quad (4.44)$$

One-sided *predictive power* is given by

$$P_k = \Phi\left(\frac{Z_k\sqrt{I_k} - z_\alpha\sqrt{I_k}}{\sqrt{I_K - I_k}}\right), \quad k = 1, \ldots, K. \quad (4.45)$$

The *futility index* is defined as 1 minus the conditional probability under H_a:

$$\mathrm{FI}_k = 1 - P_k(\theta \mid H_a). \tag{4.46}$$

Calculation of the RCI at analysis k is similar to the naive confidence interval but replacing $z_{1-\alpha}$ ($z_{1-\alpha/2}$) with C_k, the stopping boundary on the standard z-statistic. For example, CI = $d \pm z_{1-\alpha/2}\sigma$; RCI = $d \pm C_k\sigma$.

4.5.4 Bias-Adjusted Estimates

Bias-Adjusted Point Estimation The bias-adjusted estimators require evaluation under certain θ values:

$$E_\theta\left(\hat{\theta}\right) = \sum_{k=1}^{K}\left[\int_{-\infty}^{a_k} g_k(z_k;\theta)\frac{z_k}{\sqrt{I_k}}dz_k + \int_{b_k}^{\infty} g_k(z_k;\theta)\frac{z_k}{\sqrt{I_k}}dz_k\right]. \tag{4.47}$$

A typical lower integral in this sum can be written as

$$\int_{a_{k-1}}^{b_{k-1}}\int_{-\infty}^{a_k} g_{k-1}(z_{k-1};\theta)f_k(z_{k-1},z_k;\theta)\frac{z_k}{\sqrt{I_k}}dz_k dz_{k-1}, \tag{4.48}$$

$$\int_{a_{k-1}}^{b_{k-1}} g_{k-1}(z_{k-1};\theta)r_{k-1}(z_{k-1},a_k;\theta)dz_{k-1}, \tag{4.49}$$

where

$$r_{k-1}(z_{k-1},a_k;\theta) = \frac{-\sqrt{\Delta_k}}{I_k}\phi\left(\frac{a_k\sqrt{I_k} - z_{k-1}\sqrt{I_{k-1}} - \theta\Delta_k}{\sqrt{\Delta_k}}\right) + \frac{z_{k-1}\sqrt{I_{k-1}} + \theta\Delta_k}{I_k}\Phi\left(\frac{a_k\sqrt{I_k} - z_{k-1}\sqrt{I_{k-1}} - \theta\Delta_k}{\sqrt{\Delta_k}}\right). \tag{4.50}$$

We can evaluate the integral numerically as

$$\sum_{i_{k-1}=1}^{m_{k-1}} h_{k-1}(i_{k-1};\theta)r_{k-1}(z_{k-1}(i_{k-1}),a_k;\theta). \tag{4.51}$$

Stagewise-Ordering Adjusted p-Values We can adjust the stagewise-ordering p-values on the termination of a group sequential test: for example, a test with continuation regions (a_1, b_1), . . . , (a_K, b_K) for $Z_1, \ldots, Z_K$ stops after crossing the upper boundary at analysis k^* with $Z_{k^*} = z^*$. The one-sided upper p-value for testing H_0: $\theta = 0$ based on stagewise ordering is then

$$\sum_{j=1}^{k^*-1}\psi_j(a_1,b_1,\ldots,a_j,b_j;0) + \psi_{k^*}(a_1,b_1,\ldots,a_{k^*-1},b_{k^*-1},a_{k^*},z^*;0), \tag{4.52}$$

which can be calculated numerically. One-sided lower p-values are found in the same manner, and a two-sided p-value is twice the smaller of these two quantities.

5 Adaptive Trial Design

5.1 INTRODUCTION

Drug development is a sequence of complicated decision-making processes. Options are provided at each stage, and decisions depend on prior information and the probabilistic consequence of each action (decision) taken. This requires the trial design to be flexible such that it can be modified during the trial process. Adaptive design has been developed for this reason and has become very attractive to pharmaceutical firms. An adaptive design is a design that allows modifications to some aspects of a trial after its initiation, without undermining the validity and integrity of the trial. Following are examples of adaptations to a trial:

- Early stopping due to efficacy or futility
- Sample-size reestimation
- Adaptive randomization
- Dropping inferior treatment groups

Adaptive designs must often be combined with clinical trial simulation to achieve the ultimate goals because closed mathematical solutions are not always available. The overall process of adaptive design is depicted in Figure 5.1.

5.2 BASICS OF ADAPTIVE DESIGN METHODS

The three commonly used statistical methods for adaptive designs, based on the test statistic, are methods using the sum of stagewise p-values (MSP), the product of stagewise p-values (MPP), and the weighted inverse normal of stagewise p-values (MINP). A stagewise p-value is the p-value calculated on a subsample at each stage of an adaptive trial. A critical aspect for an adaptive design is to determine the stopping boundaries that ensue from type I error

---

Classical and Adaptive Clinical Trial Designs Using ExpDesign Studio™,
By Mark Chang

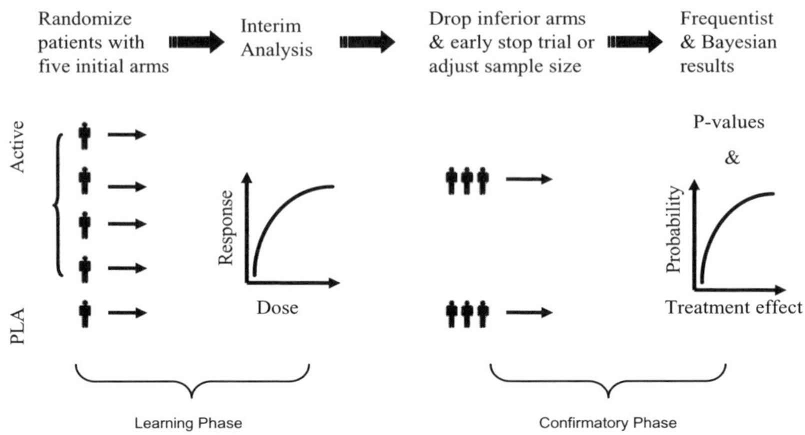

Figure 5.1 Overview of adaptive design.

control. Let's review the formulation for determining the stopping boundaries using MSP, MPP, and MINP.

The general stopping rules for a K-stage adaptive design are:

$$\begin{aligned}&\text{Stop for efficacy if } T_k \le \alpha_k,\\ &\text{Stop for futility if } T_k > \beta_k,\\ &\text{Continue and make adaptations if } \alpha_k < T_k \le \beta_k,\end{aligned} \tag{5.1}$$

where the efficacy and futility boundaries satisfy

$$\alpha_k < \beta_k\,(k = 1, \ldots, K-1) \quad \text{and} \quad \alpha_K = \beta_K. \tag{5.2}$$

For MSP, the test statistic is defined as

$$T_k = \sum_{i=1}^{k} p_i, \qquad k = 1, \ldots, K, \tag{5.3}$$

where K is the total number of stages for the trial and p_i is a stagewise p-value calculated based on a subsample from the ith stage.

The stopping boundaries for the two-stage design can be solved analytically:

$$\alpha_2 = \begin{cases} \sqrt{2(\alpha-\alpha_1)} + \alpha_1, & \text{without futility binding,} \quad (5.4)\\ \dfrac{\alpha-\alpha_1}{\beta_1-\alpha_1} + \dfrac{1}{2}(\beta_1+\alpha_1),\ \beta_1 < \alpha_2, & \text{with futility binding.} \quad (5.5)\end{cases}$$

The regulatory authorities apply the nonfutility binding rule (i.e., the futility boundaries don't have to be followed).

For MPP, the test statistic is defined as

$$T_k = \prod_{i=1}^{k} p_i, \qquad k = 1, \ldots, K. \tag{5.6}$$

The stopping boundaries for the two-stage design can be solved analytically:

$$\alpha_2 = \begin{cases} \dfrac{\alpha_1 - \alpha}{\ln \alpha_1}, & \text{without futility binding,} \quad (5.7) \\ \dfrac{\alpha - \alpha_1}{\ln \beta_1 - \ln \alpha_1}, & \text{with futility binding.} \quad (5.8) \end{cases}$$

For MINP, the test statistic is defined as

$$T_k = 1 - \Phi\left(\sum_{i=1}^{k} w_{ki} z_i \right), \qquad k = 1, \ldots, K, \tag{5.9}$$

where the constant weights $\sum_{i=1}^{k} w_{ki}^2 = 1$, $z_i = \Phi^{-1}(1 - p_i)$, and Φ is the c.d.f. of the standard normal distribution. The stopping boundaries can be calculated using numerical integrations or simulations.

ExpDesign Studio allows you to generate various adaptive trials nearly as quickly as you can in a classical design. You can use response-adaptive randomization to assign more patients to superior treatment groups or to drop a "loser" when an inferior group is identified. You may stop a trial early to claim efficacy or futility based on the data observed or the conditional power. You may modify the sample size based on the treatment difference observed. You may conduct simulations for a dose-escalation trial using Bayesian or frequentist modeling approaches. We are going to show you how to design adaptive trials using ExpDesign Studio through examples.

5.3 HOW TO DESIGN A SAMPLE-SIZE REESTIMATION TRIAL USING EXPDESIGN

Regardless of ours efforts, we often face a high degree of uncertainty about parameters when designing a trial or justifying the sample size at the design stage. This could involve initial estimates of within- or between-patient variation, a control group event rate for a binary outcome, the treatment effect sought, the recruiting pattern, or patient compliance, all of which affect the ability of a trial to address its primary objective (Shih, 2001). This uncertainty can include the correlation between measures (if a repeated-measure model is used) or among different variables (e.g., multiple endpoints, covariates). If a small uncertainty of prior information exists, a classical design can be used. However, when the uncertainty is greater, a classical design with a fixed sample size is inappropriate. Instead, it is desirable to have a trial design that allows for reestimation of the sample size in the middle of a trial based on "unblinded" data. Several different algorithms have been proposed for sample-size reestimation, including the conditional power approach and Cui-Hung Wang's approach based on the ratio of effect size observed to size expected.

5.3.1 Sample-Size Adjustment Based on the Effect-Size Ratio

The formation for sample-size adjustment based on the ratio of the initial estimate of the effect size (E_0) to the size observed (E) is given by

$$N = \left(\frac{E_0}{E}\right)^2 N_0, \tag{5.10}$$

where N is the newly estimated sample size per group (combined from the two stages) and N_0 is the initial sample size per group, which can be estimated using a classical design.

5.3.2 Sample-Size Adjustment Based on Conditional Power

The sample size per group based on conditional power for a two-stage design can be obtained analytically (M. Chang, 2007a). For MSP, the sample size per group required for a given conditional power P_c can be expressed as

$$n_2 = \frac{2\sigma^2}{\delta^2}[\Phi^{-1}(1-\max(0, \alpha_2 - p_1)) - \Phi^{-1}(1-P_c)], \qquad \alpha_1 < p_1 < \beta_1. \tag{5.11}$$

For MPP, the sample size per group can be expressed as

$$n_2 = \frac{2\sigma^2}{\delta^2}\left[\Phi^{-1}\left(1-\frac{\alpha_2}{p_1}\right) - \Phi^{-1}(1-P_c)\right], \qquad \alpha_1 < p_1 < \beta_1. \tag{5.12}$$

For MINP, the sample size per group can be expressed as

$$n_2 = \frac{2\sigma^2}{\delta^2}\left[\frac{1}{w_2}\Phi^{-1}(1-\alpha_1) - \frac{w_1}{w_2}\Phi^{-1}(1-p_1) - \Phi^{-1}(1-P_c)\right], \qquad \alpha_1 < p_1 < \beta_1. \tag{5.13}$$

Next, we illustrate how to use ExpDesign to produce adaptive designs for trials with different endpoints. The examples we discuss are acute ischemic stroke, asthma, and oncology trials.

5.3.3 Adaptive Design for an Acute Ischemic Stroke Trial

A phase III trial is to be designed for patients with acute ischemic stroke of recent onset. The primary endpoint is the composite endpoint (death or MI),

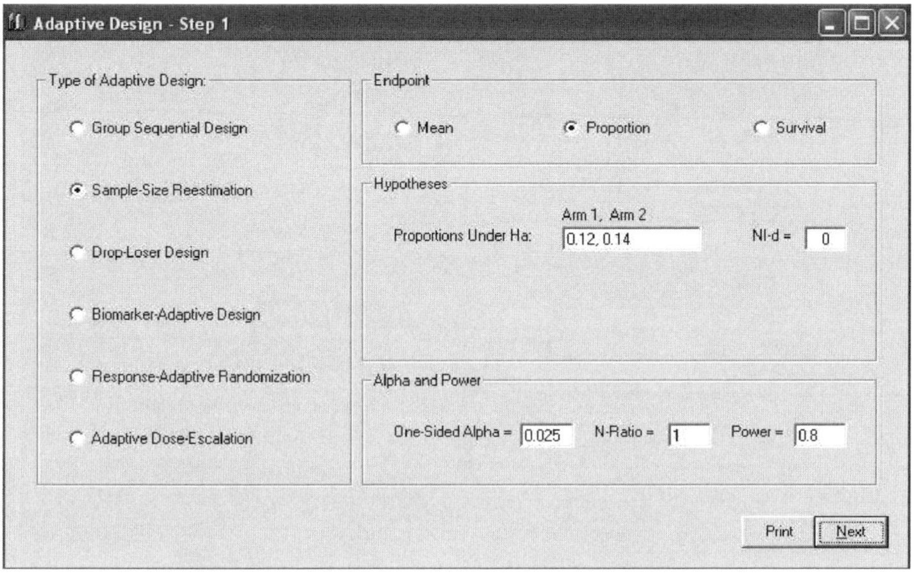

Figure 5.2 Sample-size reestimation step 1 window.

with an event rate of 14% for the control group and 12% for the test group. Based on a large-sample assumption, a sample size of 4473 for a classical design will provide 80% power to detect the difference at a one-sided α value of 0.025.

We can design an adaptive trial with sample-size reestimation using ExpDesign with the following simple steps:

- After launching ExpDesign Studio, click Adaptive Design; the **Adaptive Design–Step 1** window (Figure 5.2) will appear.

In the **Adaptive Design–Step 1** window, do the following:

- Select the **Sample-Size Reestimation** option in the **Type of Adaptive Design** panel.
- Select the **Proportion** option in the **Endpoint** window.
- Enter "0.12, 0.14" for **Response Under Ha** in the **Hypotheses** panel.
- Enter "0" for **NI-d**, the noninferiority margin, for the noninferiority trial.
- Enter "0.025" for **One-Sided Alpha** and "0.8" for **Power**.
- Click Next; the **Adaptive Design–Step 2** window will appear.

In the **Adaptive Design–Step 2** window (Figure 5.3), do the following:

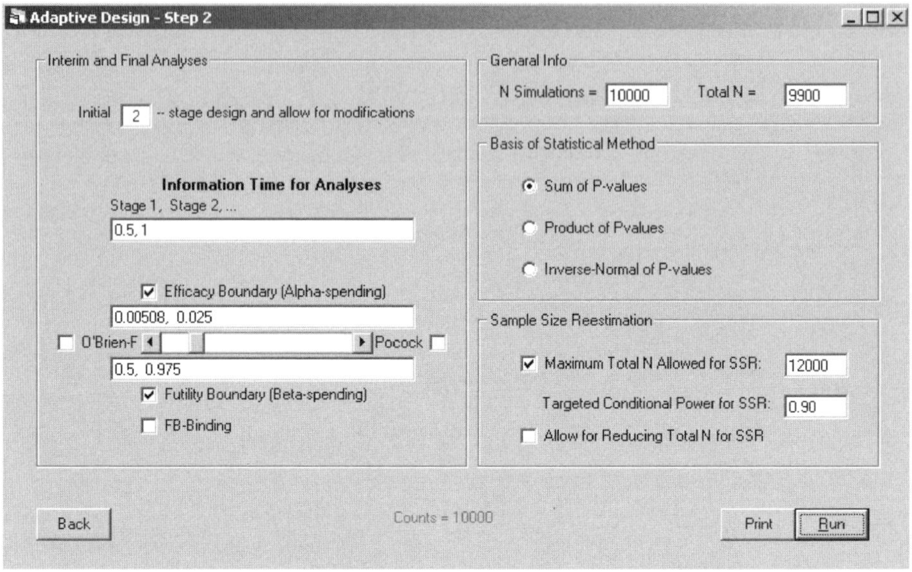

Figure 5.3 Sample-size reestimation step 2 window.

- Enter "2" for the initial number of stages.
- Enter "0.5, 1" for **Information Time for Analyses**.
- Choose stopping boundaries using the arrow near **O'Brien** or **Pocock**. Note that **O'Brien** spends less α (type I error) at the early stage than does **Pocock**.
- If you want to have futility boundaries, you can check the **Futility Boundary (Beta-spending)** checkbox. The futility boundaries are not necessarily followed. Therefore, leave **FB-Binding** unchecked. If you check the **FB-Binding** box, the stopping boundaries will change to anticonservative. Therefore, make sure that the regulatory authorities agree with the stopping boundaries in the protocol.
- Enter "10000" for **N Simulations**. 10,000 runs are suggested for a power simulation and at least 100,000 runs are suggested for an α simulation (i.e., type I error simulation).
- Enter "9900" for **Total N**, which is close to the classical design value. The sample size entered here should be around 100 to 120% of the sample size for the classical design under the same effect size.
- Select the **Sum of P-values** option in the **Basis of Statistical Method** panel. You can choose another method if you prefer.
- Enter "12000" for **Maximum Total N Allowed for SSR** and check the checkbox. If financial and other conditions permit, you can enter a larger number.

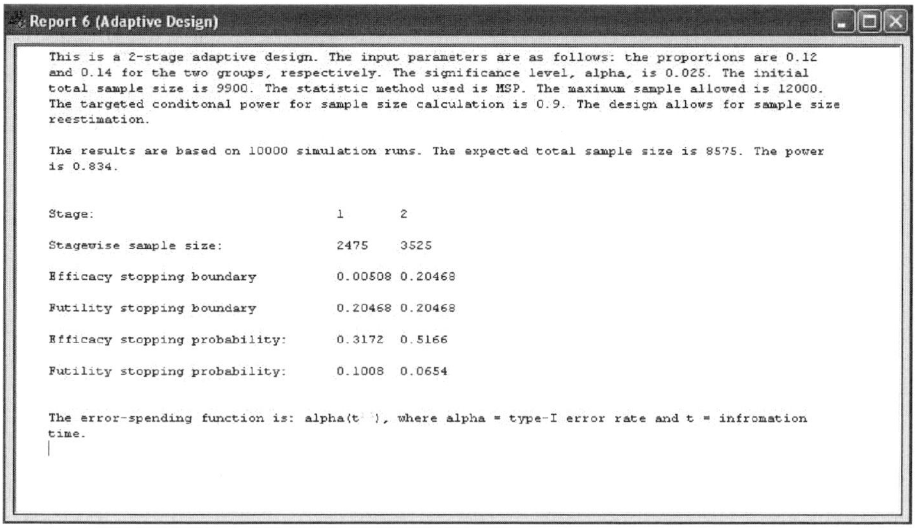

Figure 5.4 Report generated by ExpDesign.

- Enter "0.90" for **Targeted Conditional Power for SSR**. Ninety percent or higher is recommended for SSR.
- Click 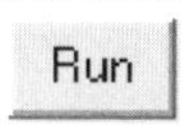

to start the simulation. It will take about 1 minute to complete a simulation with 10,000 runs.

After the simulation is completed, click 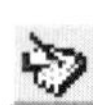 on the toolbar to view the report for the adaptive design (Figure 5.4).

To compare a group sequential design and this adaptive design, let's assume that the event rates are 0.12 and 0.138 for the groups, but that we mistakenly estimate 0.12 and 0.14. We change the event rates to "0.12, 0.138" in the **Adaptive Design–Step 1** window. Keeping everything else the same, the simulation results show that the adaptive design has 76% power. To obtain the power for a group sequential design using MSP without sample-size reestimation, we uncheck the **Maximum Total N Allowed for SSR** box. All other parameters are the same. The simulation results show that there is only 72% power. Other operating characteristics, such as average sample size, stopping boundaries, efficacy, and futility stopping probabilities are also included in the report.

5.3.4 Adaptive Design for an Asthma Study

In a phase III asthma study with two dose groups (control and active) with the primary efficacy endpoint of the percent change from baseline in FEV1, the estimated FEV1 improvement from baseline is 5% and 12% for the control and active groups, respectively, with a common standard deviation of

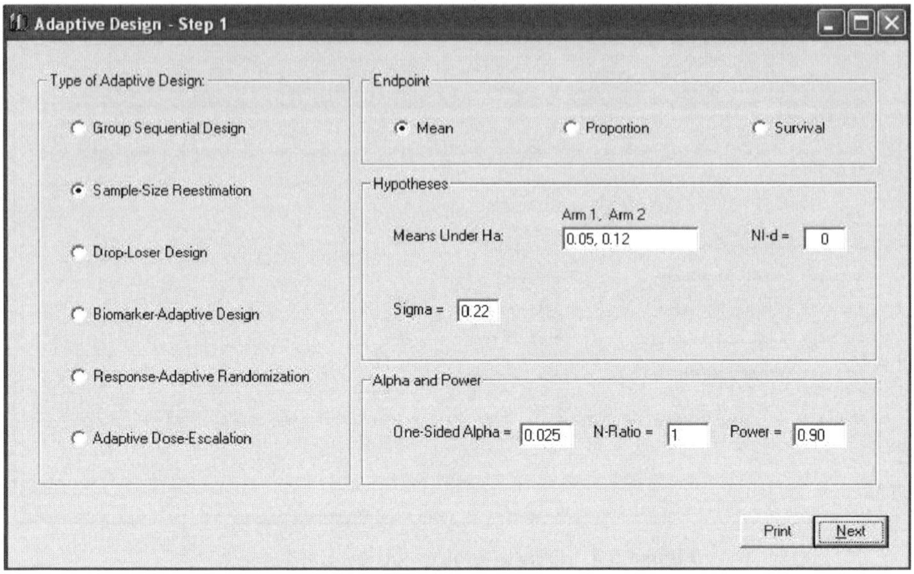

Figure 5.5 Adaptive design for asthma study.

$\sigma = 22\%$. Based on a large-sample assumption, a sample size of 208 per group in a classical design will provide 90% power to detect the difference at a one-sided α value of 0.025.

To design a two-stage adaptive trial, we use MPP this time with an interim analysis planned based on the response assessments of 50% of the patients. Following are the step-by-step design instructions using ExpDesign Studio:

- Click 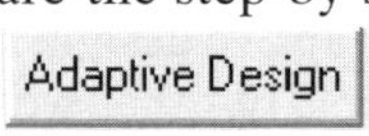

 to bring up the **Adaptive Design–Step 1** window (Figure 5.5).

In the **Adaptive Design–Step 1** window, do the following:

- Select the **Sample-Size Reestimation** option in the **Type of Adaptive Design** panel.
- Select the **Mean** option in the **Endpoint** window.
- Enter "0.05, 0.12" for the **Response Under Ha** in the **Hypotheses** panel.
- Enter "0" for **NI-d**, the noninferiority margin, because it is a superiority trial.
- Enter "0.025" for **One-Sided Alpha** and "0.9" for **Power**.
- Click 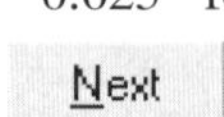

 to bring up the **Adaptive Design–Step 2** window.

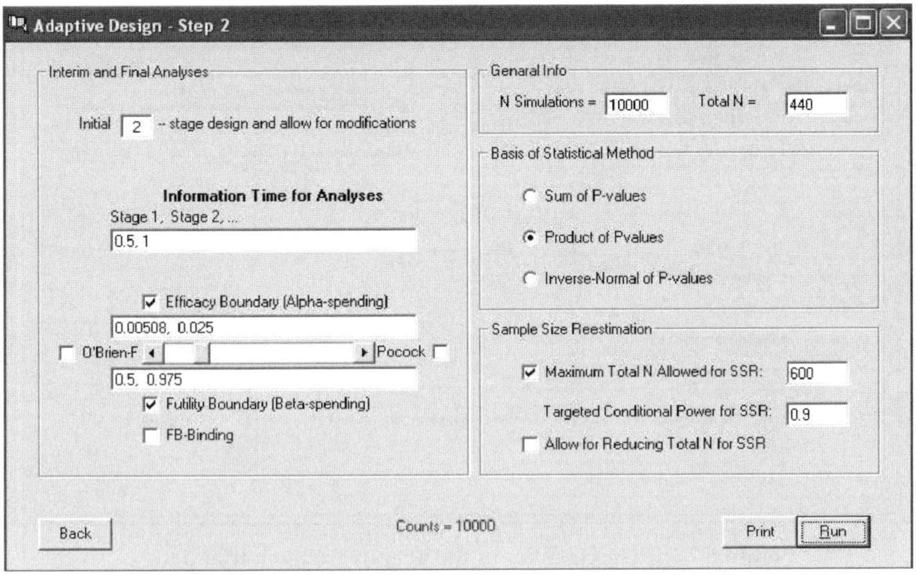

Figure 5.6 Parameters for the adaptive asthma trial.

In the **Adaptive Design–Step 2** window (Figure 5.6), do the following:

- Enter "2" for the initial number of stages.
- Enter "0.5, 1" for the **Information Time for Analyses**.
- Choose stopping boundaries using the arrow near **O'Brien** or **Pocock**.
- If you want to have futility boundaries, you can check the **Futility Boundary (Beta-spending)** checkbox.
- Enter "10000" for **N Simulations**.
- Enter "440" for **Total N**, which is close to the classical design value. Again, the sample size entered here should be 100 to 120% of the sample size for the classical design under the same effect size.
- Select the **Product of P-values** option in the **Basis of Statistical Method** panel.
- Enter "600" for **Maximum Total N Allowed for SSR** and check the box.
- Enter "0.90" for **Targeted Conditional Power for SSR**. Ninety percent or higher is recommended for SSR.
- Click 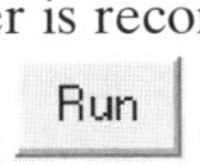

 to start the simulation.

After the simulation is completed, click 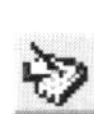 to view the report for the adaptive design (Figure 5.7). The design has 95% power with a sample size of 401 expected for each group.

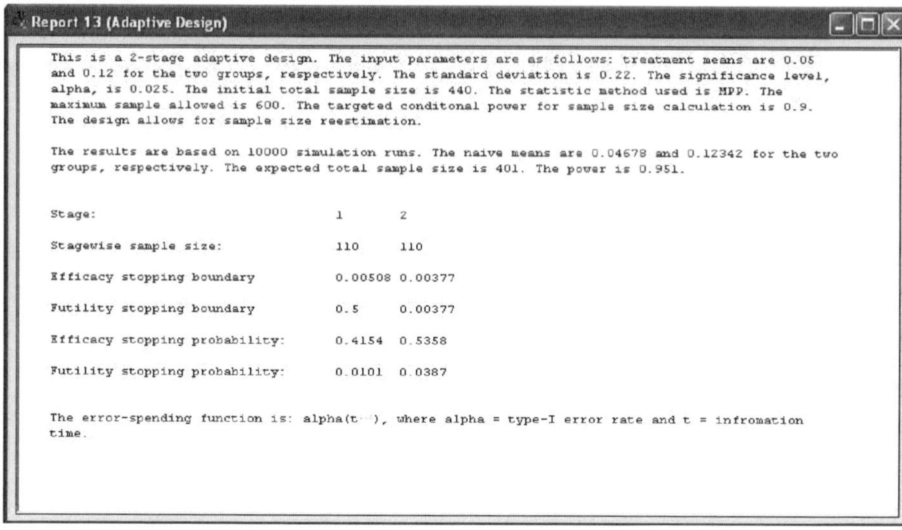
Report 13 (Adaptive Design)

This is a 2-stage adaptive design. The input parameters are as follows: treatment means are 0.05 and 0.12 for the two groups, respectively. The standard deviation is 0.22. The significance level, alpha, is 0.025. The initial total sample size is 440. The statistic method used is MPP. The maximum sample allowed is 600. The targeted conditonal power for sample size calculation is 0.9. The design allows for sample size reestimation.

The results are based on 10000 simulation runs. The naive means are 0.04678 and 0.12342 for the two groups, respectively. The expected total sample size is 401. The power is 0.951.

Stage:	1	2
Stagewise sample size:	110	110
Efficacy stopping boundary	0.00508	0.00377
Futility stopping boundary	0.5	0.00377
Efficacy stopping probability:	0.4154	0.5358
Futility stopping probability:	0.0101	0.0387

The error-spending function is: alpha(t), where alpha = type-I error rate and t = infromation time.

Figure 5.7 Characteristics of the adaptive asthma trial design.

What if the treatment is actually smaller than estimated: for example, 5% versus 11% in FEV1 change for the two groups? To answer this question, we keep everything the same but change the treatment to 5% and 11%, respectively, in the **Adaptive Design–Step 1** window. The simulation results show that the adaptive design has 88% power with an expected sample size of 444 per group, whereas a classical design with a sample size of 440 has 81% power and a group sequential design with a maximum total sample size of 440 without sample-size reestimation has 78% power. The group sequential design has an expected sample size of 370 based on MPP.

5.3.5 Adaptive Design for an Oncology Trial

In a two-arm comparative oncology trial with time to progression (TTP) as the primary efficacy endpoint, the median TTP is estimated to be 8 months (hazard rate = 0.08664) for the control group and 10.5 months (hazard rate = 0.06601) for the test group. Assume a uniform enrollment with an accrual period of 9 months and a total study duration of 24 months. An exponential survival distribution is assumed for the purpose of sample-size calculation. The classical design requires a sample size of 321 subjects per group for 85% power.

We design the trial with one interim analysis when 40% of patients have been enrolled. The interim analysis for efficacy is planned based on TTP, but it does not allow for futility stopping. Following are the steps for the trial design using ExpDesign Studio.

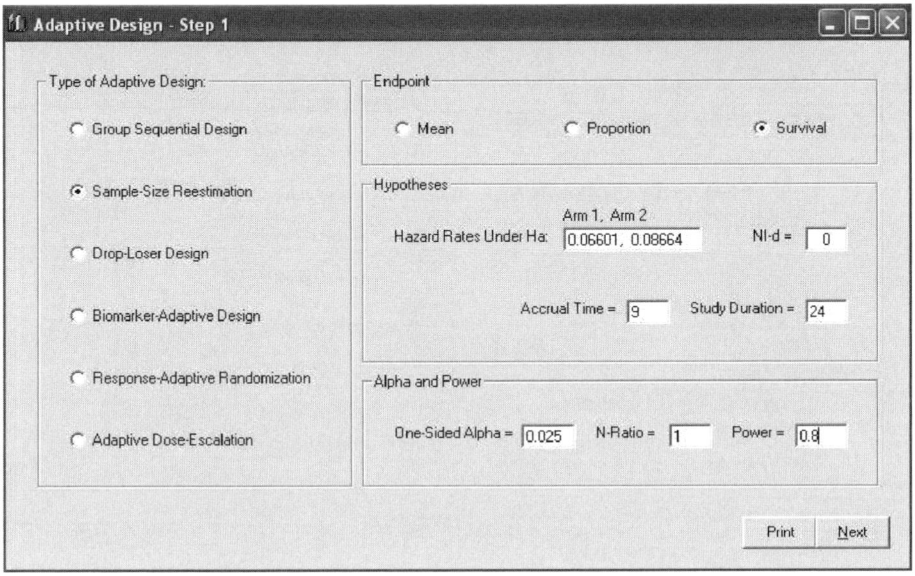

Figure 5.8 Adaptive design for the oncology trial.

- Click 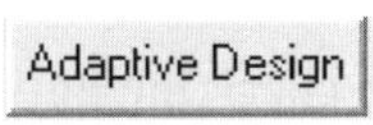

to bring up the **Adaptive Design–Step 1** window (Figure 5.8).

In the **Adaptive Design–Step 1** window, do the following:

- Select the **Sample-Size Reestimation** option in the **Type of Adaptive Design** panel.
- Select the **Survival** option in the **Endpoint** window.
- Enter "0.06601, 0.08664" for **Hazard Rates Under Ha** in the **Hypotheses** panel.
- Enter "0" for **NI-d**, the noninferiority margin, because it is a superiority trial.
- Enter "9" for **Accrual Time** and "24" for **Study Duration**.
- Enter "0.025" for **One-Sided Alpha** and "0.8" for **Power**.
- Click 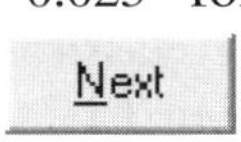

to bring up the **Adaptive Design–Step 2** window (Figure 5.9).

In the **Adaptive Design–Step 2** window, do the following:

- Enter "2" for the initial number of stages.
- Enter "0.4, 1" for **Information Time for Analyses**.
- Choose stopping boundaries using the arrow near **O'Brien** or **Pocock**.

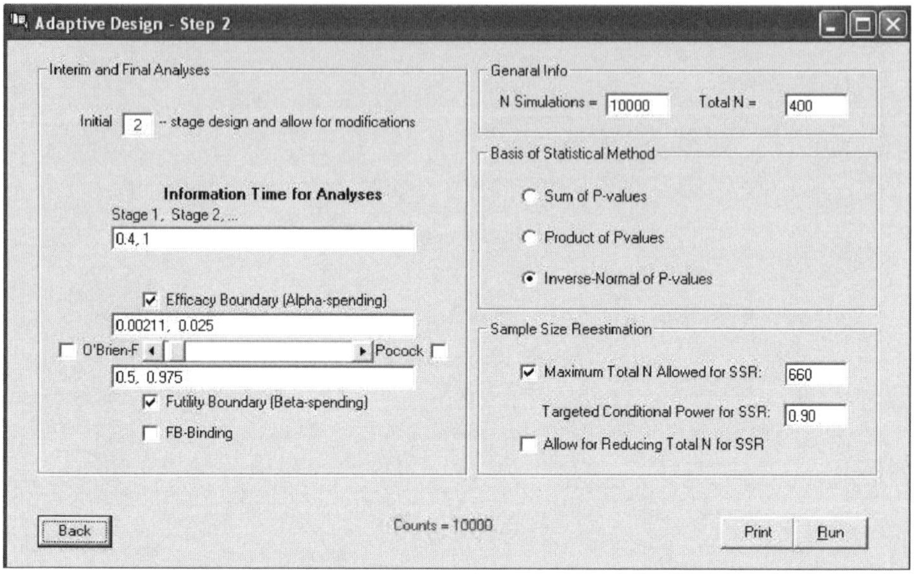

Figure 5.9 Input parameters for the adaptive oncology trial.

- If you want to have futility boundaries, you can check the **Futility Boundary (Beta-spending)** checkbox.
- Enter "100000" for **N Simulations**.
- Enter "400" for **Total N** (events).
- Select the **Inverse-Normal of P-values** option in the **Basis of Statistical Method** panel.
- Enter "660" for **Maximum Total N Allowed for SSR** (this is the number of events for a survival endpoint) and check the box.
- Enter "0.90" for the **Targeted Conditional Power for SSR**.
- Click Run to start the simulation.

After the simulation is completed, you can click 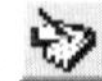 to view the design report (Figure 5.10). We can see that the sample size expected is 616 under the alternative hypothesis and the power is 87.4%. The classical design has 83.5% power with the same sample size. When the median TTP is 10 months instead of 10.5, this adaptive design will still have 73% power, whereas the classical design has only 70% power.

5.3.6 Noninferiority Design with a Binary Endpoint

A phase III trial is to be designed for patients with acute ischemic stroke of recent onset. The primary endpoint is defined as the composite endpoint

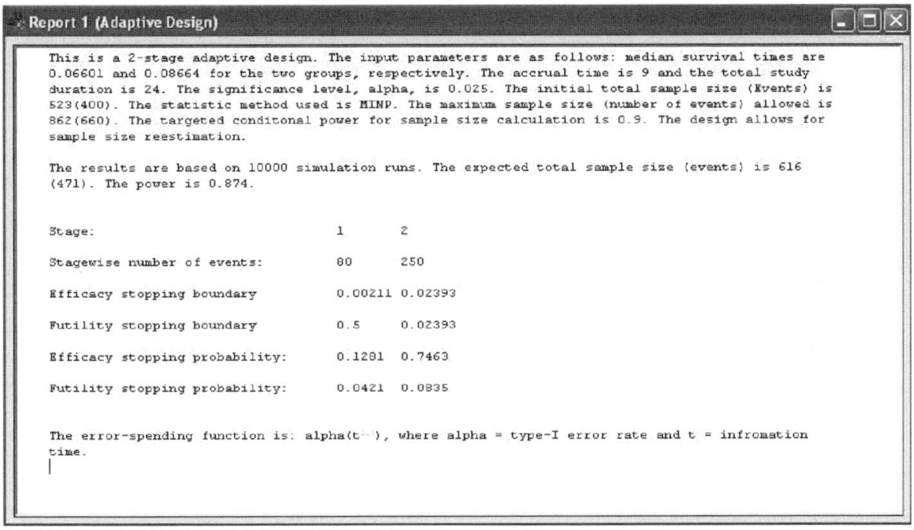

Figure 5.10 Characteristics of the adaptive oncology trial design.

(death or MI) with an estimated event rate 14% for the control group and 12% for the test group. Based on a large-sample assumption, the sample size for a classical design is 4437 per group, which provides 80% power to detect the difference at a one-sided α value of 0.025 (the superiority test).

If superiority is not achieved, a noninferiority test will be performed. Because of the closed testing procedure, no α adjustment is required for the two hypothesis tests. The noninferiority boundary is determined to be 0.5%. We are going to use three-stage adaptive design for the noninferiority trial. The futility stopping boundaries are also used for cost savings. We follow the steps below to design an adaptive trial using ExpDesign Studio:

- Click Adaptive Design to bring up the **Adaptive Design–Step 1** window (Figure 5.11).

In the **Adaptive Design–Step 1** window, do the following:

- Select the **Sample-Size Reestimation** option in the **Type of Adaptive Design** panel.
- Select the **Proportion** option in the **Endpoint** window.
- Enter "0.12, 0.14" for **Proportions Under Ha** in the **Hypotheses** panel.
- Enter "0.005" for **NI-d**, the noninferiority margin, for the noninferiority trial.
- Enter "0.025" for **One-Sided Alpha** and "0.8" for **Power**.
- Click Next to bring up the **Adaptive Design–Step 2** window.

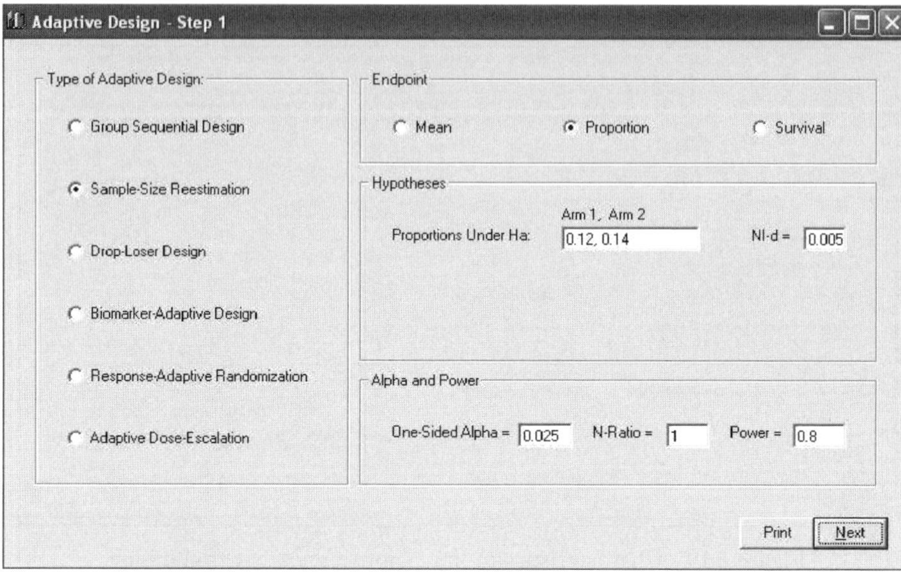

Figure 5.11 Adaptive design for the noninferiority trial.

In the **Adaptive Design–Step 2** window (Figure 5.12), do the following:

- Enter “3” for the initial number of stages.
- Enter “0.33, 0.67, 1” for **Information Time for Analyses**.
- Choose stopping boundaries by the arrow near **O’Brien** or **Pocock**.
- If you want to have futility boundaries, you can check the **Futility Boundary (Beta-spending)** checkbox.
- Enter “10000” for **N Simulations**.
- Enter “9000” for **Total N**, which is close to the classical design value.
- Select the **Inverse-Normal of P-values** option in the **Basis of Statistical Method** panel.
- Enter “12000” for **Maximum Total N Allowed for SSR** and check the box.
- Enter “0.02” for **DuHa**, the estimated treatment difference.
- Click 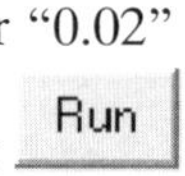

 to start the simulation.

After the simulation is completed, you can click  to view the report (Figure 5.13). We can see that the adaptive design has an expected sample size of 6977 with 96% power. To see if the adaptive design protects the power, let’s assume that the event rate is 0.14 versus 0.128. We change the responding inputs to “0.14, 0.128” for the **Proportions Under Ha** in the

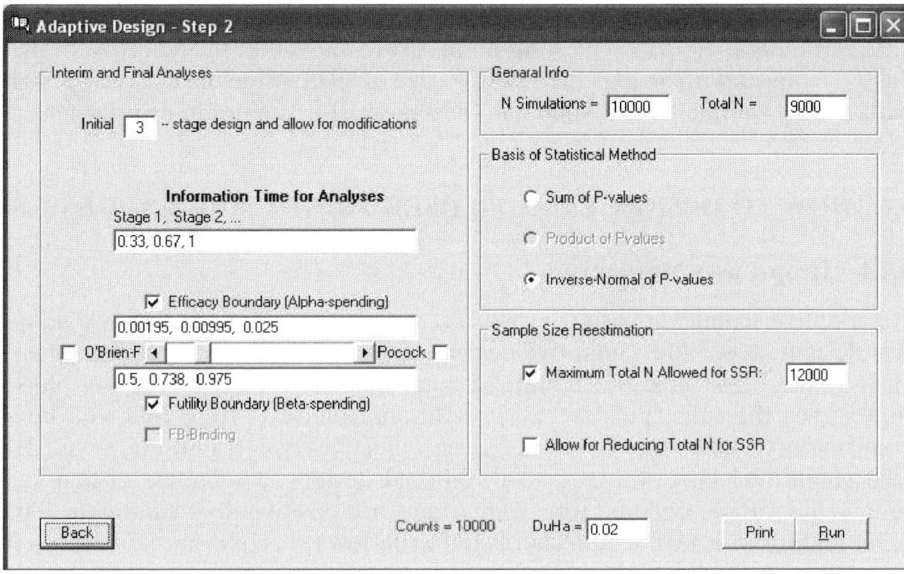

Figure 5.12 Input parameters for the adaptive noninferiority trial design.

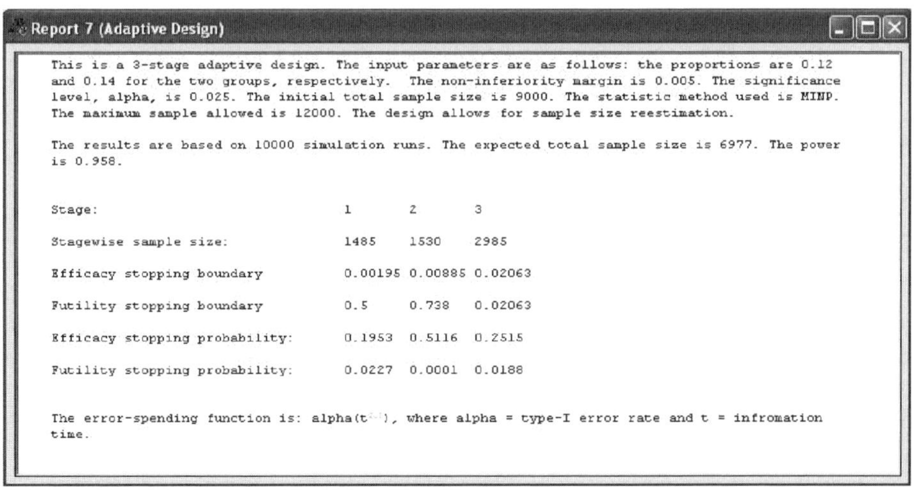

Figure 5.13 Characteristics of the adaptive noninferiority trial design.

Adaptive Design–Step 1 window. Keep everything else the same (DuHa = 0.02, not DuHa = 0.012). The simulation results show that the adaptive design has 72% power with an expected sample size of 8988, while the classical design with a fixed sample size of 9000 has 65% power for the noninferiority test.

5.4 HOW TO DESIGN A DROP-LOSER TRIAL USING EXPDESIGN

5.4.1 Drop-Loser Mechanism

An adaptive seamless phase II or III design is one of the most attractive adaptive designs. A seamless adaptive design is a combination of traditional phase II and phase III trials. In seamless design, there is usually a learning phase that serves the same purpose as a traditional phase II trial, followed by a confirmatory phase that serves the same objectives as a traditional phase III trial (Figure 11.1). Compared to traditional designs, a seamless design can reduce the sample size and time to market for a positive drug candidate. The main feature of a seamless design is the drop-loser mechanism. Sometimes it also allows for adding new treatment arms. A seamless design usually starts with several arms or treatment groups. At the end of the learning phase, inferior arms (losers) are identified and dropped from the confirmatory phase (M. Chang, 2007a).

Hung and co-workers at the FDA (2006) suggest that it may be advisable to redistribute the remaining planned sample size of a terminated arm to the remaining treatment arms for comparison so that coupled with use of a proper valid adaptive test, one may enhance the statistical power of the design to detect a dose that is effective.

5.4.2 Seamless Design of an Asthma Trial

The objective of this trial in an asthma patient is to confirm the sustained treatment effect of a new compound, measured as the FEV1 change from baseline to one year of treatment. Initially, patients are equally randomized to four doses of the compound and a placebo. Based on early studies, the estimated FEV1 changes at week 4 are 6%, 12%, 13%, 14%, and 15% (with a pooled standard deviation of 18%) for the placebo (dose level 0) and dose levels 1, 2, 3, and 4, respectively. One interim analysis is planned when 50% of patients have the efficacy assessments. The interim analysis will lead to either picking the winner (the arm with the best observed response) or stopping the trial for efficacy or futility. The winner and placebo will be used at stage 2. The final analysis will be based on the product of the stagewise p-values from both stages. At the final analysis, if $p_1p_2 \leq \alpha_2$, claim efficacy; otherwise, claim futility. For the weak control, $p_1 = \hat{p}_1$, where $\hat{p}_1$ is the naive stagewise p-value from a contrast test based on a subsample from stage 1. For

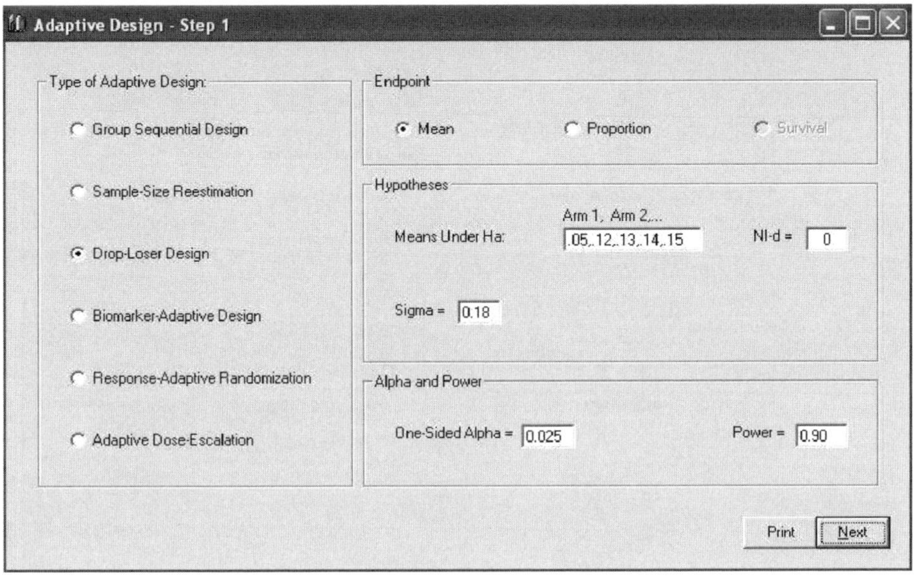

Figure 5.14 Drop-loser design.

the strong control, p_1 is the adjusted p-value (i.e., $p_1 = 4p_{\min}$), where $p_{\min}$ is the smallest p-value among the four comparisons.

To do an adaptive design with ExpDesign, follow the steps below.

- Click 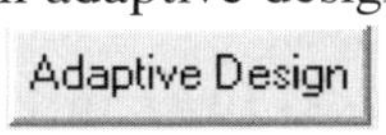

 to bring up the **Adaptive Design–Step 1** window (Figure 5.14).

In the **Adaptive Design–Step 1** window, do the following:

- Select the **Drop-Loser Design** option in the **Type of Adaptive Design** panel.
- Select the **Mean** option in the **Endpoint** window.
- Enter "0.05, 0.12, 0.13, 0.14, 0.15" for **Mean Under Ha** and 0.18 for sigma in the **Hypotheses** panel.
- Enter "0" for **NI-d**, the noninferiority margin, for the noninferiority trial.
- Enter "0.025" for **One-Sided Alpha** and "0.90" for **Power**.
- Click 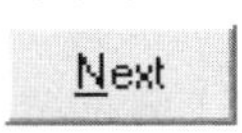

 to bring up the **Adaptive Design–Step 2** window (Figure 5.15).

In the **Adaptive Design–Step 2** window, do the following:

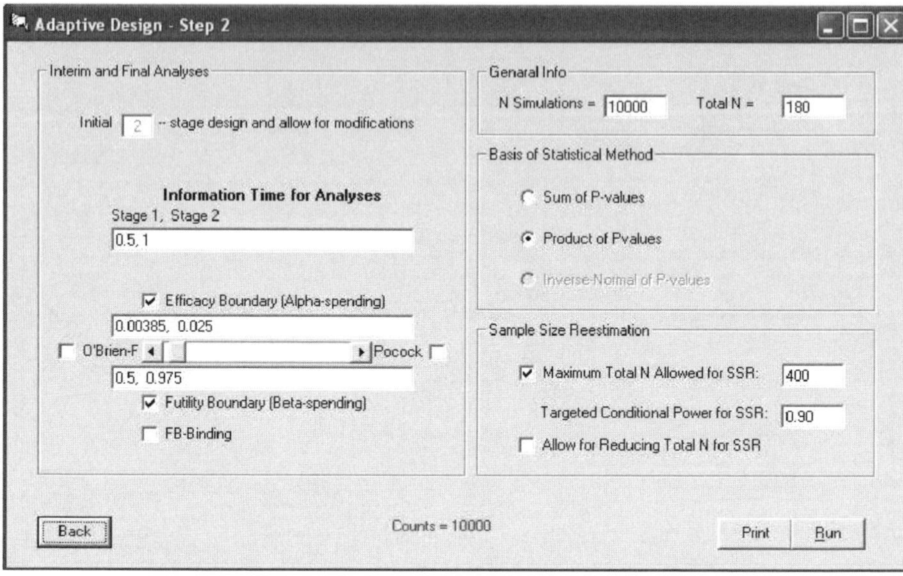

Figure 5.15 Input parameters for the drop-loser design.

- Enter “2” for the initial number of stages.
- Enter “0.5, 1” for **Information Time for Analyses**.
- Choose stopping boundaries by the arrow near **O’Brien** or **Pocock**.
- If you want to have futility boundaries, you can check the **Futility Boundary (Beta-spending)** checkbox.
- Enter “10000” for **N Simulations**.
- Enter “180” for **Total N**, which is close to the classical design.
- Select the **Product of P-values** option in the **Basis of Statistical Method** panel.
- Enter “400” for **Maximum Total N Allowed for SSR** and check the box.
- Enter “0.90” for **Targeted Conditional Power for SSR**, the estimated treatment difference.
- Click Run to start the simulation.

After the simulation is completed, you can click to view the report (Figure 5.16). The design has 95% power for the given dose–response relationship. Because the adaptive also allows for sample-size reestimation, when the responses in arms 2 through 5 decrease to 0.12, the design still has 80% power with the expected sample size of 287—a very robust design.

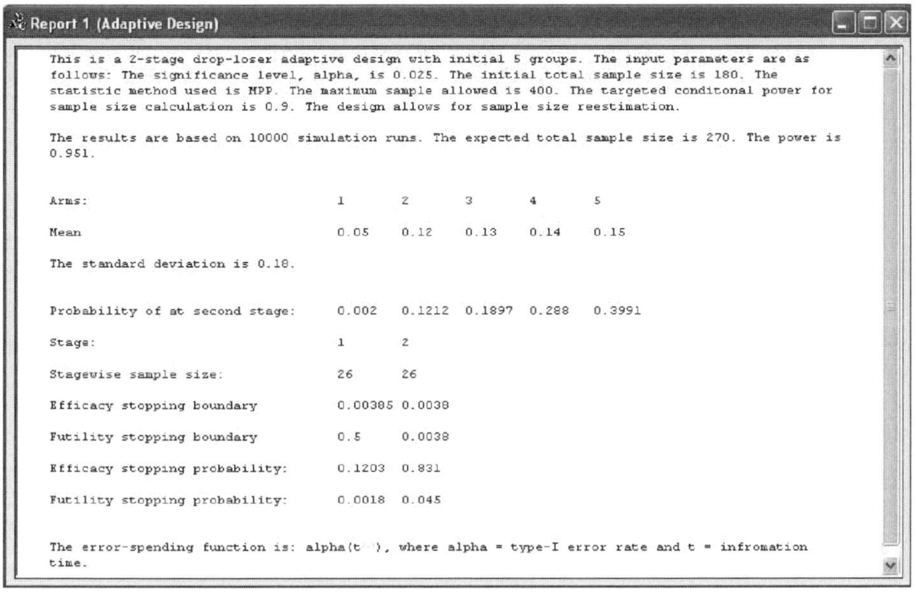

Report 1 (Adaptive Design)

This is a 2-stage drop-loser adaptive design with initial 5 groups. The input parameters are as follows: The significance level, alpha, is 0.025. The initial total sample size is 180. The statistic method used is MPP. The maximum sample allowed is 400. The targeted conditonal power for sample size calculation is 0.9. The design allows for sample size reestimation.

The results are based on 10000 simulation runs. The expected total sample size is 270. The power is 0.951.

Arms:	1	2	3	4	5
Mean	0.05	0.12	0.13	0.14	0.15

The standard deviation is 0.18.

Probability of at second stage:	0.002	0.1212	0.1897	0.288	0.3991

Stage:	1	2
Stagewise sample size:	26	26
Efficacy stopping boundary	0.00385	0.0038
Futility stopping boundary	0.5	0.0038
Efficacy stopping probability:	0.1203	0.831
Futility stopping probability:	0.0018	0.045

The error-spending function is: alpha(t), where alpha = type-I error rate and t = infromation time.

Figure 5.16 Characteristics of the drop-loser design.

5.5 HOW TO DESIGN A TRIAL USING A CLASSIFIER BIOMARKER

5.5.1 Biomarker Classifications

Compared to a true endpoint such as survival, biomarkers can often be measured earlier, more easily, and more frequently; are less subject to competing risks; and are less confounded. Utilization of a biomarker will lead to a better target population with a larger effect size, a smaller required sample size, and faster decision making. With advancements in proteomic, genomic, and genetic technologies, personalized medicine—the right drug for the right patient—becomes possible.

As mentioned earlier, a classifier biomarker is a marker (e.g., a DNA marker) that usually does not change over the course of a study. A classifier biomarker can be used to select the most appropriate target population or even for personalized treatment. For example, a study drug is expected to have effects on a population with a biomarker, which is only 20% of the overall patient population. Because the sponsor suspects that the drug may not work for the overall patient population, it may be efficient and ethical to run a trial only for subpopulations with the biomarker rather than for the general patient population. On the other hand, some biomarkers, such as RNA markers, are expected to change over the course of a study. This type of marker can be either a prognostic or a predictive marker.

A *prognostic biomarker* informs the clinical outcomes, independent of treatment. Biomarkers provide information about the natural course of a disease in persons who have or have not received the treatment under study. Prognostic markers can be used to separate good- and poor-prognosis patients at the time of diagnosis. If an expression of the marker clearly separates patients with an excellent prognosis from those with a poor prognosis, the marker can be used to aid the decision as to how aggressive the therapy needs to be.

A *predictive biomarker* informs the treatment effect on the clinical endpoint. Compared to a gold-standard endpoint such as survival, a biomarker can often be measured earlier, more easily, and more frequently. A biomarker is less subject to competing risks and less affected by other treatment modalities, which may reduce sample size due to a larger effect size. A biomarker could lead to faster decision making (M. Chang, 2007a).

Let the hypothesis test for a biomarker-positive subpopulation at the first stage (size = n_1/group) be

$$H_0\colon \delta_+ = 0 \tag{5.14}$$

and the hypothesis test for overall population (size = N_1/group) be

$$H_0\colon \delta = 0 \tag{5.15}$$

with the corresponding stagewise p-values, p_{1+} and p_1, respectively. These stagewise p-values should be adjusted. A conservative approach is to use the Bonferroni method or a method similar to the Dunnett method, which takes the correlation into consideration. For a Bonferroni-adjusted p-value and MSP, the test statistic is $T_1 = 2\min(p_{1+}, p_1)$ for the first stage. The population with a smaller p-value will be chosen for the second stage, and the test statistic for the second stage is defined as $T_2 = T_1 + p_2$, where p_2 is the stagewise p-value from the second stage.

5.5.2 Biomarker-Adaptive Design

Suppose that in an active-control trial, the estimated treatment difference is 0.2 for the biomarker-positive population (BPP) and 0.1 for the biomarker-negative population (BNP), with a common standard deviation of $\sigma = 1.4$. Following are the steps for a trial simulation using ExpDesign Studio.

- Click [Adaptive Design] to bring up the **Adaptive Design–Step 1** window.

In the **Adaptive Design–Step 1** window, do the following:

- Select the **Biomarker-Adaptive Design** option in the **Type of Design** panel. The **Biomarker-Adaptive Design** window will appear.
- Enter "0.2" for Mean **Difference with Biomarker**.
- Enter "0.1" for Mean **Difference without Biomarker**.

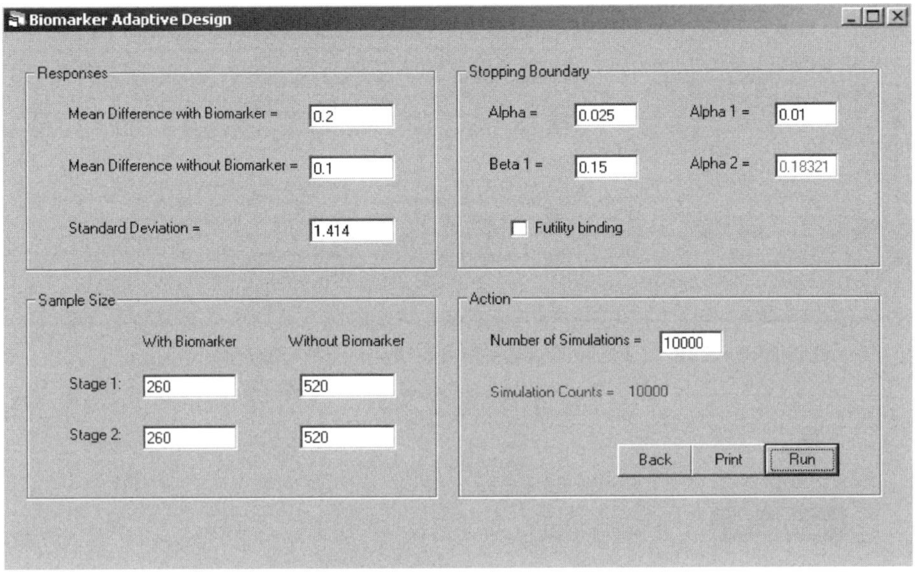

Figure 5.17 Biomarker-adaptive design.

- Enter "1.414" for **Standard Deviation**.
- Enter "0.025" or other desired value for the efficacy stopping boundary, **Alpha 1**.
- Enter "0.15" or other desired value for the futility stopping boundary, **Beta 1**.
- Enter "10000" or other desired value for the **Number of Simulations**.
- Enter the desired numbers for the sample sizes for different stages with and without a biomarker, as shown in Figure 5.17.
- Click 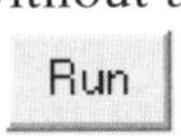

to start the simulation.

After the simulation is completed, you can click 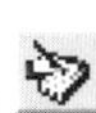 to view the report for the adaptive design (Figure 5.18). We see that the power of the overall significance is 91%. The power to claim efficacy is 32% for the biomarker group and 59% for the combined group.

5.6 HOW TO DESIGN A PLAY-THE-WINNER TRIAL USING EXPDESIGN

The randomized play-the-winner (RPW) model is a simple probabilistic model used to randomize subjects sequentially in a clinical trial (Wei and Durham, 1978; Coad and Rosenberger, 1999). The RPW model can be used

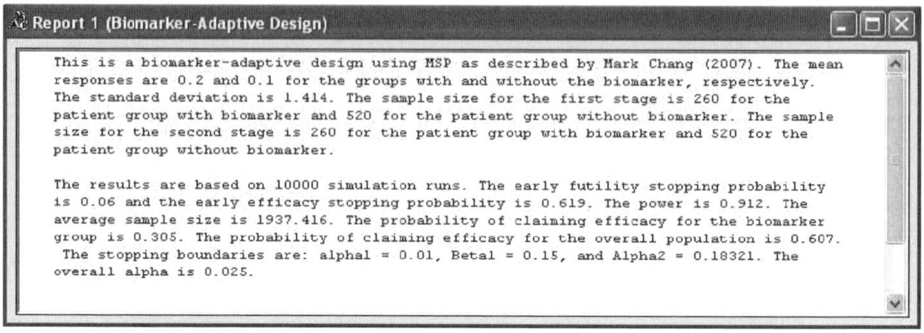
Report 1 (Biomarker-Adaptive Design)

This is a biomarker-adaptive design using MSP as described by Mark Chang (2007). The mean responses are 0.2 and 0.1 for the groups with and without the biomarker, respectively. The standard deviation is 1.414. The sample size for the first stage is 260 for the patient group with biomarker and 520 for the patient group without biomarker. The sample size for the second stage is 260 for the patient group with biomarker and 520 for the patient group without biomarker.

The results are based on 10000 simulation runs. The early futility stopping probability is 0.06 and the early efficacy stopping probability is 0.619. The power is 0.912. The average sample size is 1937.416. The probability of claiming efficacy for the biomarker group is 0.305. The probability of claiming efficacy for the overall population is 0.607. The stopping boundaries are: alpha1 = 0.01, Beta1 = 0.15, and Alpha2 = 0.18321. The overall alpha is 0.025.

Figure 5.18 Characteristics of the biomarker-adaptive design.

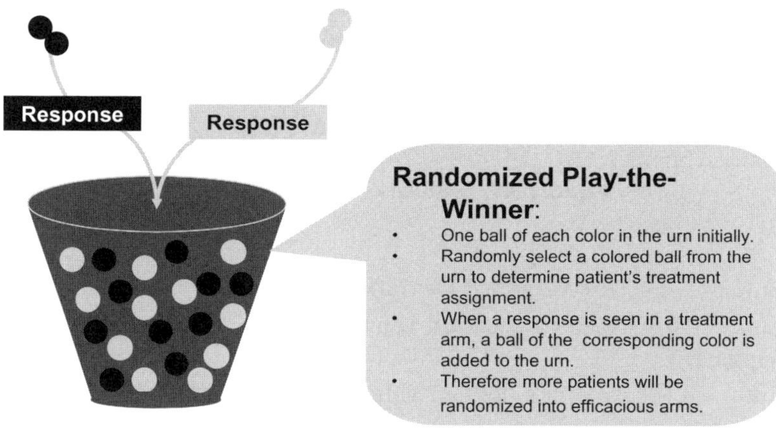

Figure 5.19 Randomized play-the-winner: Wei's (1978) urn model.

for randomized clinical trials with a binary endpoint. In the RPW model it is assumed that the previous subject's outcome will be available before the next patient is randomized. At the start of the clinical trial, an urn contains a_0 balls representing treatment A and b_0 balls representing treatment B, where a_0 and b_0 are positive integers. We denote these balls as either type A or type B balls. When a subject is recruited, a ball is drawn and replaced. If it is a type A ball, the subject receives treatment A; if it is a type B ball, the subject receives treatment B. When a subject's outcome is available, the urn is updated as follows: Success on treatment A (B) or a failure on treatment B (A) will generate additional a_1 (b_1) type A (B) balls in the urn. In this way the urn builds up more balls, representing the more successful treatment (Figure 5.19).

5.6.1 Randomized Play-the-Winner Design

Suppose that we are designing an oncology clinical study with tumor response as the primary endpoint. The response rate is estimated to be 0.3 in the control

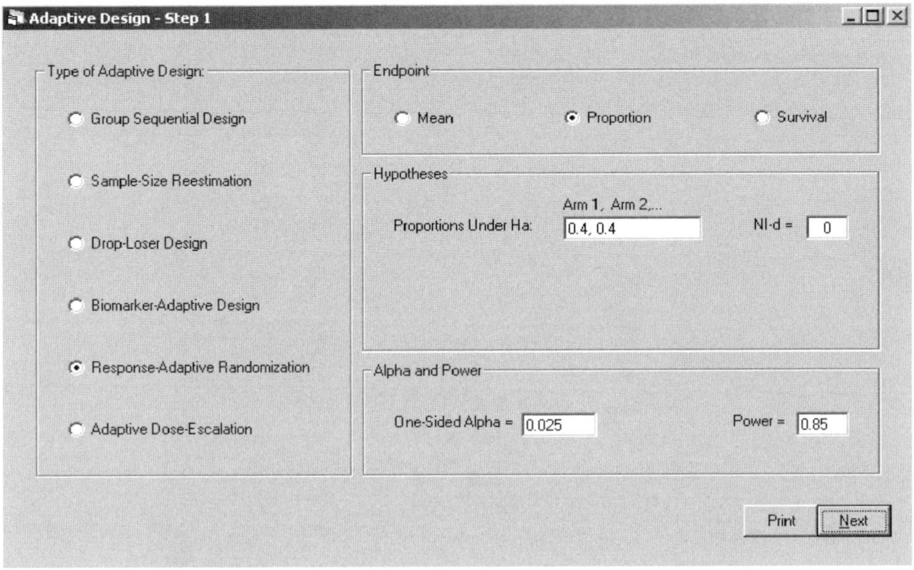

Figure 5.20 Response-adaptive randomization design.

group and 0.5 in the test group. The response rate is 0.4 in both groups under the null condition. We want to design the trial with about 80% power at a one-sided α value of 0.025.

We first check the type I error of a classical two-group design with $n = 200$ (100 per group), which is the sample size required for 83% power using a classical design. We now use the RPW design as specified in the following steps.

- Click 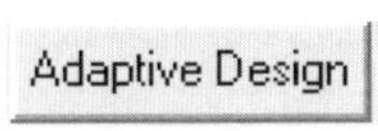

 to bring up the **Adaptive Design–Step 1** window (Figure 5.20).

In the **Adaptive Design–Step 1** window, do the following:

- Select the **Response-Adaptive Randomization** option in the **Type of Adaptive Design** panel.
- Select the **Proportion** option in the **Endpoint** window.
- Enter "0.4, 0.4" for **Proportions Under Ha** in the **Hypotheses** panel.
- Enter "0" for **NI-d**, the noninferiority margin, because it is a superiority trial.
- Enter "0.025" for **One-Sided Alpha** and any decimal value for **Power** (no effect in this version).
- Click 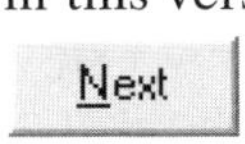

 to bring up the **Response-Adaptive Randomization** window (Figure 5.21).

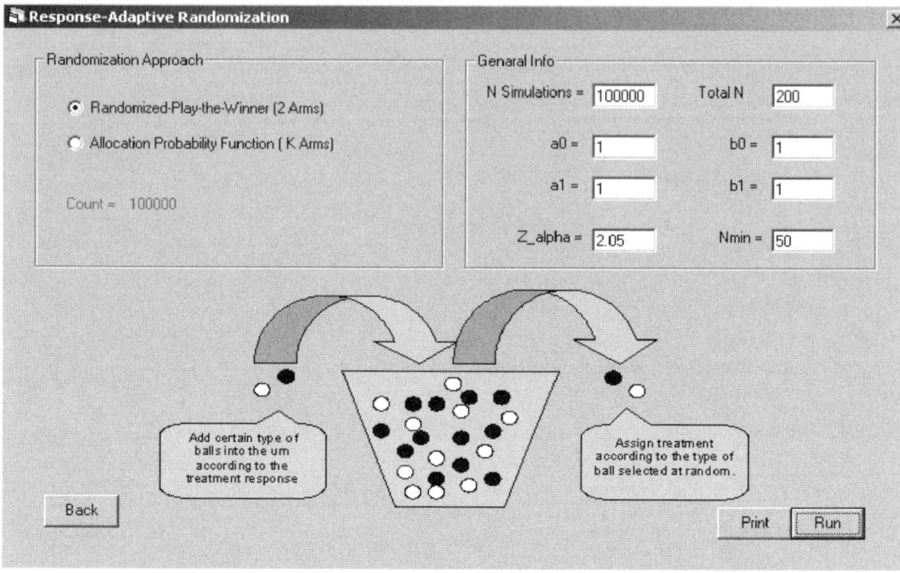

Figure 5.21 Input parameters for the binary RAR design.

- Enter "100000" for **N Simulations** in the **General Info** panel.
- Enter "200" for **Total N**, which is based on a classical design for 83% power.
- Enter "1" for the four randomization parameters: **a0, b0, a1**, and **b1**.
- Enter "2.06" for the critical value **Z_alpha**. You may have to try difference numbers until the simulated power is equal to 0.025, the α level.
- Click 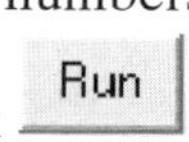 to start the simulation.
- When the simulation is finished, click 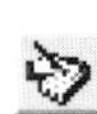 to view the results (Figure 5.22).

To simulate the power and other characteristics under the alternative hypothesis, enter "0.3, 0.5" for **Proportions Under Ha** in the **Hypotheses** panel. Keep other inputs unchanged. The results show that there is 74% power for the adaptive design with 200 patients. The classical design has 83% power to detect the difference with 200 patients (Figure 5.23).

5.6.2 Adaptive Randomization with a Normal Endpoint

The objective of this trial in asthma patients is to confirm a sustained treatment effect, measured as FEV1 change from baseline to one year of treatment. Initially, patients are equally randomized to four doses of the new compound

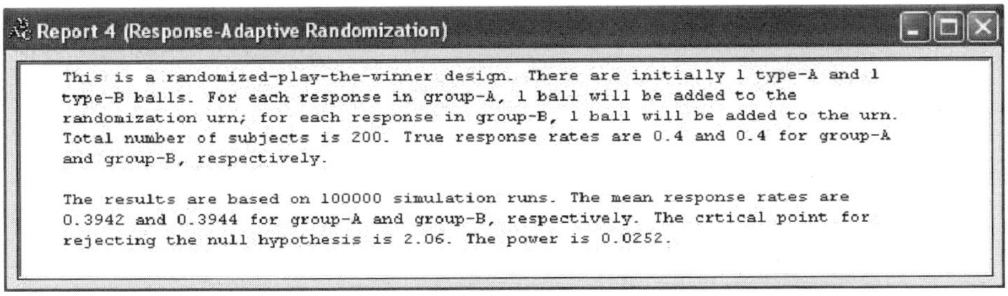

Figure 5.22 Determination of rejection region–based type I error.

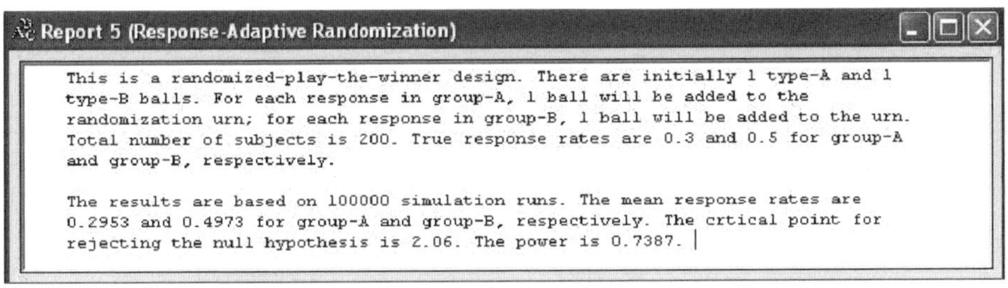

Figure 5.23 Simulation of power for the RAR design.

and a placebo. Based on early studies, the estimated FEV1 changes at week 4 are 6%, 12%, 13%, 14%, and 15% (with a pooled standard deviation of 18%) for the placebo and dose levels 1, 2, 3, and 4, respectively.

Following are the steps to design an adaptive trial using ExpDesign.

- Click 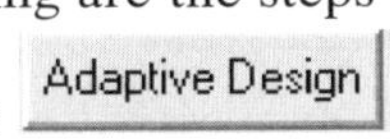

to bring up the **Adaptive Design–Step 1** window (Figure 5.24).

In the **Adaptive Design–Step 1** window, do the following:

- Select the **Response-Adaptive Randomization** option in the **Type of Adaptive Design** panel.
- Select the **Mean** option in the **Endpoint** window.
- Enter “0.06, 0.06, 0.06, 0.06, 0.06” for **Means Under Ha** in the **Hypotheses** panel.
- Enter “0.18” for **Sigma**, the standard deviation.
- Enter “0” for **NI-d**, the noninferiority margin, because it is a superiority trial.
- Enter “0.025” for **One-Sided Alpha** and any decimal value for **Power** (no effect in this version).

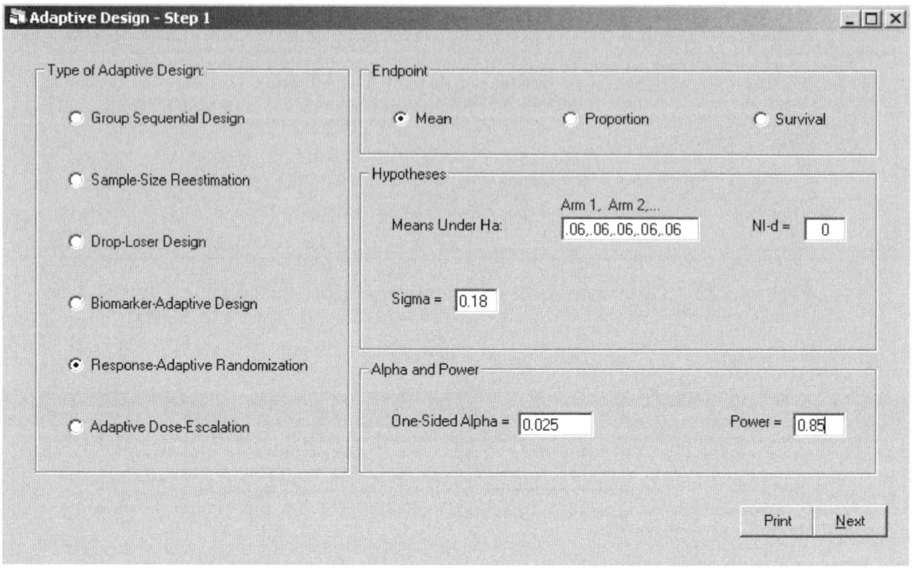

Figure 5.24 RAR design with normal endpoint.

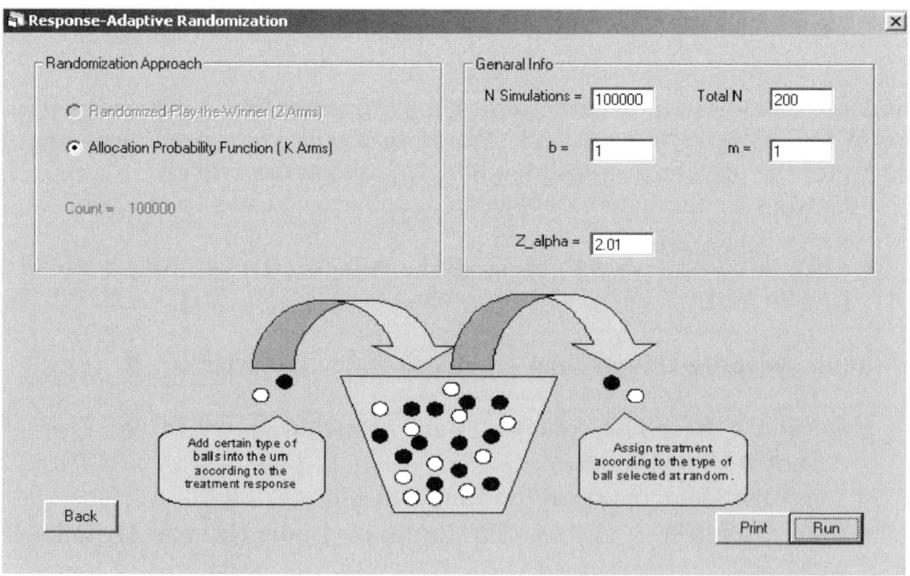

Figure 5.25 Input parameters for the normal RAR design.

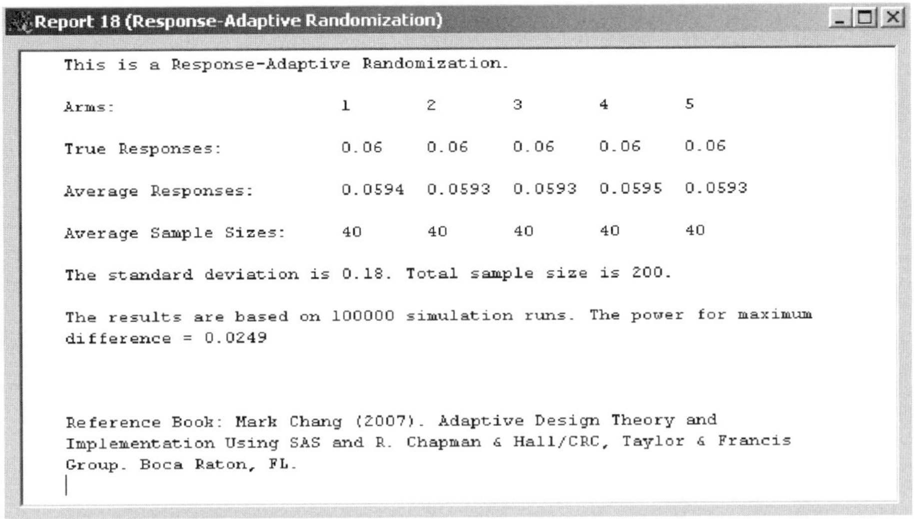

Figure 5.26 Characteristics of the RAR under the null condition.

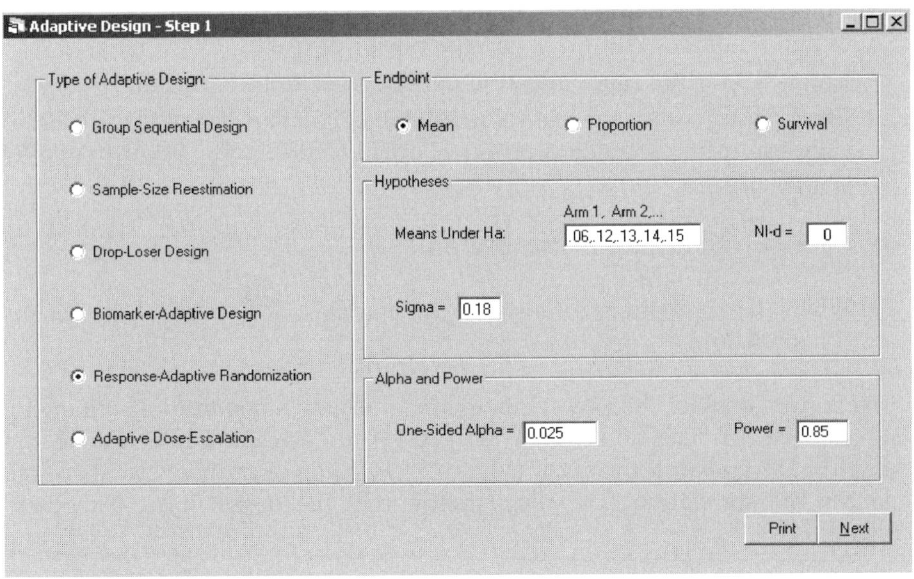

Figure 5.27 Input Parameters of RAR design for the alternative condition.

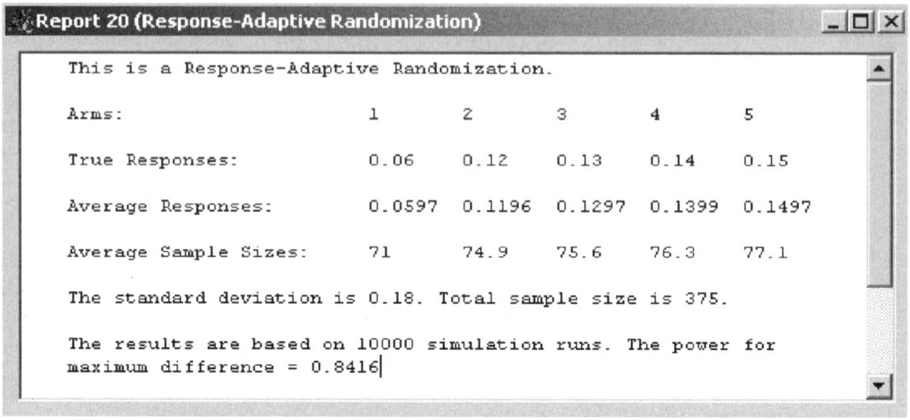

Figure 5.28 Characteristics of the RAR under the null condition.

- Click 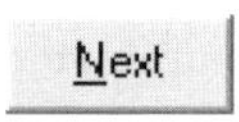

 to bring up the **Adaptive Design–Step 2** window (Figure 5.25).
- Enter "100000" for **N Simulations**.
- Enter "200" for **Total N**. You may need to use a trial-and-error method to find a number that gives you the power devised.
- Enter "1" for the randomization parameter **b** and "1" for **m**.
- Enter "2.01" for the critical value **Z_alpha**. You may have to try different values until the simulated power is equal to 0.025, the α level (weakly controlled).
- Click 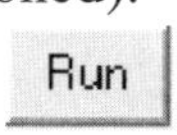

 to start the simulation.
- When the simulation is finished, you can click 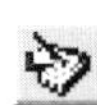 to view the results (Figure 5.26).

Next, we simulate the power under the alternative condition by changing the response to "0.06, 0.12, 0.13, 0.14, 0.15" for **Means Under Ha** in the **Adaptive Design–Step 1** window (Figure 5.27). Keep everything else the same and run the simulation. The results show that the design has 84% power (Figure 5.28).

6 Adaptive Trial Monitoring

6.1 INTRODUCTION

In this chapter we discuss the very important aspect of adaptive design: trial monitoring. Our discussion focuses on how to use statistical tools such as stopping boundaries, boundary-crossing probabilities, conditional power, and the futility index. We illustrate how to use ExpDesign to predict the probability of success, to calculate the conditional power, to reestimate the sample size, and to change the number and timing of the analyses. Using ExpDesign to perform these tasks is pretty straightforward. However, we first review the techniques for monitoring so that we can use them appropriately.

6.2 ERROR-SPENDING APPROACH

There are often changes in the information time for the interim analyses (IAs). The reason may, for example, be slow enrollment, but the DMC is not able to change their meeting schedule due to other commitments. As a result, the information time for the interim analyses moves back. There are also other reasons for a sponsor to change the information timing ($t = n/N$, the sample-size fraction at an interim analysis or the fraction of deaths) and number of analyses. When using MPP or MSP, interim analyses can be made any time without inflating the type I error rate because these two methods do not require prespecification of the time for IAs. MSP and MPP require only mutual independence of stagewise p-values, and they are either distributed uniformly or are larger. To change the number of IAs, we can use recursive two-stage adaptive designs (see M. Chang, 2007a, Chap. 8). For MINP, the recursive approach can be used, but more often the error-spending method is adopted.

Deviations in timing and number of analyses from the original design will affect the stopping boundaries in classical group sequential design. Therefore, the original stopping boundaries cannot be used, and new stopping

---

boundaries have to be recalculated based on a prespecified error-spending function. An error-spending function $\pi^*(t)$ is a cumulative error spent up to information time t. The α or error spent at a typical stage k can be expressed as $\pi^*(t_k) - \pi^*(t_{k-1})$, where t_k is the information time at stage k. Because $\pi^*(t)$ is a monotonically increasing function $(0 \le t \le 1)$ with $\pi^*(t_0) = 0$ and $\pi^*(t_k) = \pi^*(1) = \alpha$, the total error rate is

$$\sum_{k=1}^{K}[\pi^*(t_k) - \pi^*(t_{k-1})] = \pi^*(t_K) = \alpha. \tag{6.1}$$

The p-value (unadjusted) at the kth stage is compared against the stopping boundary on the p-scale, but not against the spending function, to determine whether or not to reject the null hypothesis.

There are at least three types of commonly used error-spending functions: O'Brien–Fleming-like, Pocock-like, and power-family error-spending functions.

1. The O'Brien–Fleming-like error-spending function is given by

$$\pi^*(t) = 2\left[1 - \Phi\left(\frac{z_{1-\alpha/2}}{\sqrt{t}}\right)\right], \tag{6.2}$$

where Φ is the c.d.f. of the standard normal distribution.

2. The Pocock-like error-spending function is given by

$$\pi^*(t) = \alpha \log[1 + (e - 1)t]. \tag{6.3}$$

3. The power-family (PF) error-spending function is given by

$$\pi^*(t) = \alpha t^b, \tag{6.4}$$

where t is the information time and b is a constant.

The various error-spending functions are compared in Figure 6.1. We can see that the power-family function provides a nice range of stopping boundaries. The Pocock-like function spends more α at early stages than does the O'Brien–Fleming-like function, while the linear function (PF with $b = 1$) is somewhere in between. The power family will spend more α at early stages when the parameter b decreases.

From Figure 6.1 and Table 6.1 we can see that the O'Brien–Fleming boundary with (an infinite number of) equal information intervals can be well approximated by both OF-like function (6.2) and the power-family function

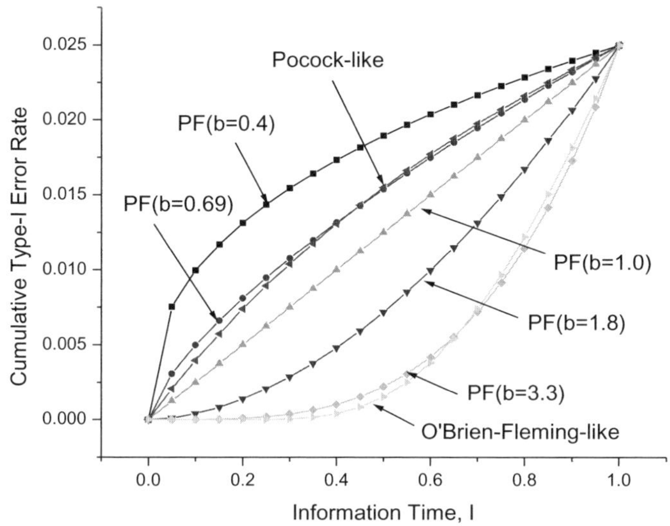

Figure 6.1 Error-spending functions.

with b = 3.3, as can a Pocock boundary with equal information intervals by a Pocock-like or power-family function with b = 0.688. Yet the Wang–Tsiatis boundary with Δ = 0.25 can be approximated by the power-family function with b = 2. The reason that using an error-spending function is preferable to traditional group sequential design is that the former makes it possible to change the number and timing of analyses without inflating the type I error. With a prespecified error-spending function, the stopping boundaries can be recalculated when there is a change in the number or timing of the analyses.

6.3 HOW TO RECALCULATE STOPPING BOUNDARIES USING EXPDESIGN

As mentioned earlier, the determination of stopping boundaries is necessary at the trial design and monitoring stages. In ExpDesign Studio, the power function is used for error spending in the adaptive design module. The O'Brien–Fleming spending function can be approximated by the power-family function $\pi^*(t) = \alpha t^{3.3}$ or the O'Brien–Fleming-like function (6.1). The Pocock spending function can be approximated by $\pi^*(t) = \alpha t^{0.688}$ or (6.2). To use function (6.2), click the Adaptive Trial Monitor icon 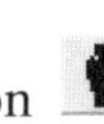; then check the **O'Brien-F** checkbox in the **Adaptive Trial Monitor** window. To use the Pocock-like function, check the **Pocock** checkbox.

TABLE 6.1 Comparison of Cumulative Error Rates[a]

Information Time t	OF	OF-like	PF (b = 3.3)	WT (Δ = 0.25)	PF (b = 2)	PK	PK-like	PF (b = 0.688)
0.1	0.0000	0.0000	0.0000	0.0000	0.0003	0.0067	0.0040	0.0051
0.2	0.0000	0.0000	0.0001	0.0004	0.0010	0.0109	0.0074	0.0083
0.3	0.0000	0.0000	0.0005	0.0016	0.0023	0.0139	0.0104	0.0109
0.4	0.0004	0.0004	0.0012	0.0036	0.0040	0.0163	0.0131	0.0133
0.5	0.0016	0.0015	0.0025	0.0063	0.0063	0.0182	0.0155	0.0155
0.6	0.0039	0.0038	0.0046	0.0094	0.0090	0.0199	0.0177	0.0176
0.7	0.0074	0.0074	0.0077	0.0129	0.0123	0.0214	0.0197	0.0196
0.8	0.0122	0.0122	0.0120	0.0167	0.0160	0.0227	0.0216	0.0214
0.9	0.0181	0.0182	0.0177	0.0208	0.0203	0.0239	0.0234	0.0233
1.0	0.0250	0.0250	0.0250	0.0250	0.0250	0.0250	0.0250	0.0250

[a] OF = WT(Δ = 0), OF-like = Eq. (6.2), PK = WT(Δ = 0.5), PK-like = Eq. (6.3). WT cumulative error rate = stopping probability from the ExpDesign classical design module when the two groups have the same means (*H*o).

Example: Changing the Timing of Interim Analysis Suppose that we are monitoring a two-stage adaptive design with the power-family ($b = 1.93$) spending function featuring an interim analysis on 50% of the patients (i.e., information $t = 0.5$), which was expected one year after the trial started. However, due to slow enrollment, the newly projected time line will be 20 months from the beginning of the trial (i.e., 8 months later than the earlier projection). This setback will have a negative impact on the study and the company.

However, it will also not be helpful if the interim analysis is performed too early on the original projected calendar schedule because only a little information is available. A reasonable approach is to perform the interim analysis at 16 months after the trial started and when 40% patients would have the data. After the IDMC agree on the meeting date, the actual stopping boundaries have to be calculated based on the actual number of patients in the interim analysis. Assume that the company was to collect data on 40% patients for the interim analysis. The stopping boundary can be recalculated using ExpDesign:

1. Click the adaptive trial monitor icon 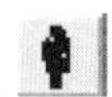 to bring up the **Adaptive Trail Monitor** window (Figure 6.2).
2. Select the recompute stopping boundary in the **Objective** panel. The **Adaptive Trial Monitor** window will appear (Figure 6.3).
3. Enter the "2" for **Number of Stages** and "0.4, 1" for **Information time for Analyses**.

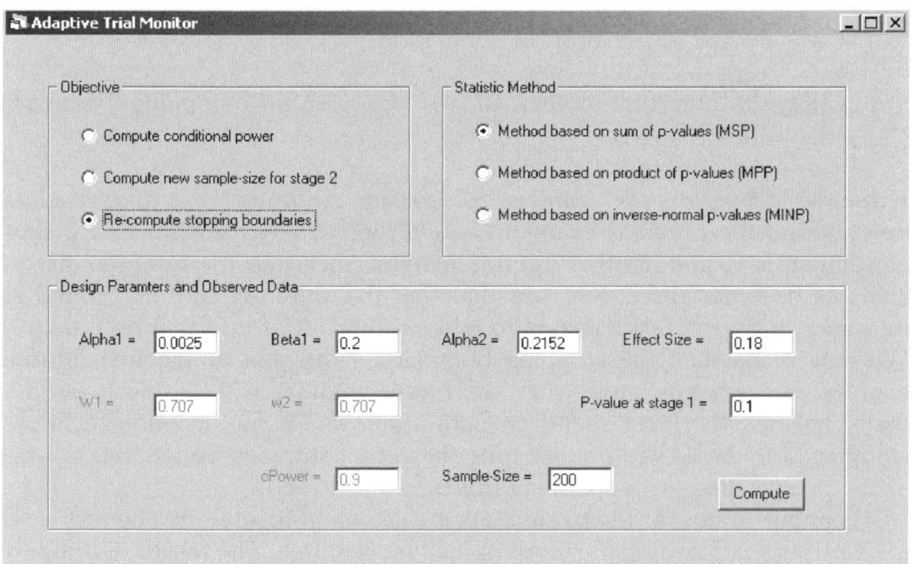

Figure 6.2 Adaptive trial monitor window.

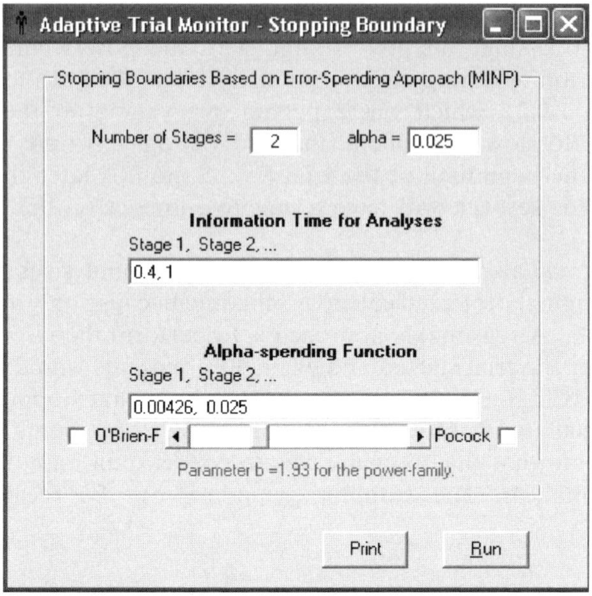

Figure 6.3 Calculation of stopping boundary.

4. Set the same spending function for the stopping boundary by either checking the checkbox or using the scrollbar. In the current case, check the **O'Brien–F** checkbox.
5. Click Run to perform the simulation.
6. Click  on the toolbar to see the resulting stopping boundary (Figure 6.4).

Example: Changing the Number of Interim Analyses For the problem described in the previous example, an alternative way to adapt to the slow enrollment is to add another interim analysis, such that the total number of analyses becomes three. Suppose that the first were actually performed at information time 0.3. We decide to add another IA at information time 0.7. We now recalculate the stopping boundary. Note that at the first interim analysis, we may not know when the future analyses will be, but it doesn't mater because the error-spending method allows for modification of future stopping boundaries without affecting the earlier stopping boundaries as long as the prespecified error-spending function is followed.

The input values for the parameters are shown in Figure 6.5. The rest steps are very straightforward, as shown in the first example. The resulting stopping boundaries on the p-scale are 0.00245, 0.01099, and 0.01892 for the three analyses, respectively.

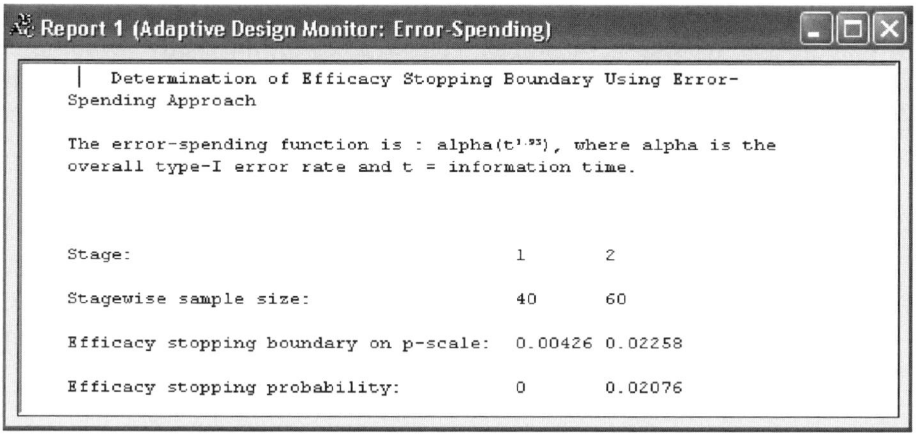

Figure 6.4 Resulting stopping boundary.

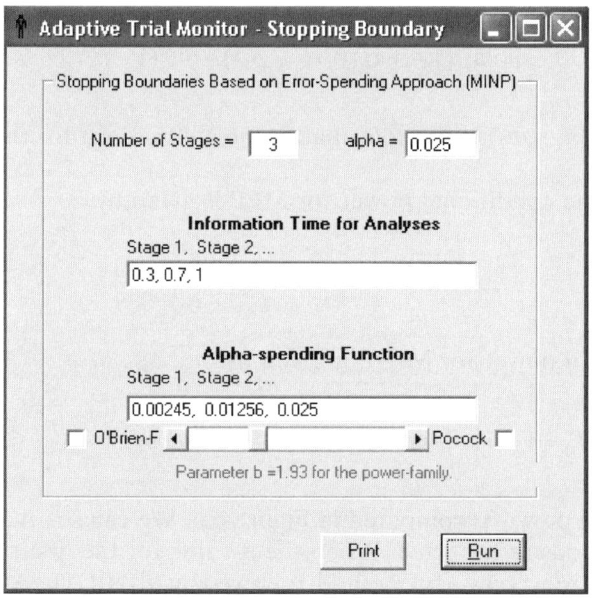

Figure 6.5 Redesigning the trial as a three-stage design.

6.4 CONDITIONAL POWER AND THE FUTILITY INDEX

The *conditional power* is the probability that the null hypothesis will eventually be rejected given the data observed at the moment. Therefore, the conditional power is dependent on the data observed, but is also dependent on the adaptive methods used in the trial. The *futility index* is defined as the probability that the null hypothesis will not be rejected when the alternative hypothesis is true. Hence, the futility index can be defined as 1 – conditional power if both use the same estimate for the parameter δ.

The conditional power for MSP is given by

$$P_c = 1 - \Phi\left(\Phi^{-1}(1 - \max(0, \alpha_2 - p_1)) - \frac{\delta}{\sigma}\sqrt{\frac{n_2}{2}}\right), \tag{6.5}$$

where $\alpha_1 < p_1 \leq \beta_1$; α_1 and β_1 are the efficacy and futility stopping boundaries, respectively; n_1 is the sample size at the first stage, the effect size; and δ/σ can be estimated using the $\hat{\delta}$ and $\hat{\sigma}$ observed for two groups or using p_1:

$$\frac{\delta}{\sigma} = \Phi^{-1}(1 - p_1)\sqrt{\frac{2}{n_1}}. \tag{6.6}$$

Therefore Eq. (6.5) can be written as

$$P_c = 1 - \Phi\left(\Phi^{-1}(1 - \max(0, \alpha_2 - p_1)) - \Phi^{-1}(1 - p_1)\sqrt{\frac{1}{t_1} - 1}\right), \tag{6.7}$$

where $t_1 = n_1/(n_1 + n_2)$ is the information time (fraction) for the first interim analysis.

Similarly, the conditional power for MPP is given by

$$P_c = 1 - \Phi\left(\Phi^{-1}\left(1 - \frac{\alpha_2}{p_1}\right) - \frac{\delta}{\sigma}\sqrt{\frac{n_2}{2}}\right). \tag{6.8}$$

The conditional power for MINP is given by

$$P_c = 1 - \Phi\left(\frac{1}{w_2}\Phi^{-1}(1 - \alpha_1) - \frac{w_1}{w_2}\Phi^{-1}(1 - p_1) - \frac{\delta}{\sigma}\sqrt{\frac{n_2}{2}}\right). \tag{6.9}$$

Conditional power is compared in Figure 6.6. We can see that it differs for different methods as expected. When the p-value for the first stage is around 0.1, MSP is the most powerful method, followed by MINP. The MPP and MINP methods perform better at the two extremes when the p-value p_1 is either very small or very large.

An interesting question is: When will the p-value be rounded to 0.1? Here is a common scenario: At the design stage, the standard effect size was estimated to be 0.25, and about 254 subjects per group are needed for 90% power. At the interim analysis the effect size observed (standardized) based on 50% of the subjects is 0.164 (only 65.6% of the original estimation). The reason that we observed 0.164 could be because the drug is truly less effective, or because, just by chance, we observed a lower effect or a combination the two. In such

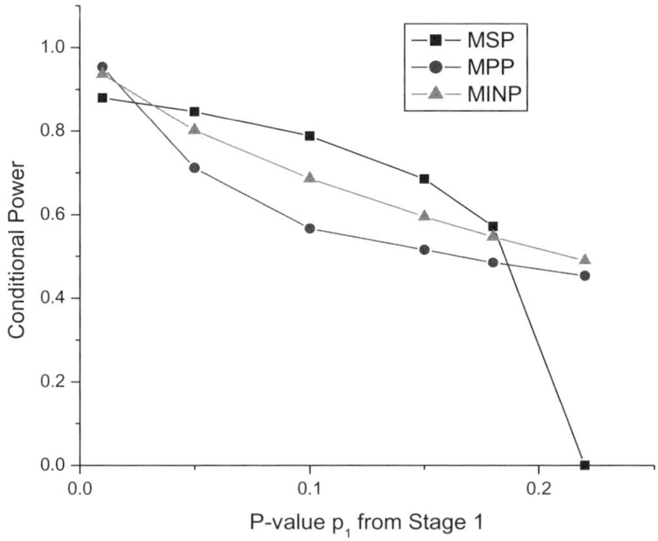

Figure 6.6 Comparisons of conditional power.

a case the p-value at the interim analysis is $p_1 = 0.1$. It is not uncommon at all to estimate the treatment effect by 30% or more at the design stage. Also, more than one-third of phase III trials failed. It is reasonable to believe that 33% p-values > 0.025 at the final analysis (most of the trials are fixed-sample-size designs). Therefore, it is also not unreasonable to say that the p-value based on interim analyses would be larger that 0.025 ($z = 1.96$) or somewhere larger than 0.083 ($z = 1.96/2^{0.5}$). Note that the commonly used group sequential design is a special case of MINP. For details, see the book *Adaptive Design Theory and Implementation Using SAS and R* (M. Chang, 2007a).

An interesting way to monitor an adaptive trial informally is the ESP (expected sample path) approach (Figure 6.7), in which several critical lines are drawn on an information-Z plan. We first draw the stopping boundary specified in the protocol and several lines for ESP with different powers. When the data become available, we draw the actual sample path.

The expected or average sample path is the z-value when the alternative condition H_a for sample size calculation is true. Mathematically, we can write the z-value at information time t as

$$z(t) = Z(1)\sqrt{t}. \tag{6.10}$$

The power in Figure 6.7 is the power for the trial. From the figure we can see that when the trial has 90% power, the ESP crosses the boundaries at about $t = 0.6$; when it has 80% power, it crosses at about $t = 0.7$. If the effect size is overestimated such that the trial has only 50% power, ESP touch as the

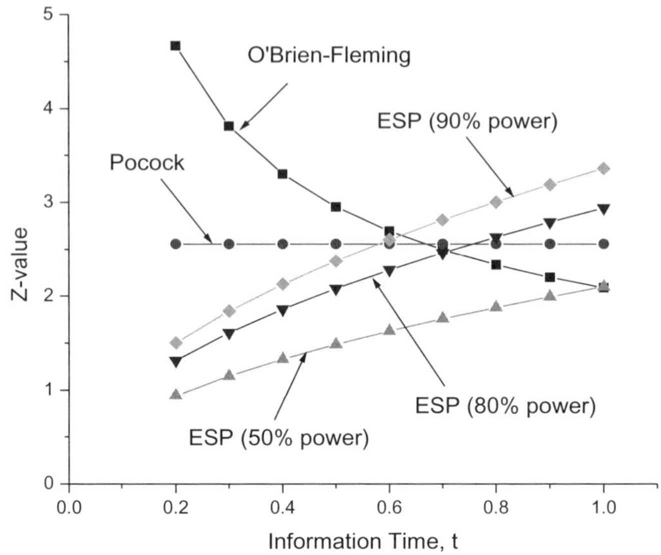

Figure 6.7 Stopping boundaries and expected sample paths.

boundary at $t = 1$ (i.e., the end of the trial). If the sample path is observed above the ESP for 90% power, the trial is very promising; on the other hand, if the actual sample path is below ESP for the 50% power, we are probably going to fail the trial.

6.5 HOW TO REESTIMATE SAMPLE SIZE USING EXPDESIGN

6.5.1 Calculating Conditional Power Using ExpDesign

Calculation of conditional power using ExpDesign is straightforward, as illustrated in the following example. Suppose that a two-stage adaptive trial was designed using MSP with stopping boundaries $\alpha_1 = 0.0025$, $\beta_1 = 0.2$, and $\alpha_2 = 0.2152$. The sample size for the interim analysis $n_1 = 100$ per group. The sample size (not cumulative) for the second stage $n_2 = 200$ per group. Assume that $p_1 = 0.1$, $n_1 = 100$, and the effect size (treatment difference divided by standard deviation) observed can be calculated using Eq. (6.5) in Section 6.3:

$$\frac{\hat{\delta}}{\hat{\sigma}} = \Phi^{-1}(0.9)\sqrt{\frac{2}{100}} = 1.2816\sqrt{\frac{2}{100}} = 0.18.$$

This is the default value in ExpDesign and is available by clicking the **Default** checkbox next to it.

Here are the steps to obtaining the conditional power:

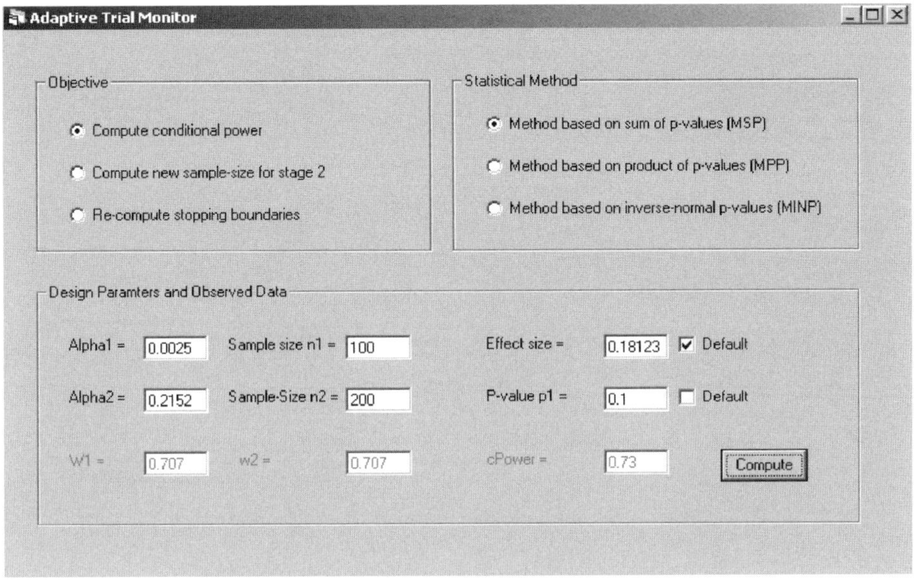

Figure 6.8 Conditional power with MSP.

1. Click the adaptive trial monitor icon  to bring up the **Adaptive Trial Monitor** window (Figure 6.2).
2. Select the **Compute conditional power** option in the **Objective** panel.
3. Select the **MSP** option in the **Statistical Method** panel.
4. Enter the values "0.0025, 0.2152, 0.2, 0.1, 200" for α_1, α_2, β_1, and sample size, respectively.
5. Click the **Default** checkbox next to **Effect Size**; "0.18123" will fill into the corresponding textbox.
6. Click Run; a conditional power of 0.73 is obtained from the textbox labeled as **cPower** (Figure 6.8).

6.5.2 Reestimating Sample Size Using ExpDesign

This conditional power 73% is considered too low. We may decide to increase the sample size to retain 80% (conditional) power. Use the following steps to estimate the new sample size required for the second stage with 80% conditional power (Figure 6.9):

1. Select the **Compute new sample-sign for stage 2** option in the **Objective** panel.
2. Select the **MSP** option in the **Statistical Method** panel.

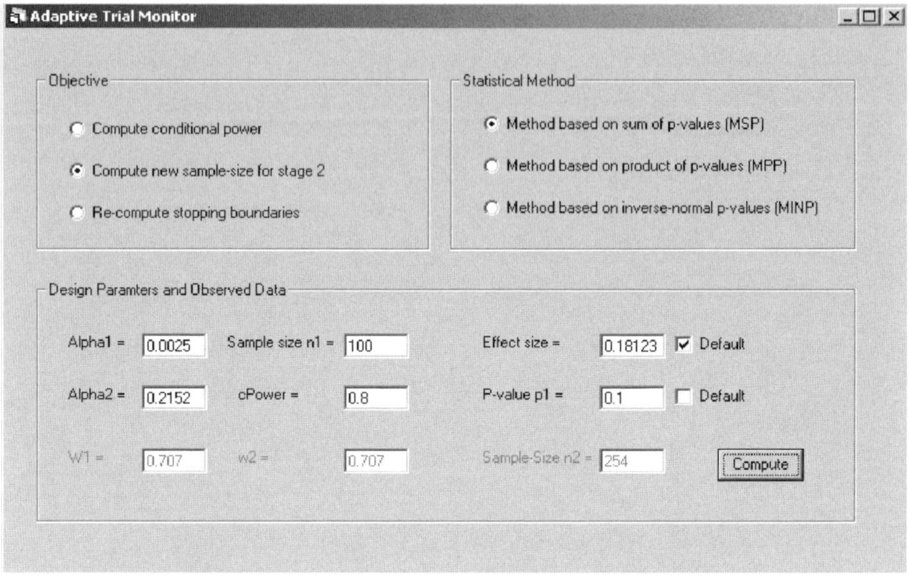

Figure 6.9 Sample size based on conditional power.

3. Enter "0.0025, 0.2152, 0.1, 200" for α_1, α_2, p_1, and the sample size.
4. Click the **Default** checkbox next to **Effect size**; "0.18123" will fill into the corresponding textbox.
5. Click Compute; the required sample size is $n_2 = 254$ per group for the second stage, as shown in Figure 6.9.

The procedures to obtain the conditional power and new sample size with MPP and MINP are similar; you can try this yourself.

6.6 TRIAL EXAMPLES

6.6.1 Changes in Number and Timing of the Analyses

"In the 1970s, it was thought that blockade of the beta-adrenergic receptors might be beneficial for patients with myocardial infarction. This led to the conduct of several clinical trials. Some of these trials treated patients with intravenous beta-blockers at the time of the acute MI; others began treatment intravenously at the time of the acute event and continued with oral beta-blockers after hospital discharge; still others began long-term oral treatment of patients after the acute recovery phase. Relevant to the development of the Beta-Blocker Heart Attack Trial (BHAT) were concerns that the long-term trials that had been conducted were inconclusive. In particular, some were underpowered, one used a beta-blocker that had unexpected serious toxicity, and some may have used inadequate doses of medication. Therefore, a workshop conducted by the National Heart, Lung, and Blood Institute (NHLBI) recommended that another long-term trial with a sufficiently large sample size and using appropriate doses of a beta-blocker with which there was considerable experience and a known toxicity profile, such as propranolol, be conducted" (DeMets, 2006).

Patients aged 30 to 69 years who had had a myocardial infarction 5 to 21 days prior to randomization were to be enrolled. The primary objective of the study was to determine if long-term administration of propranolol would result in a difference in all-cause mortality. The group sequential design with six interim analyses (O'Brien–Fleming boundary with equal information intervals) was used for BHAT. The actual trial path (z-values) is presented in Figure 6.10.

A total of 4040 patients were to enroll. Participant enrollment began in 1978; a total of 3837 participants were actually enrolled. This trial of 1884 survivors of an acute myocardial infarction showed a statistically significant reduction in all-cause mortality, from 16.2% to 10.4%, during a mean follow-up of 17 months. At this point, BHAT was no longer enrolling patients, but follow-up was continuing.

We are now ready to reproduce the group sequential design and than change to a more flexible or adaptive design. For the latter we discuss how to monitor and take adaptations according to the data observed. For a group sequential design with seven analyses with equal intervals and O'Brien–Fleming boundaries, 4040 patients will have 89.3% power (using either ExpDesign 5.0 or East 4.1) to detect a 28% relative change in mortality, from a three-year rate of 17.46% in the control (placebo) group to 13.75% in the intervention group, which was estimated from previous studies.

Suppose that we originally use an error-spending approach with an O'Brien–Fleming-like spending function featuring seven analyses at equal information intervals. After the third analysis, we find that the efficacy results are somewhat promising, and the trend (Figure 6.10) shows that the trial is likely be successful at the fifth interim analysis. Therefore, we want to do one more analysis (final analysis) for the study and eliminate the rest of the interim analyses. The final analysis is scheduled at the time for the original fifth interim analysis. Therefore, we calculate the stopping boundary using the same OF error-spending function but with four analyses at information time: 1/7, 2/7, 3/7, and 1 (Figures 6.11 and 6.12).

The new final stopping boundary is naive p-value ≤ 0.0248 ($z = 1.9634$) using the distribution calculator in ExpDesign (Figure 6.13). The observed p-values at the first three IAs are 0.0465 ($z = 1.68$), 0.0125 ($z = 2.24$), and 0.0089 ($z = 2.37$), respectively. We want to check if the new design has sufficient power. If not, a sample-size reestimation may be required. We can accomplish this with ExpDesign as specified in the following steps:

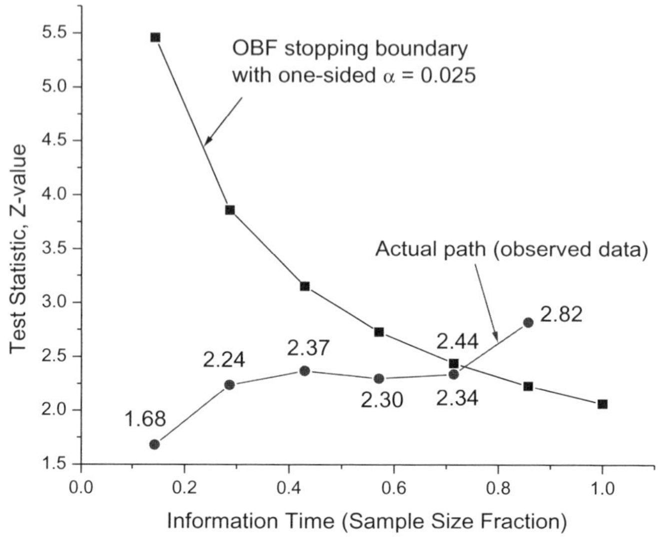

Figure 6.10 BHAT stopping boundary and actual path. (Data from DeMets et al., 2006.)

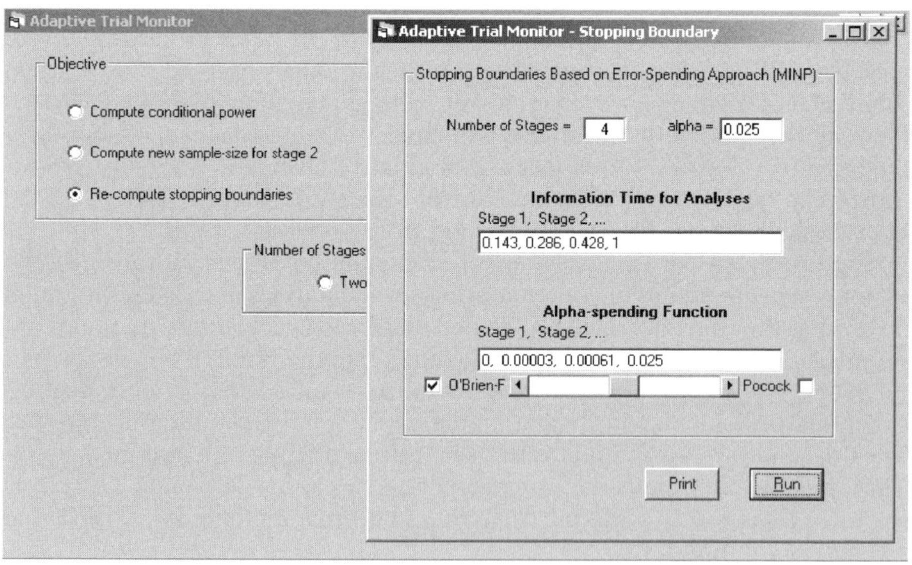

Figure 6.11 Stopping boundary for the BHAT trial.

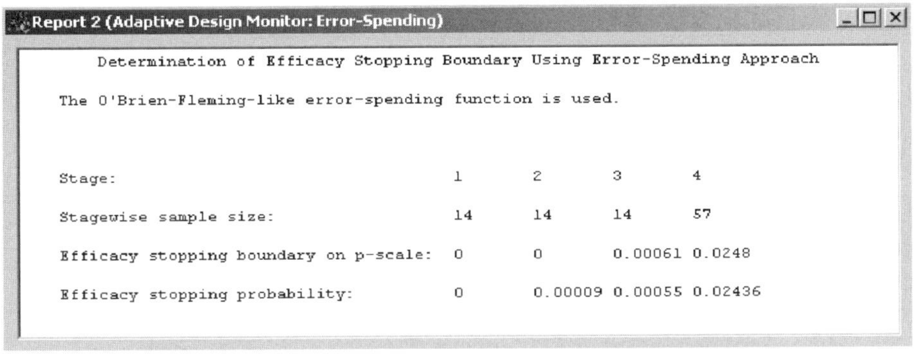

Figure 6.12 New stopping boundary for the BHAT trial.

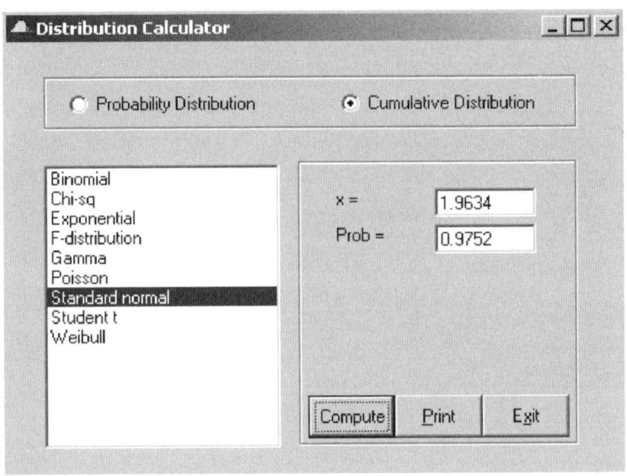

Figure 6.13 Assist from ExpDesign probability calculator.

1. Click the adaptive trial monitor icon  to bring up the **Adaptive Trial Monitor** window (Figure 6.14).
2. Select the **Compute conditional power** option in the **Objective** panel and **K-stage** in the **Number of Stages** panel.
3. Select the **MSP** option on the **Statistical Method** panel.
4. Enter "577, 1154, 1731, 4040" for the stagewise sample sizes; "0.0, 0.0, 0.00061, 0.0248" for the efficacy boundary on the p-scale; "1, 1, 1, 1" for the futility boundary on the p-scale; and "0.0465, 0.0125, 0.0089" for the stagewise p-values observed, respectively.
5. Click 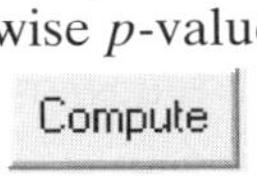

 (Figure 6.15).

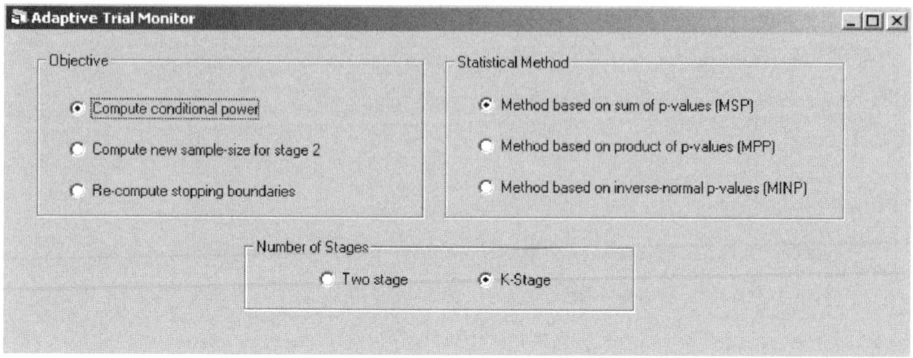

Figure 6.14 ExpDesign adaptive trial monitor.

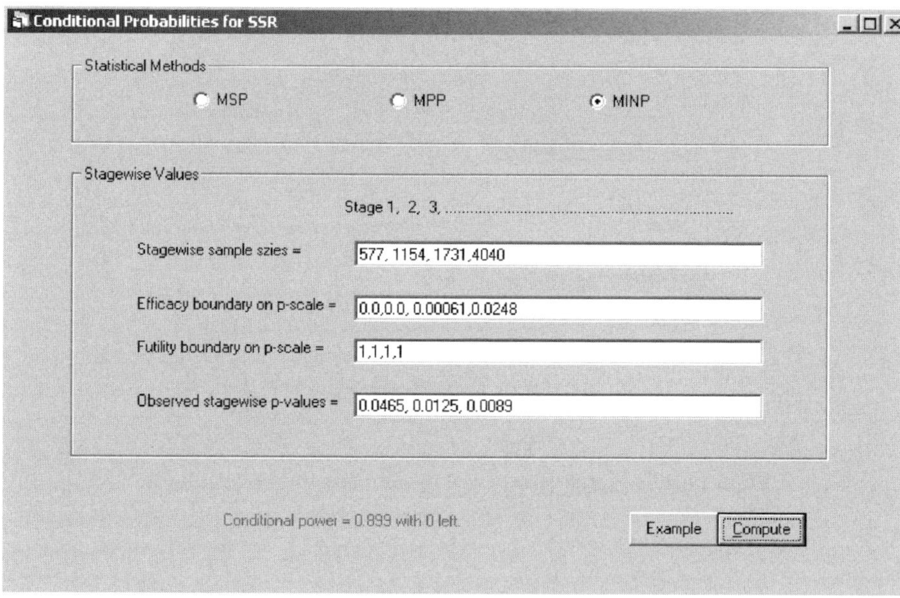

Figure 6.15 Conditional power calculation with ExpDesign.

The conditional power of rejecting the null hypothesis at the final step turns out to be 0.899; with such high power the sample size does not need to be adjusted. The timing of the analysis is one year earlier than the original schedule planned for the final analysis.

We now do the final analysis. The observed test statistic $z = 2.34$ or p-value $= 0.0096 < 0.0248$ (the stopping boundary); therefore, the null hypothesis is rejected. From this example we can see that the adaptive design has advantages over the classical group sequential design.

Note that the timing of the analyses is assumed to be independent of interim data. However, practically, we want to change the timing based on the data observed. Fortunately, the potential type I error rate inflation due to the data-dependent timing is small (<10%) (Proschan et al., 2006).

6.6.2 Recursive Two-Stage Adaptive Design

Let's use the recursive two-stage adaptive design (M. Chang, 2007a, Chap. 8) to redesign the example of Section 6.6.1. The conditional error principle allows one to redesign a two-stage trial at every analysis as long as the conditional error is retained at each stage. Following are the steps for performing the recursive two-stage design on the fly:

1. Initiate the first two-stage trial.
2. After looking at the IA data, decide whether to keep the original design or redesign a two-stage trial using the conditional error function.
3. If a decision not to change the design is made, it is straightforward adaptive design.
4. If a decision to redesign the two-stage trial is made, the conditional error function is calculated as $A = \alpha_2 - p_1$ and the new two-stage trial design is based on the new type I error rate: $\alpha = A$.
5. Repeat steps 2 to 4 until the trial eventually stops.

See M. Chang (2007a, Chap. 8) for a trial example.

6.6.3 Conditional Power and Sample-Size Reestimation

"The Randomized Aldactone Evaluation Study (RALES) was a randomized double-blind placebo-controlled trial designed to test the hypothesis that addition of daily spironolactone to standard therapy would reduce the risk of all-cause mortality in patients with severe heart failure as a result of systolic left ventricular dysfunction. The Data Safety Monitoring Board (DSMB) for RALES reviewed data on safety and efficacy throughout the trial using pre-specified statistical stopping boundaries for efficacy. To ensure that the data were complete, the DSMB requested successive 'mortality sweeps.' At the time of these sweeps, all RALES investigators determined the vital status of participants at their clinics. Therefore, the data that the DSMB saw included a much higher percentage of the deaths than would have been observed without these sweeps. At the DSMB's fifth meeting, the data showed 351 deaths in the placebo group and 269 in the spironolactone group, for an estimated hazard ratio of 0.78 (p 0.00018). The board recommended early termination of the trial because the observed Z-value of 3.75 exceeded the pre-specified critical value of 2.79 and the data on mortality showed consistency among subgroups and across time. The sweeps had identified 31deaths that likely would not have

TABLE 6.2 *p*-Values Observed in the Aldactone Study[a]

IA Time	Death Placebo/Test	Hazard Ratio	*p*-Value	Stopping Boundary on *p*-Scale	Conditional Power
(8/96)	70/52	0.76	0.11	0.0000	
(3/97)	136/109	0.83	0.092	0.0000	
(8/97)	224/175	0.80	0.11	0.0002	
(3/98)	304/241	0.81	0.0026	0.0009	
(8/99)	351/269	0.78	0.00018	0.0026	0.00824
				0.0054	0.05669
				0.0092	0.25458
				0.0137	0.38956
				0.0188	0.22647

Source: Wittes et al. (2005).

[a]First patient in March 24, 1995.

been reported by the time of the meeting. Subsequent data collection identified an additional 46 deaths that had occurred by the time the study ended. Even when the endpoint of a randomized clinical trial is mortality, routine methods of data collection and reporting are unlikely to identify all events in a timely manner. The experience from RALES provides an example of the importance of active follow-up of patients to ensure that a DSMB is observing a high proportion of the events that have actually occurred" (Wittes et al., 2005).

The first patient was randomized on March 24, 1995 and the planned end of the trial was December 31, 1999. Thus, the trial was now based on calendar time instead of total events. Consequently, calculations for the interim analysis had to be based on an unknown total number of deaths. The *p*-values observed are presented in Table 6.2.

Suppose that the hazard ratio is 1.25 between the treatment groups; $\ln(1.25) = -0.22314$. To calculate the number of events needed, we can use normal endpoint design with mean = $\ln(0.8)$ and standard deviation = 1. Redesign an adaptive design with 90% power and nine interim analyses of the OF boundary for the trial. The number of events required is 874 (Figure 6.16).

As an exercise, draw the ESP (90% power) and ESP (50% power); calculate the conditional power at each stage up to the fourth stage and adjust the sample size to 95% conditional power at the fourth stage if it is lower than that. The conditional efficacy stopping probabilities for stages 5 to 9 are 0.00824, 0.05669, 0.25458, 0.38956, and 0.22647, respectively. The overall conditional power at stage 4 is 0.936 (Figure 6.17).

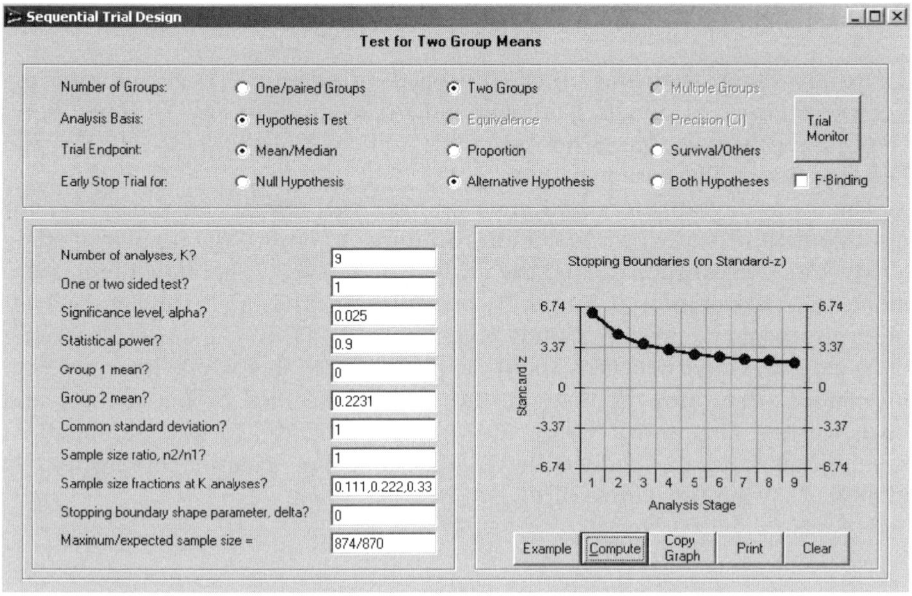

Figure 6.16 Using a normal endpoint to mimic a design with a survival endpoint.

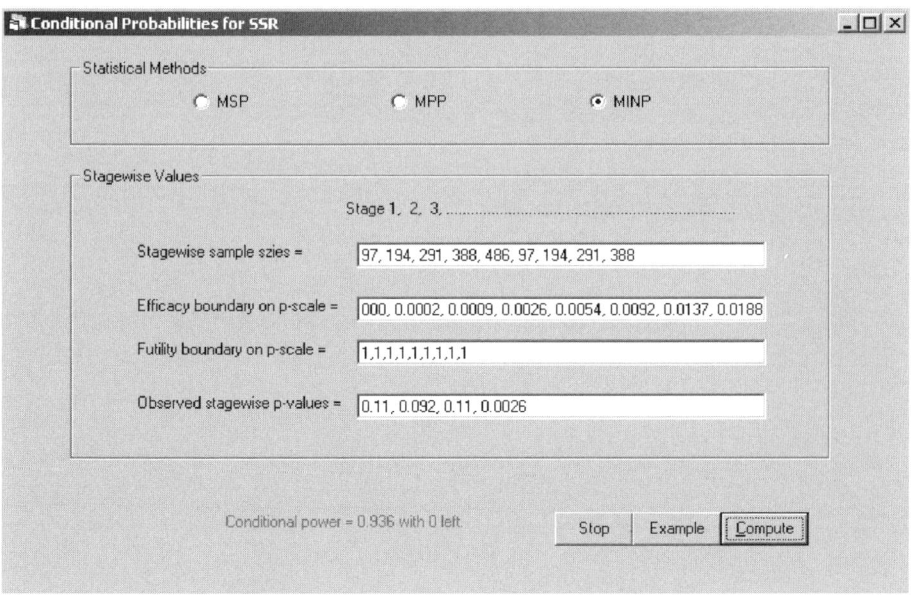

Figure 6.17 Conditional power calculation.

REMARKS

There are theoretical and practical aspects of adaptive design monitoring. For the theoretical details I recommend Proschan, Lan and DeMets' book (2006); for practical aspects books on this topic by Ellenberg et al. (2002) and DeMets et al. (2006) are excellent.

The study investigators and sponsor have the primary responsibility for development of study protocol and procedures to ensure the quality of study conduct in many instances, and the DMC will be asked to review these documents prior to initiation of a trial. By providing an advisory review of the draft of the protocol and proposed study procedures, the DMC can ensure that none of its members have concerns about the planned trial that would interfere with the ability to monitor the study in the manner specified by the sponsor and investigators. This initial review also allows the DMC to give independent scientific guidance and reduce the risk that ethical or scientific flaws would be identified during the course of the study.

7 Oncology Adaptive Trial Design

7.1 MULTISTAGE TRIAL DESIGN

7.1.1 Introduction

Multistage designs represent a specific category of sequential design where the response is binary in nature and the statistical method used is exact in terms of binomial distribution. Multistage design is often used in a phase I or II clinical trial where a single-arm trial is utilized to determine whether an experimental treatment holds sufficient promise to warrant further study. The number of patients is usually not very large, and normal approximation may not be applicable. The initial design for two-stage phase II cancer clinical trials proposed by Gehan (1961) provided the minimum number of patients required to enter in stage 1, such that if all patients were nonresponders, the therapy could be discontinued from further study with a given chance of rejection error. Given P_0, a response rate that is not of interest for conducting further studies, and P_1, a response rate of definite interest ($P_1 > P_0$), Fleming developed two- and three-stage designs for testing hypotheses about the true response rate p. Fleming's designs allow for early termination with acceptance or rejection of the new therapy at each stage. The plans preserved (approximately) the size and power of a single-stage procedure for testing the hypotheses. Simon (1989) modified Fleming's plans by considering two-stage procedures that permitted rejection of a therapy at either of the two stages but acceptance only at the final stage. The rationale was that stopping a study early was undesirable when a therapy appeared to be effective, but desirable when the treatment seemed to be ineffective. Simon's design is optimal in that it minimizes the expected sample size when the true response rate $p = P_0$ at given levels of significance and power. Also, he proposed a design that minimizes the maximum number of patients required. Ensign et al. (1994) proposeda three-stage design that permits early stopping when a moderately long sequence of initial failures occurs.

ExpDesign has implemented Simon's two-stage design and generalized Ensign et al.'s three-stage design, which permit early stopping for futility. The resulting designs have controlled the overall type I error rate. There are three

Classical and Adaptive Clinical Trial Designs Using ExpDesign Studio™,
By Mark Chang

types of optimal designs in ExpDesign: MinMaxSize, MinExpSize, and MaxUtility. *MinMaxSize design* minimizes the maximum sample size when the trial goes through all the stages, *MinExpSize design* minimizes the expected sample size when the null hypothesis is true, and *MaxUtility design* maximizes the utility that is defined as a composite index combining the expected sample size and maximum sample size, and then normalized such that the corresponding classical design has a utility of 1.

7.1.2 How to Design a Multistage Design Using ExpDesign

Let's explain the steps in designing a multistage trial through an example. Suppose that we are planning a phase II trial with a single group of cancer patients to investigate the efficacy and safety of an experimental drug called AntiGen. The primary endpoint is cancer response (complete response + partial response). It is specified that if the response rate is less that 5%, the trial will not be continued, and if the response rate is greater than 20%, investigation will continue. The company recognizes the importance of stopping the trial early if the testing drug is not promising, but is willing to spend more if the drug is very promising. More specifically, the importance of minimizing the sample size expected under the null hypothesis is rated 8 on a 10-point scale, and the importance of minimizing the maximum sample size is rated 2. For this reason we are going to generate two- and three-stage designs and select the final design that meets our needs through comparisons. Note that $\alpha = 0.1$ and power = 0.9 are common in a phase II oncology study. However, a trial designer can use other settings as long as justifications are provided.

We now use Expdesign to generate two-stage designs as follows. Click Multistage Design. Based on the information provided in the example, we select the option **2-stage design**. Enter "0.05" for **Proportion for Ho**, "0.20" for **Proportion for Ha**, "0.05" for **Alpha**, and "0.8" for **Power**. Suppose that we believe that minimizing the sample size expected is more important than minimizing the maximum sample size, and as an example, we enter "2, 8" for the utility weights (see Figure 7.1). Click Compute to generate a two-stage design and click 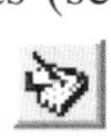 on the toolbar to review the design report reviewed below.

Two-Stage Design Testing (One-Sided) for a Single Proportion Featuring Early Stopping for Futility Common settings for the three designs (MinMaxSize, MinExpSize, and MaxUtility) are: level of significance $\alpha = 0.05$, power = 0.8, proportion for the null hypothesis $P_0 = 0.05$, and proportion for the alternative hypothesis $P_a = 0.2$.

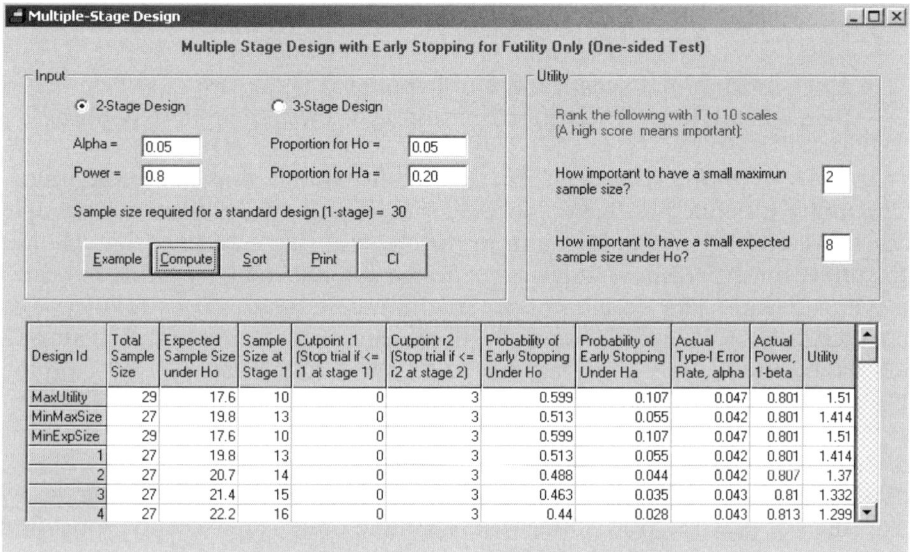

Figure 7.1 Example of two-stage design.

MinMaxSize Two-Stage Design The MinMaxSize design minimizes the maximum size required. The design characteristics are summarized as follows: The cumulative sample size at stage 1 = 13, the cumulative sample size at stage 2 = 27, the actual type I error rate $\alpha = 0.042$, the actual power = 0.801, and the utility index is 1.414 for the design.

The stopping rules are as follows:

- *Stage 1:* Stop and accept the null hypothesis if the response rate is less than or equal to 0/13. Otherwise, continue on to stage 2. The probability of stopping for futility is 0.513 when H_0 is true and 0.055 when Ha is true.
- *Stage 2:* Stop and accept the null hypothesis if the response rate is less than or equal to 3/27. Otherwise, stop and reject the null hypothesis.

MinExpSize Two-Stage Design The MinExpSize (optimal) design minimizes the sample size expected. The design characteristics are summarized as follows: The cumulative sample size at stage 1 = 10, the cumulative sample size at stage 2 = 29, the actual type I error rate $\alpha = 0.047$, the actual power = 0.801, and the utility index is 1.51 for the design.

The stopping rules are as follows:

- *Stage 1:* Stop and accept the null hypothesis if the response rate is less than or equal to 0/13. Otherwise, continue on to stage 2. The probability of stopping for futility is 0.599 when H_0 is true and 0.107 when H_a is true.

- *Stage 2:* Stop and accept the null hypothesis if the response rate is less than or equal to 3/29. Otherwise, stop and reject the null hypothesis.

MaxUtility Two-Stage Design The MaxUtility design maximizes the utility. The utility is defined as (0.8 × expected sample size + 0.2 × maximum sample size) divided by the sample size from the classical single-stage design. Hence, the utility for the classical single-stage design is 1, and a higher utility indicates a better design. The design characteristics are summarized as follows: The cumulative sample size at stage 1 = 10, the cumulative sample size at stage 2 = 29, the actual type I error rate $\alpha = 0.047$, the actual power = 0.801, and the utility index = 1.51 for the design.

The stopping rules are as follows:

- *Stage 1:* Stop and accept the null hypothesis if the response rate is less than or equal to 0/13. Otherwise, continue on to stage 2. The probability of stopping for futility is 0.599 when H_0 is true and 0.107 when *Ha* is true.
- *Stage 2:* Stop and accept the null hypothesis if the response rate is less than or equal to 3/29. Otherwise, stop and reject the null hypothesis.

Note: There are more than three designs generated by ExpDesign (see the spreadsheet in Figure 7.1). All meet the desired α and power values. You can sort the designs by any of the headers; just click the header and click [Sort].

Alternatively, we can generate three-stage designs. To do that we specify the input as follows: three-stage design, proportion for $H_0 = 0.05$, proportion for $H_a = 0.20$, $\alpha = 0.05$, power = 0.8, and 2 and 8 for the utility weights (see Figure 7.2). Click [Compute] to generate the two-stage designs and click 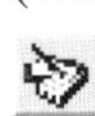 on the toolbar to review the following report.

Three-Stage Design Testing (One-Sided) for a Single Proportion Featuring Early Stopping for Futility Common settings for the three designs (MinMaxSize, MinExpSize, and MaxUtility) are: level of significance $\alpha = 0.05$, power = 0.8, proportion for the null hypothesis $P_0 = 0.05$, and proportion for the alternative hypothesis $P_a = 0.2$.

MinMaxSize Three-Stage Design The MinMaxSize design minimizes the maximum size required. The design characteristics are summarized as follows: The cumulative sample size at stage 1 = 14, the cumulative sample size at stage 2 = 20, the cumulative sample size at stage 3 = 27, the actual type I error rate $\alpha = 0.041$, the actual power = 0.801, and the utility index = 1.5.

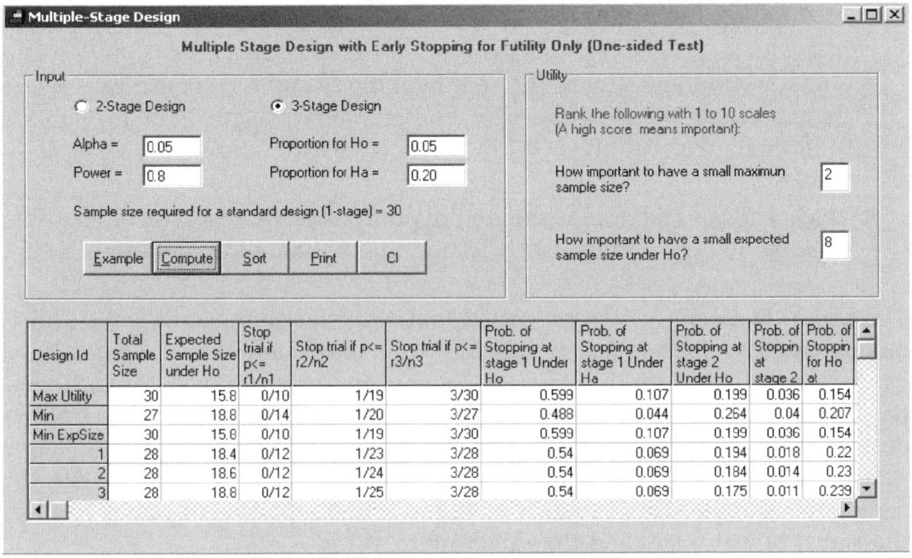

Design Id	Total Sample Size	Expected Sample Size under Ho	Stop trial if p<= r1/n1	Stop trial if p<= r2/n2	Stop trial if p<= r3/n3	Prob. of Stopping at stage 1 Under Ho	Prob. of Stopping at stage 1 Under Ha	Prob. of Stopping at stage 2 Under Ho	Prob. of Stoppin at stage 2	Prob. of Stoppin for Ho at
Max Utility	30	15.8	0/10	1/19	3/30	0.599	0.107	0.199	0.036	0.154
Min	27	18.8	0/14	1/20	3/27	0.488	0.044	0.264	0.04	0.207
Min ExpSize	30	15.8	0/10	1/19	3/30	0.599	0.107	0.199	0.036	0.154
1	28	18.4	0/12	1/23	3/28	0.54	0.069	0.194	0.018	0.22
2	28	18.6	0/12	1/24	3/28	0.54	0.069	0.184	0.014	0.23
3	28	18.8	0/12	1/25	3/28	0.54	0.069	0.175	0.011	0.239

Figure 7.2 Example of three-stage design.

The stopping rules are as follows:

- *Stage 1:* Stop and accept the null hypothesis if the response rate is less than or equal to 0/14. Otherwise, continue on to stage 2. The probability of stopping for futility is 0.488 when H_0 is true and 0.044 when H_a is true.
- *Stage 2:* Stop and accept the null hypothesis if the response rate is less than or equal to 1/20. Otherwise, continue on to stage 3. The probability of stopping for futility is 0.264 when H_0 is true and 0.04 when H_a is true.
- *Stage 3:* Stop and accept the null hypothesis if the response is less than or equal to 3/27. Otherwise, stop and reject the null hypothesis.

MinExpSize Three-Stage Design The MinExpSize (optimal) design minimizes the sample size expected. The design characteristics are summarized as follows: The cumulative sample size at stage 1 = 10, the cumulative sample size at stage 2 = 19, the cumulative sample size at stage 3 = 30, the actual type I error rate α = 0.048, the actual power = 0.8, and the utility index = 1.6.

The stopping rules are as follows:

- *Stage 1:* Stop and accept the null hypothesis if the response rate is less than or equal to 0/14. Otherwise, continue on to stage 2. The probability of stopping for futility is 0.599 when H_0 is true and 0.107 when H_a is true.

- *Stage 2:* Stop and accept the null hypothesis if the response rate is less than or equal to 1/19. Otherwise, continue on to stage 3. The probability of stopping for futility is 0.199 when H_0 is true and 0.036 when H_a is true.
- *Stage 3:* Stop and accept the null hypothesis if the response is less than or equal to 3/30. Otherwise, stop and reject the null hypothesis.

MaxUtility Three-Stage Design The MaxUtility design maximizes the utility, defined as (0.8 × expected sample size + 0.2 × maximum sample size) divided by the sample size from the classical single-stage design. Hence, the utility for the classical single-stage design is 1 and a higher utility indicates a better design. The design characteristics are summarized as follows: The cumulative sample size at stage 1 = 10, the cumulative sample size at stage 2 = 19, the cumulative sample size at stage 3 = 30, the actual type I error rate $\alpha = 0.048$, the actual power = 0.8, and the utility index = 1.6.

The stopping rules are as follows:

- *Stage 1:* Stop and accept the null hypothesis if the response rate is less than or equal to 0/14. Otherwise, continue on to stage 2. The probability of stopping for futility is 0.599 when H_0 is true and 0.107 when H_a is true.
- *Stage 2:* Stop and accept the null hypothesis if the response rate is less than or equal to 1/19. Otherwise, continue on to stage 3. The probability of stopping for futility is 0.199 when H_0 is true and 0.036 when H_a is true.
- *Stage 3:* Stop and accept the null hypothesis if the response is less than or equal to 3/30. Otherwise, stop and reject the null hypothesis.

Final Design We now discuss how to select the final design. Since the utility is specified, we should use the maximum utility design. Comparing three- and two-stage design, three-stage design provides a larger utility value (1.6) than that of two-stage design (1.5). However, three-stage design requires a maximum of 30 patients (15.8 patients expected), and two-stage design requires a maximum of 29 patients (17.6 expected). The main concern is that the three-stage design is more complicated and requires more effort to implement, partially because when the interim analysis is done, all patients would have been enrolled in the trial. Therefore, the two-stage maximum utility design is chosen for the trial. The stopping rules are specified as follows: At stage 1, stop the trial and accept the null hypothesis if the response rate is less than or equal to 0/13; otherwise, continue on to stage 2. At stage 2, accept the null hypothesis if the response rate is less than or equal to 3/29; otherwise, reject the null hypothesis.

7.2 DOSE-ESCALATION TRIAL DESIGN

7.2.1 Introduction

Objectives of a Phase I Clinical Trial The goal of a phase I trial is to define and characterize the new treatment in humans to set the basis for later investigations of efficacy and superiority. Therefore, the safety and feasibility of the treatment are at the center of interest. A positive risk–benefit judgment should be expected such that the possible harm of the treatment is outweighed by the possible gain in cure, suppression of the disease and its symptoms, and an improved quality of life and survival.

For example, in a cancer study, beginning treatment at a low dose is very likely to be safe (starting dose). Small cohorts of patients are treated at progressively higher doses (dose escalation) until drug-related toxicity reaches a predetermined level [dose-limiting toxicity (DLT)]. The objective is to determine the maximum tolerated dose (MTD) of a drug for a specified mode of administration and to characterize the DLT. The goals in phase I trials can be stated as follows (Crowley, 2001):

1. Establishment of an MTD
2. Determination of the toxicity profile
3. Characterization of the DLT
4. Identification of antitumor activity
5. Investigation of basic clinical pharmacology
6. Recommendation of a dose for phase II studies

Population for Treatment The phase I trial should define a standardized treatment schedule to be applied safely to humans and worth being investigated further for efficacy. For non-life-threatening diseases, phase I trials are usually conducted on human volunteers, at least as long as the expected toxicity is mild and can be controlled without harm. In life-threatening diseases such as cancer and AIDS, phase I studies are conducted with patients because of the aggressiveness and possible harmfulness of cyrostatic treatments, because of possible systemic treatment effects, and the high interest in the new drug's efficacy in those patients directly.

Dose-Limited Toxicity and Maximum Tolerated Dose Drug toxicity is considered to be tolerable if the toxicity is acceptable, manageable, and reversible. Drug safety has now been standardized for oncological studies by establishment of the common toxicity criteria (CTC) by the U.S. National Cancer Institute (NCI). This is a large list of adverse events (AEs) subdivided into organ and symptom categories that can be related to anticancer treatment. Each AE has been categorized into five classes:

1. CTC grade 0: no AE, or normal
2. CTC grade 1: mild (elevated/reduced)
3. CTC grade 2: moderate
4. CTC grade 3: serious/severe
5. CTC grade 4: very serious or life threatening

A toxicity of grade 3 or 4 is usually considered dose limiting. In other words, any AE of grade 3 or higher related to treatment is considered a DLT. Often, a judgment of "possible" or higher is considered as drug-related toxicity and called an *adverse drug reaction* (ADR). The *maximum tolerated dose* (MTD) is defined as a dose level at which DLTs occur at least with a certain frequency. For example, at least one out of three patients has one grade 3 or higher CTC, or two of three patients have grade 2 or higher CTC.

Dose–Toxicity Modeling Most designs for dose finding in phase I trials assume a monotone dose–toxicity relationship and a monotone dose–response (tumor response) relationship (Figure 7.3). Ideally, the relationship can be described as "biologically inactive dose < biologically active dose < highly toxic dose." The choice of an appropriate dose–toxicity model is important not only for the planning, but also for the analysis of phase I data. Most applications use an extended logit model and apply the logistic regression because of its flexibility, the ease of accounting for patient covariates (e.g., pretreatment. disease staging. performance), and the availability of computing software. A

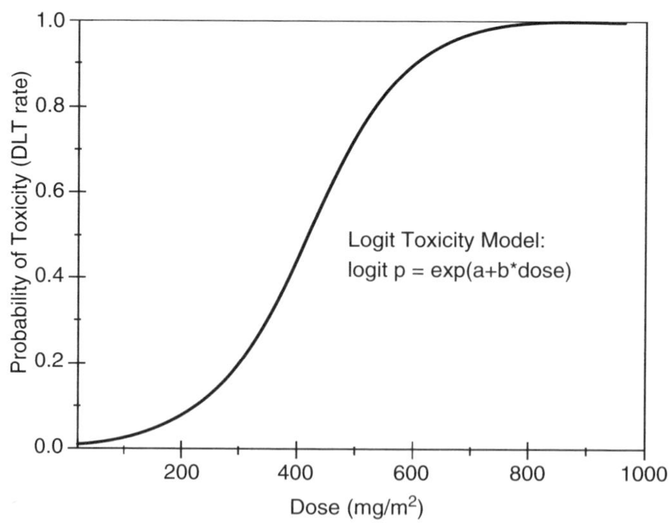

Figure 7.3 Logistic toxicity model.

general class of toxicity models is a two-parameter family in which the toxicity rate or probability of toxicity is given by

$$\psi(x, a) = F(a_0 + a_1 h(x)), \tag{7.1}$$

where x is the dose and a_0 and a_1 are considered as constants to be determined in a frequentist approach. In Bayesian approaches, these parameters have distributions that are updated constantly based on cumulative information. Various functions $F(\cdot)$ and $h(x)$ can be chosen to fit particular needs. In frequentist approaches, the parameters a_0 and a_1 can be determined based on data from the trial. Once the constants are determined and the toxicity rate θ at the MTD is defined, the MTD can easily be solved:

$$\text{MTD} = \frac{1}{a_1}[F^{-1}(\theta) - a_0]. \tag{7.2}$$

The commonly used functions for F are probit(x) or inverse Gaussian, logit(x): $1/[1 - \exp(x)]$, and hyperbolic tangent(x): $[(\tanh x + 1)/2>)]^{-a}$. The choice of θ depends on the nature of the DLT and the type of target tumor. For an aggressive tumor and a transient and non-life-threatening DLT, θ could be as high as 0.5. For persistent DLT and less aggressive tumors, it could be as low as 0.1 to 0.25. A commonly used value ranges from 0 to 1/3 (= 0.33).

ExpDesign allows users to select three different toxicity models (dose–response models):

$$\text{Linear model: } p = a + bx \tag{7.3}$$

$$\text{Logistic model: } p = \frac{1}{1 + b\exp(-ax)} \tag{7.4}$$

$$\text{Log-logit model: } p = \frac{1}{1 + b\exp(-a\ln x)}, \tag{7.5}$$

where x is the actual dose or a function of dose [such as dose levels (integers)]; p is the toxicity rate, probability of toxicity, or DLT; and a and b are constants determined by the starting dose level, the DLT rate at that level, the estimated MTD, and the DLT rate at the MTD. The DLT rate at the MTD commonly used for oncology trials varies from 20 to 50%, depending on the disease states.

Dose-Level Selection An inadequate dose range could totally ruin a clinical trial, because it does not cover the biologically active dose or requires too many dose escalations to reach the target dose level. The initial dose given to the first patients in a phase I study should be low enough to avoid severe toxicity but high enough for a chance of activity and potential efficacy in humans. Extrapolation from preclinical animal data focused on the lethal dose 10%

(LD_{10}) of the mouse (dose with 10% drug-induced deaths) converted into equivalents in units of mg/m^2 of body surface area. The standard starting dose became 1/10 of the minimal effective dose level for 10% deaths ($MELD_{10}$) of the mouse after verification that no lethal and no life-threatening effects were seen in another species (e.g., rats, dogs). Earlier recommendations had used higher portions of the $MELD_{10}$ (mouse) or other characteristic doses, as, for example, the lowest dose with toxicity (toxic dose low) in mammals (Crowley, 2001).

The highest dose level should be selected that covers the biologically active dose but remains lower than a toxic dose. A pharmacokinetically guided dose escalation (PGDE) was proposed based on the equivalence of drug blood levels in mice and humans and on the pharmacodynamic hypothesis that equal toxicity is caused by equal drug plasma levels. It postulates that the DLT is determined by plasma drug concentrations and that AUC is a measure that holds across species. The AUC calculated at the MTD for humans was found to be fairly equal to the AUC for mice if calculated at the LD_{10} (in mg/rn^2 equivalents, $MELD_{10}$).

Subsequent dose levels can be determined by using the additive set,

$$x_i = x_{i-1} + \Delta x \qquad i = 1, 2, \ldots, \tag{7.6}$$

or the multiplicative set,

$$x_i = f_{i-1} x_{i-1} \qquad i = 0, 1, \ldots, \tag{7.7}$$

where f_i is the dose-escalation factor. Popular dose-escalation factors are the Fibonacci number (2, 1.5, 1.67, 1.60, 1.63, 1.62, 1.62, . . .) and modified Fibonacci schemes (2, 1.65, 1.52, 1.40, 1.33, 1.33, . . .).

ExpDesign has five different dose interval sequences for users to choose from: Fibonacci and modified Fibonacci sequence, constant-dose-increment sequence, constant-multiple-factor sequence, and a customized sequence that allow users to specify any sequence they like.

Dose-Escalation Schemes After dosage levels are determined, the next step in designing a phase I trial consists of the establishment of a rule by which the doses are assigned to patients. Proceeding from a starting dose, the sequence of dosing has to be fixed in advance in a *dose-escalation rule*. The most common dose-escalation rules are the *traditional escalation rules* (TERs), also known as *3 + 3 rules*, because it became common practice to enter three patients at a new dose level and when any toxicity was observed, to enter a total of six patients at that dose level before deciding to stop at that level or to increase the dose. Two versions of the 3 + 3 rule are TER and strict TER (STER). TER does not allow you to deescalate the dose, but STER does when two of three patients had the DLT rate (Figure 7.4). The stochastic approximation method (SA) has no fixed dose level. Instead, the level is determined

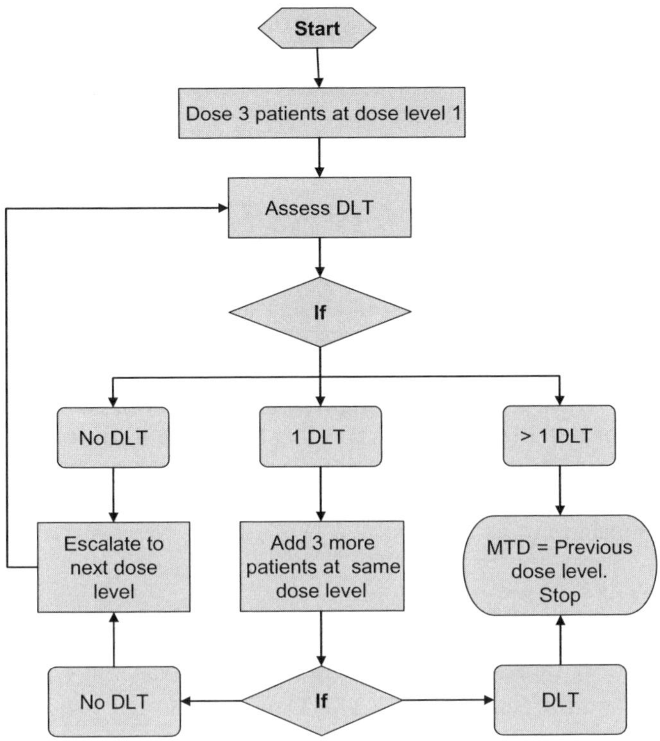

Figure 7.4 3 + 3 Traditional dose-escalation algorithm.

not only by the toxicity from the last dose level but also the total cumulative toxicity. The continual reassessment method (CRM), a Bayesian approach, can be generalized for combination therapies where dose escalation takes place in several dimensions.

The 3 + 3 TER and STER can be generalized to $A + B$ TER and STER. To introduce the $A + B$ escalation rule, let A, B, C, D, and E be integers. The notation A/B indicates that there are A toxicity incidences out of B subjects, and $>A/B$ means that there are more than A toxicity incidences out of B subjects.

$A + B$ Escalation Without Dose Deescalation General $A + B$ designs without dose deescalation can be described as follows. Suppose that there are A patients at dose level i. If fewer than C/A patients have DLTs, the dose is escalated to the next dose level, $i + 1$. If more than D/A (where $D \geq C$) patients have DLTs, the previous dose (or current dose level) will be considered the MTD. If no fewer than C/A but no more than D/A patients have DLTs, B more patients are treated at this dose level, i. If no more than E (where $E \geq$ D) of the total of $A + B$ patients experience DLTs, the dose is escalated. If more than E of the total of $A + B$ patients have DLT, the previous dose,

$i - 1$, will be considered the MTD. It can be seen that the traditional 3 + 3 design without dose deescalation is a special case of the general $A + B$ design with $A = B = 3$ and $C = D = E = 1$. Closed forms of operating characteristics are given by Lin and Shih (2001).

The escalation probability from one dose level to the next is given by

$$\Pr(\text{escalation}) = (1-p)^3 + 3p(1-p)^5, \tag{7.8}$$

where p is the DLT rate at the current dosage level. The 3 + 3 TER, STER, $A + B$ TER, two-stage accelerated dose escalation, and CRM have been implemented in ExpDesign Studio (see Figure 7.6).

Evaluation of Dose-Escalation Algorithms All dose-escalation schemes have advantages and disadvantages. For example, the traditional 3 + 3 escalation is easy to apply, but the MTD estimation is usually biased, especially when there are many dose levels. The criteria for evaluation of an escalation scheme used in ExpDesign are as follows:

- Number of DLTs
- Number of patients
- Number of patients dosed above MTD
- Accuracy and precision of the MTD prediction

ExpDesign allows users to do simulations under various scenarios and provides evaluations based on the foregoing criteria. For details on oncology dose-escalation trials, see the *Handbook of Statistics in Clinical Oncology* (Crowley, 2001).

7.2.2 Bayesian Continual Reassessment Method

The continual reassessment method (CRM) is a model approach in which the parameters in the model for the response are updated continually based on the response data observed. The method used to update the parameters can be either the frequentist or Bayesian approach. CRM was initially proposed by O'Quigley (O'Quigley et al., 1990; O'Quigley and Shen, 1996; Babb and Rogatko, 2004) for oncology dose-escalation trials, but it can be extended to other types of trials (M. Chang and Chow, 2006). In CRM the dose–response relationship is reassessed continually based on accumulative data collected from the trial. The next patient who enters the trial is then assigned to the currently estimated MTD or lower dose level, for safety consideration's. The CRM escalation rules are presented in Figure 7.5 and described below.

First, dose (assume that $k = 1$) the patient at the first dose level; the DLT is assessed for the patient and the MTD is predicted using the Bayesian CRM. If the value closest to the predicted MTD (PMTD) is higher than the current

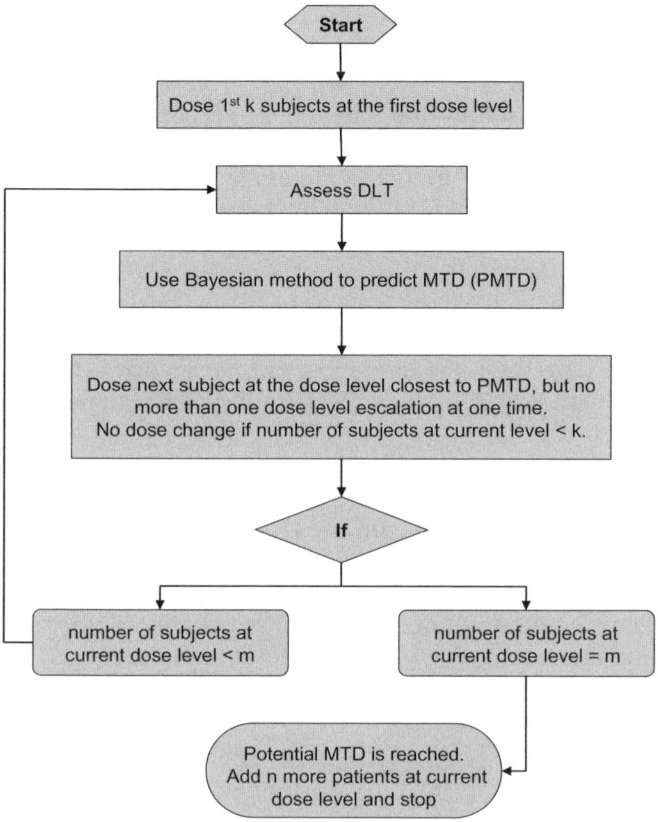

Figure 7.5 CRM escalation rules.

dose level, escalate the next scheduled level. If the closest dose level is lower than the current level, deescalate to that level. This process continues until there are m (a value of 4 to 8 seems a good choice for m). CRM is more efficient than TER with respect to finding the MTD. CRM can also be used for other dose-finding trials.

7.2.3 How to Design a Dose-Escalation Trial Using ExpDesign

Suppose that we design a phase I oncology trial whose primary objective it is to determine the MTD for new test drug ABC. Based on the animal studies, it is estimated that the toxicity (the DLT rate) is 1% for the starting dose 25 mg/m^2 (1/10 of the lethal dose). The DLT rate at MTD is defined as 0.25 and the MTD is estimated to be 150 mg/m^2.

Based on the information provided above, we can use ExpDesign to do the simulations and select an optimal design. As an illustration, we first do a one-stage trial simulation with TER and two-stage design simulation with single-patient escalation at the first stage and 3 + 3 TER at the second stage. A logistic toxicity model is chosen for the simulations.

Single-Stage Design Simulation In the **ExpDesign Studio** window, click Dose-Escalation; select the option **Single-Stage Traditional Escalation** in the window and specify the following parameters for the one-stage design with ExpDesign: the number of stages = 1, the number of simulations = 5000, the starting dose = 25, the DLT rate at the starting dose = 0.01, the MTD = 150, the DLT rate at MTD = 0.25, the number of dose levels = 7, and the maximum deescalations allowed = 0. Select the customized sequence (2, 1.67, 1.33, 1.33, 1.33, 1.33, 1.33, 1.33, 1.33), the logit model in the **Toxicity (Response) Model** panel, and the standard 3 + 3 rule (STER) in the **Escalation Scheme** panel (Figure 7.6). Clicking Compute to run the simulation. When it is finished, click  on the toolbar to bring up the simulation results described below.

Single-Stage Dose-Escalation Design: Computer Simulation by ExpDesign See Table 7.1. The simulation parameter settings are: the number of simulations = 5000, the number of stages = 1, the number of dose levels = 7, the maximum deescalations allowed = 0, the true maximum tolerated dose (MTD) = 150, the DLT rate at MTD = 0.25, the starting dose = 25, and the DLT rate at the starting dose = 0.01. The dose interval sequence is chosen to be the customized

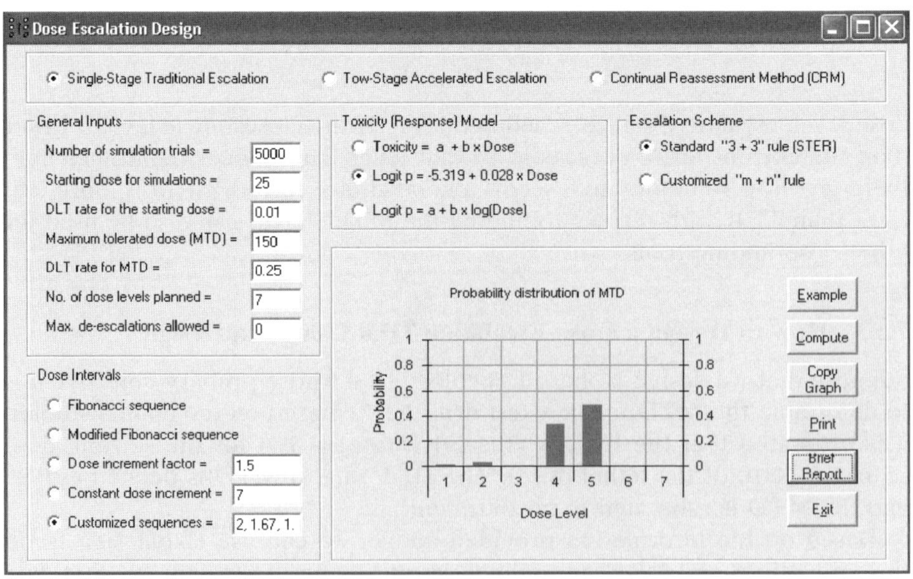

Figure 7.6 Simulations of single-stage dose-escalation design.

TABLE 7.1

	Dose Level						
	1	2	3	4	5	6	7
Dose	25	50	83.5	111.1	147.7	196.4	261.3
Toxicity rate	0.01	0.02	0.049	0.1	0.238	0.552	0.884
Mean no. patients	3.1	3.2	3.4	3.6	3.7	2.2	0.2
Mean no. DLTs	0.03	0.06	0.16	0.37	0.87	1.2	0.2
Percent MTDs	0.006	0.024	0.095	0.323	0.48	0.073	0

dose increment sequence (increment factors = 2, 1.67, 1.33, 1.33, 1.33, 1.33, 1.33, 1.33, 1.33); the 3 + 3 strict traditional rule is used; and the true toxicity rates are defined by logit $p = -5.319 + 0.028 \times \text{dose}$.

Simulation results are given as follows: the mean MTD = 130.4477, the standard deviation of the MTDs predicted = 31.1, the mean number of patients treated above the true MTD = 2.434, the mean number of patients treated under the true MTD = 16.959, the mean number of overshoots in a trial = 0, the mean number of undershoots in a trial = 0.001, the number of patients expected = 19.393, and the number of DLT patients expected = 2.901.

Note: If overshooting, MTD is set conservatively to the highest planned dose. If undershooting, the lowest scheduled dose is chosen as MTD. An *overshoot* is defined as an attempt to escalate to a dose level higher than the highest level planned. An *undershoot* is defined as an attempt to deescalate to a dose level lower than the starting dose level. The dispersion of predicted MTDs is measured by the average distance between the true and predicted MTDs. The percent MTDs for a dose level k is the probability of dose level k being the MTD based on simulations.

Two-Stage Design Simulation In the **Dose-Escalation** window, select the two-stage design option. The rest of the parameter specifications are the same as those for single-stage dose escalation (Figure 7.7). Click 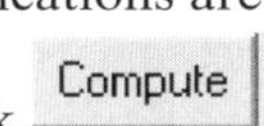

and click 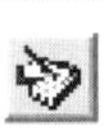 after the simulation is finished. The results described below will be displayed.

Two-Stage Dose-Escalation Design—Computer Simulation by ExpDesign See Table 7.2. The simulation parameter settings are: the number of simulations = 5000, the number of stages = 2, the number of dose levels = 7, the maximum deescalations allowed = 0, the true MTD = 150, the DLT rate at MTD = 0.25, the starting dose = 25, and the DLT rate at the starting dose = 0.01. The dose interval sequence is specified as the customized dose-increment sequence (increment factors = 2, 1.67, 1.33, 1.33, 1.33, 1.33, 1.33, 1.33, 1.33). The 3 + 3

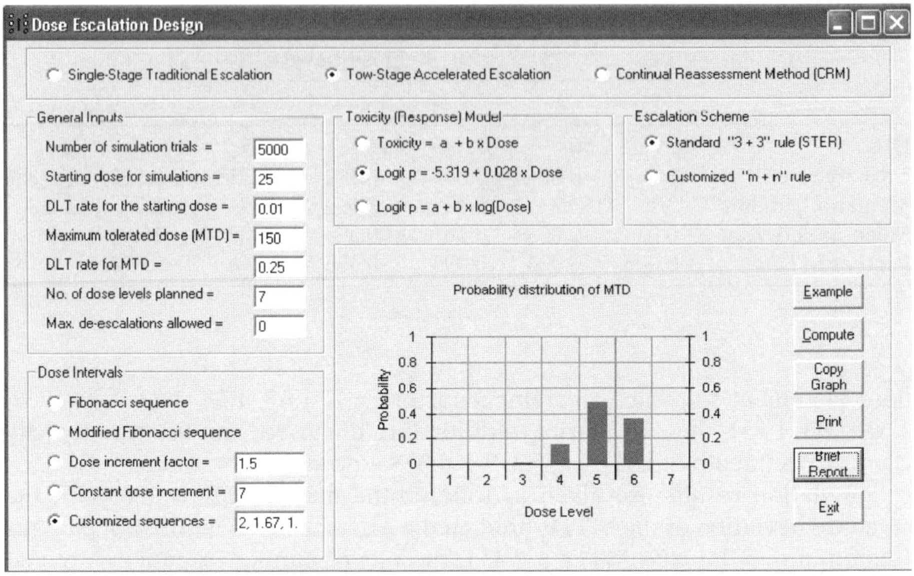

Figure 7.7 Simulations of two-stage dose escalation design.

TABLE 7.2

	Dose Level						
	1	2	3	4	5	6	7
Dose	25	50	83.5	111.1	147.7	196.4	261.3
Toxicity rate	0.01	0.02	0.049	0.1	0.238	0.552	0.884
Mean no. patients	1	1	1.1	1.3	2	2.8	2.3
Mean no. DLTs	0	0	0.01	0.04	0.29	1.23	1.8
Percent MTDs:	0	0.002	0.014	0.149	0.479	0.355	0

strict traditional rule is used. The true toxicity rates are defined by logit $p = -5.319 + 0.028 \times \text{dose}$.

Simulation results are given as follows: the mean MTD = 158.5057, the standard deviation of the MTDs predicted = 31.4, the mean number of patients treated above the true MTD = 6.071, the mean number of patients treated under the true MTD = 6.457, the mean number of overshoots in a trial = 0, the mean number of undershoots in a trial = 0, the number of patients expected = 11.652, the number of DLT patients expected = 5.197, the number of patients expected to be treated at stage 1 is 5.641, and the number of patients expected to be treated at stage 2 is 6.887.

CRM Design Simulation In the **Dose-Escalation** window, select **Continual Reassessment Method (CRM)** and specify the parameters as follows: the

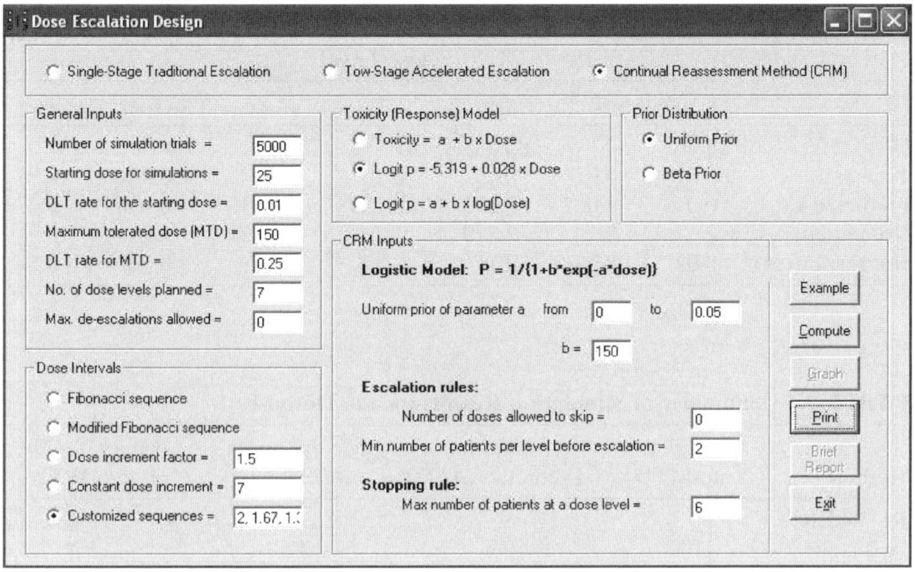

Figure 7.8 Dose–escalation design with CRM.

number of simulations = 5000, the starting dose = 25, the DLT rate at the starting dose = 0.01, the MTD = 150, the DLT rate at the MTD = 0.25, and the number of dose levels = 7. Select the customized dose sequence and logist model in the **Toxicity (Response) Model** panel. Select CRM for the simulation, and enter 0 and 0.05 as the prior's for parameter a, and set b = 150 in the logistic model. Enter 0 for the number of dose levels allowed for a skip, 2 for the minimum number of patients required at a dose level before escalation, and 6 for the maximum number of patients at a dose level for the stopping rule (Figure 7.8). Click 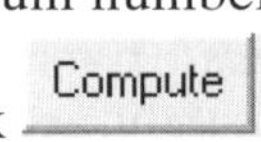

and click 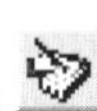 after the simulation is finished. The results described below will be displayed.

Simulation Results Using the Continual Reassessment Method See Table 7.3. The input parameters are specified as follows. The true MTD is 150 with a rate of 0.25. The stopping rule specified comes into play if the maximum number of patients at a dose level reaches 6. The dose-escalation rules are: (1) require a minimum of two patients treated at the current level before escalating to the next dose level; and (2) the number of dose levels allowed to be skipped = 0.

Simulation results are shown as follows: the mean MTD = 140.8864, the standard deviation of the MTD = 31.2, the mean MTD level = 4.7496, the average total number of patients = 15.47, and the expected number of responses = 2.48. The model used for the dose–response relationship is: response rate =

TABLE 7.3

	Dose Level						
	1	2	3	4	5	6	7
Dose	25	50	83.5	111	148	196	261
True rate	0.01	0.02	0.05	0.10	0.24	0.55	0.88
Predicted rate	0.013	0.027	0.073	0.150	0.310	0.546	0.772
No. patients	2	2	2.279	3.7092	3.72	1.55	0.21
No. responses	0.02	0.04	0.11	0.37	0.89	0.86	0.19

TABLE 7.4 Summary of Simulation Results for the Designs

Method	Assumed True MTD	Mean Predicted MTD	Mean Number of Patients	Mean Number of DLTs
3 + 3 TER	100	86.7	14.9	2.8
Two-stage		106	10.9	5.4
CRM		99.2	13.4	2.8
3+3 TER	150	125	19.4	2.9
Two-stage		159	11.6	5.2
CRM		141	15.5	2.5
3+3 TER	200	169	22.4	2.8
Two-stage		192	11.5	4.4
CRM		186	16.8	2.2

$1/[1 + 150 \exp(-a \text{ dose})]$, where the prior for parameter a is a uniform prior in (0, 0.05).

Comparison of Escalation Methods Evaluations of the escalation designs are based on the following criteria: safety, accuracy, and efficiency. Simulation results for all three methods for three different MTD scenarios are summarized in Table 7.4.

In this example, we can see if the true MTD is 150 mg/m^2. The TER underestimates the MTD (125 mg/m^2), and the two-stage accelerated escalation overestimates the MTD (159 mg/m^2). CRM also slightly underpredicts the MTD (141 mg/m^2). The average number of patients required is 19.4, 11.6, and 15.5 for TER, two-stage, and CRM, respectively. From a safety perspective, the average number of DLTs is 2.9, 5.2, and 2.5 per trial for TER, two-stage, and CRM, respectively. Further comparisons are summarized in Table 7.4. From the simulation results, CRM seams preferable.

Customization of Escalation Rules As mentioned earlier, STER has been implemented in ExpDesign, which allows you to set a limit for the maximum

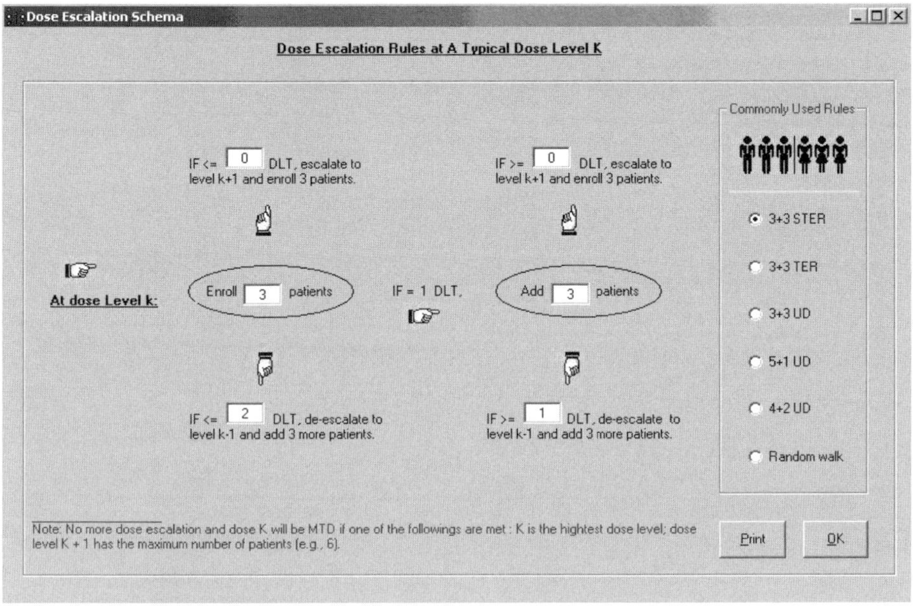

Figure 7.9 Customized dose-escalation design window.

dose levels allowed to deescalate. For example, if **Max. de-escalations allowed** is set to 1, deescalation is allowed from level 4 to level 3 and again from level 5 to level 4, but is not allowed from level 5 to level 4 and continues for deescalation to level 3. ExpDesign also allows you to design a general $m + n$. To customize the dose escalations, simply choose the option **Customized "m+n" rule** in the Escalation Scheme panel. The **Dose-Escalation Scheme** window will appear (Figure 7.9). You can specify the escalation by typing in values in the textboxes or by selecting the commonly used escalation rules in the panel and clicking 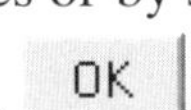. The rest is the same as for a 3 + 3 TER design.

Remark on CRM ExpDesign allows uniform and beta prior selection. The prior, the CRM model (different values of b_0), and dose intervals for the escalation all affect the outcome. These parameters should be adjusted carefully so as to produce reasonable outcomes for a wide range of scenarios (e.g., different assumed MTDs).

7.3 DOSE-ESCALATION TRIAL MONITORING USING CRM

Unlike the traditional escalation design, CRM requires dynamic randomization (i.e., the next patient assignment is based on the newly predicted MTD). Figure 7.3 illustrates the trial monitoring process.

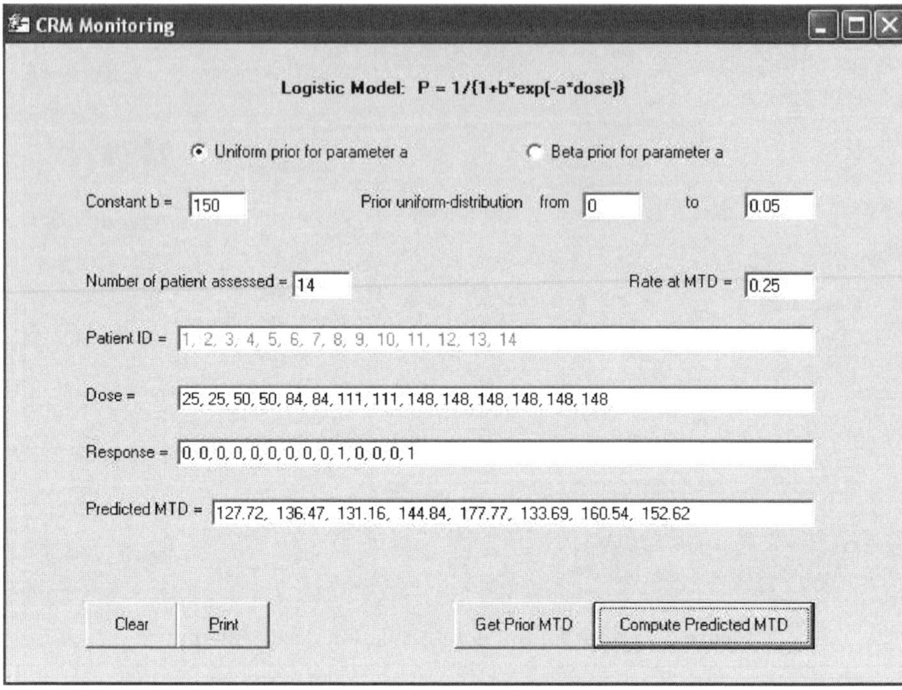

Figure 7.10 Example of CRM monitoring.

We now discuss the steps for running and monitoring a CRM trial (see the example in Section 7.2.3) using ExpDesign. The DLT observed is hypothetical. The model used is given by

$$p = \frac{1}{1 + 150e^{-ax}} \tag{7.9}$$

where the prior for parameter a is uniform in (0, 0.05).

1. Click [Dose-Escalation Trial Monitoring] (Figure 7.10).
2. Enter "150" for b, "0, 0.05" for the prior, and "0.25" for the DLT rate for the MTD.
3. Click [Get Prior MTD] to get the prior MTD (128 mg/m^2).
4. Enter "2" for the number of patients assessed (there is a minimum of two patients for each level), "25, 25" for the dose level for the two patients, and "0, 0" for their DLT (i.e., there is no DLT for either of them).

TABLE 7.5 Example of CRM Monitoring

	Patient													
	1	2	3	4	5	6	7	8	9	10	11	12	13	14
PMTD	128	128	136	136	131	131	145	145	178	178	134	134	161	161
Dose	25	25	50	50	84	84	111	111	148	148	148	148	148	148
DLT	0	0	0	0	0	0	0	0	0	1	0	0	0	1

5. Click 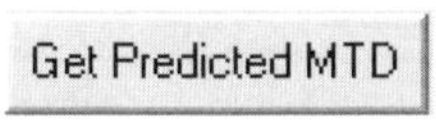

to get the MTD predicted, 136 mg/m^2.
6. The dose 111 mg/m^2 is closest to 137 mg/m^2, but one level of escalation is allowed; hence, the next two patients should be dosed with 50 mg/m^2.
7. Enter "4" for the number of patients assessed. Enter (Add) "50, 50" to the textbox for the dosage. Suppose that they are nonresponders, so add "0, 0" to the textbox for the response.
8. Click 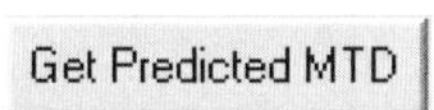

to get the MTD predicted, 131 mg/m^2. Therefore, the next two patients should be dosed at 84 mg/m^2.

This process continues until there are six patients at level. Table 7.5 summarizes the entire process.

The final MTD predicted is 153 mg/m^2 (not in Table 7.5), which can be used to design the next phase of the clinical trial. You may choose to add more patients to get a more precise estimation of the confidence interval for the DLT rate at the potential MTD.

7.4 MATHEMATICAL NOTES ON MULTISTAGE DESIGN

7.4.1 Decision Tree for a Multistage Trial

For a multistage trial regarding the hypotheses $H_0 : \theta = \theta_0$ versus $H_a : \theta = \theta_a$, we can draw a diagram known as a *decision tree* (Figure 7.11). The probabilities of accepting and rejecting the null hypothesis under θ at stage k can be expressed, respectively, as

$$P_{\text{accept } H_0}(\theta) = \prod_{j=1}^{k-1} P_{cj} P_{ak} \quad \text{and} \quad P_{\text{reject } H_0}(\theta) = \prod_{j=1}^{k-1} P_{cj} P_{rk} \qquad k = 1, 2, \ldots, K \tag{7.10}$$

The type I and II errors at stage k are written, respectively, as

$$\beta_k = P_{\text{accept } H_0}(\theta_a) \quad \text{and} \quad \alpha_k = P_{\text{reject } H_0}(\theta_0) \qquad k = 1, 2, \ldots, K \tag{7.11}$$

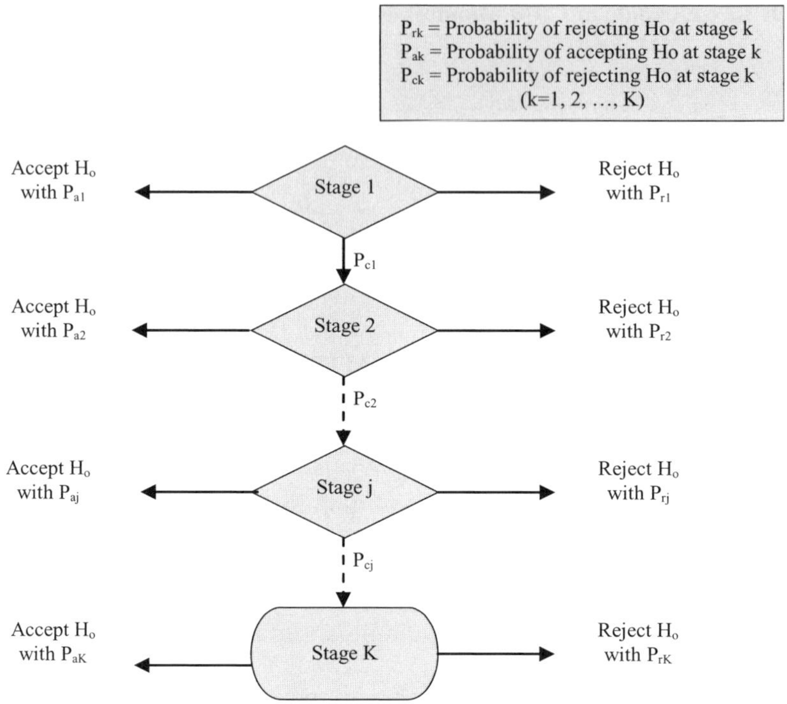

Figure 7.11 Decision tree for a multistage trial.

Sum up these to obtain the overall type I and II error rates, $\alpha = \sum_{k=1}^{K} \alpha_k$ and $\beta = \sum_{k=1}^{K} \beta_k$.

7.4.2 Two-Stage Design

The most commonly used two-stage design in phase II cancer trials is probably Simon's optimal two-stage design (Simon, 1989). The concept of Simon's optimal two-stage design is to permit early stopping when a moderately long sequence of initial failures occurs. Thus, under a two-stage trial design, the hypotheses of interest are

$$H_0: p \le p_0 \text{ versus } H_a: p > p_1, \tag{7.12}$$

where p_0 is the undesirable response rate and p_1 is the desirable response rate ($p_1 > p_0$). If the response rate of a test treatment is at an undesirable level, one may reject it as an ineffective treatment with high probability, and if its response rate is at a desirable level, one may not, with high probability, reject it as a promising compound. Note that under the hypotheses above, the usual type I error is a false positive in accepting an ineffective drug, and the type II error is a false negative in rejecting a promising compound.

Let n_1 and n_2 be the number of subjects in the first and second stages, respectively. Under a two-stage design, n_1 patients are treated in the first stage. If there are fewer than $r_1 + 1$ responses, the trial is stopped. Otherwise, additional n_2 patients are recruited and tested at the second stage. A decision regarding whether the test treatment is promising is then made based on the response rate of the $n = n_1 + n_2$ subjects. Note that the rejection of H_0 (or H_a) means that further study of the test treatment should (or should not) be carried out. Simon (1989) proposed selecting the optimal two-stage design that achieves the minimum expected sample size under the null hypothesis. Let n_{exp} and p_{et} be the expected sample size and the probability of early termination after the first stage. Thus, we have

$$n_{\text{exp}} = n_1 + (1 - p_{\text{et}})n_2. \tag{7.13}$$

At the end of the first stage, we would terminate the trial early and reject the null hypothesis if r_1 or fewer responses were observed. As a result, p_{et} is given by

$$p_{\text{et}} = B_c(r_1; n_1, p), \tag{7.14}$$

where $B(r_1; n_1, p)$ denotes the cumulative binomial distribution that $x \le r_1$. Thus, we reject the test treatment at the end of the second stage if r or fewer responses are observed. The probability of rejecting the test treatment with success probability p is then given by

$$B(r_1; n_1, p) + \sum_{x=r_1+1}^{\min(n_1, r)} b(x; n_1, p)B(r - x; n_2, p), \tag{7.15}$$

where $b(x; n_1, p)$ denotes the binomial probability mass function. For specific values of p_0, p_1, α, and β, Simon's optimal two-stage design can be obtained as the two-stage design that satisfies the error constraints and minimizes the sample size expected when the response rate is p_0.

7.4.3 Three-Stage Design

The decision rules for three-stage design are as follows:

- *Stage 1:* If $x_1 \le r_1$, accept H_0; otherwise, continue to stage 2.
- *Stage 2:* If $x_1 + x_2 \le r_2$, accept H_0; otherwise, continue to stage 3.
- *Stage 3:* If $x_1 + x_2 + x_3 \le r_3$, accept H_0, otherwise, reject H_0.

To determine n_1, r_1, n_2, r_2, n_3, and r_3 for a given α and β, it is convenient to define

$$\begin{aligned}\beta_1(p) &= \Pr(x_1 \le r_1 \mid p),\\ \beta_2(p) &= \Pr(x_1 > r_1 \cap x_1 + x_2 \le r_2 \mid p),\\ \beta_2(p) &= \Pr(x_1 > r_1 \cap x_1 + x_2 > r_2 \cap x_1 + x_2 + x_3 \le r_3 \mid p).\end{aligned} \tag{7.16}$$

Denoting binomial p.m.f. and c.d.f. by $b(x; n, p)$ and $B(x; n, p)$, respectively, we have

$$\begin{aligned}b(x; n, p) &= \binom{n}{x} p^x (1-p)^{n-x},\\ \beta_1(p) &= B(r; n_1, p),\\ \beta_2(p) &= \sum_{x_1 = r_1 + 1}^{\min(n_1, r_2)} b(x_1; n_1, p) B(r_2 - x_1; n_2, p),\\ \beta_3(p) &= \sum_{x_1 = r_1}^{\min(n_1, r_3)} \sum_{x_2 = r_2 - x_1 + 1}^{\min(n_2, r_3 - x_1)} b(x_1; n_1, p) b(x_2; n_2, p) B(r_3 - x_1 - x_2; n_3, p).\end{aligned} \tag{7.17}$$

Since the β_i represent the probabilities of accepting the null hypothesis at stage i, we can obtain the overall acceptation probability as

$$\Pr(\text{accept } H_0 \mid p) = \beta(p) = \beta_1(p) + \beta_2(p) + \beta_3(p). \tag{7.18}$$

The type II error rate is given by $\beta = \beta(p_a)$; the type I error rate is given by $\alpha = 1 - \beta(p_0)$; and the expected sample size under p is given by

$$\mathrm{EN}(p) = n_1 + n_2[1 - \beta_1(p)] + n_3[1 - \beta_1(p) - \beta_2(p)]. \tag{7.19}$$

7.5 MATHEMATICAL NOTES ON THE CRM

The continual reassessment method (CRM) is a model approach in which the parameters in the model for the response are updated continually based on the response data observed using the Bayesian method.

7.5.1 Probability Model for Dose–Response

Let x be the dose or dose level and $p(x)$ be the probability of response or response rate. The commonly used model for dose–response is a logistic model in which the probability of response (toxicity) is

$$p(x) = \frac{1}{1 + be^{-ax}}, \tag{7.20}$$

where b is usually a predetermined constant and a is a parameter to be updated based on data observed.

7.5.2 Prior Distribution of a Parameter

The Bayesian approach requires the specification of prior probability distribution of the unknown parameter a:

$$a \sim g_0(a) \tag{7.21}$$

where $g_0(a)$ is the prior probability distribution. When very limited knowledge about the prior is available, a noninformative prior can be used.

7.5.3 Likelihood Function

The next step is to construct the likelihood function. Given n observations with $y_i(i = 1, \ldots, n)$ associated with dose x_{m_i}, the likelihood function can be written as

$$f_n(r|a) = \prod_{i=1}^{n} [p(x_{m_i})]^{r_i} [1 - p(x_{m_i})]^{1-r_i}, \tag{7.22}$$

where

$$r_i = \begin{cases} 1, & \text{if response observed for } x_{m_i} \\ 0, & \text{otherwise.} \end{cases}$$

7.5.4 Reassessment of a Parameter

The key is to estimate the parameter a in the response model (7.20). For a Bayesian approach, it leads to the posterior distribution of a. The posterior probability of parameter a can be obtained as follows:

$$g_n(a|r) = \frac{f_n(r \mid a) g_0(a)}{\int f_n(r \mid a) g_0(a) da}. \tag{7.23}$$

After having obtained $g_n(a|r)$, we can update the predictive probability using

$$p(x) = \int \frac{1}{1 + be^{-ax}} g_n(a \mid r) da. \tag{7.24}$$

7.5.5 Assignment of the Next Patient

The updated dose–toxicity model is usually used to choose the dose level for the next patient. In other words, the next patient enrolled in the trial is assigned to the currently estimated MTD based on the dose–response model or predictive probability. Practically, this assignment is subject to safety constraints such as limited dose jump. Assignment of patients to the most updated MTD is intuitive. In this way, the majority of patients will be assigned to dose levels near the MTD, which allows for a more precise estimation of the MTD with a minimal number of patients.

8 Adaptive Trial Simulator

8.1 ADJUSTING THE CRITICAL REGION METHOD

The **ExpDesign adaptive design simulator** (a beta version appears in ExpDesign 5.0) allows you to simulate trials with very complex adaptive designs, which can be combinations of adaptations such as response-adaptive randomization, dropping losers, early efficacy or futility stopping, and sample-size reestimation. It can be a Bayesian or frequentist modeling or a nonparametric approach. In the simulator, the adjusting critical region (ACR) method is used, in which the critical region is determined by running simulations under null condition(s) so that the simulated power is equal to the type I error rate, α. Next, run simulations under the alternative condition using the critical region to obtain the power and other operating characteristics of the design. The approach is very flexible, but it may be difficult to get approval from regulatory agencies because they are not yet ready for very complicated adaptive designs. Therefore, it is not recommended for pivotal phase III trials. There are eight simple steps to setting up your simulations. Depending on the user's experience level (see Figure 8.1), there may be fewer steps.

Step 1: Trial Objective The simulator allows for two possible trial objectives: (1) to find the dose or treatment with the maximum response rate, such as the cured rate or the survival rate (1 – death rate), and (2) to find a dose with a target rate (e.g., the maximum tolerated dose, defined by the dose with a given toxicity rate). The response rate or probability is defined as $\Pr(u \geq c)$, where u is the utility index and c is a threshold. The utility index is the weighting average of trial endpoints, such as safety and efficacy. The weights and the threshold are often determined by experts in the relevant field. If only a single binary efficacy or safety response is concerned, the utility index u is either 0 for nonresponders or 1 for responders, and the response rate is simply $\Pr(u = 1)$.

Step 2: Global Settings Enter the number of simulations you want to run, the number of subjects for each trial, and the number of dose levels, with

---

Classical and Adaptive Clinical Trial Designs Using ExpDesign Studio™,
By Mark Chang

corresponding doses and response rates. Click the Arrow button to navigate among different dose levels. The (true) response rates can be estimated from information available. You can also input any response rates for a sensitivity analysis.

Step 3: Response Model The response rate can be modeled using the hyper-logistic function, the E_{max} model, or any user-defined function of at most five parameters (a_1, a_2, a_3, a_4, a_5). You must use *xx* as the independent variable or dose in your model specification. It is critical to set appropriate parameter ranges for your model, since it will directly affect the accuracy and precision of the modeling. You can use the Graphic Calculator on the toolbar to assist you in determining the ranges by plotting the functions. It is recommended that as few parameters as possible be used, as that will greatly improve the modeling precision. You can choose a parameter as the Bayesian parameter by checking the corresponding box next to the parameter. The response model will be updated whenever the response data become available.

Step 4: Randomization Rules It is desirable to randomize more patients to superior treatment groups. This can be accomplished by increasing the probability of assigning a patient to a treatment group when there is evidence of responsive rate increases in a group. You can choose (1) randomized-play-the-winner, or (2) the utility offset model. The cluster size is used when there is a delayed response (i.e., randomizing the next patient before knowing the responses of previous patients). A cluster size of 1 indicates no response delay. If desired, you can perform response-adaptive randomization at the time of interim analyses by setting the cluster size to the increment of patients between two analyses. However, it is not a cluster randomization, because the basic randomization unit is an individual patient, not a cluster of patients.

Step 5: Stopping Rules It is desirable to stop a trial when the efficacy or futility of the test drug becomes obvious during the trial. To stop a trial prematurely, one has to provide a threshold for the number of subjects randomized and at least one of the following:

- *Utility rules.* The difference in response rate between the most responsive group and the control (dose level 1) exceeds a threshold, and the corresponding two-sided 95% naive confidence interval lower bound exceeds a threshold.
- *Futility rules.* The difference in response rate between the most responsive group and the control (dose level 1) is lower than a threshold, and the corresponding two-sided 90% naive confidence interval upper bound is lower than a threshold.

Step 6: Dropping a Loser In addition to the response-adaptive randomization, you can improve the efficiency of a trial design by dropping some inferior groups (losers) during the trial. To drop a loser, you have to provide thresholds for (1) the maximum difference in response rate between any two dose levels, and (2) the corresponding two-sided 90% naive confidence lower bound. You may choose to retain all the treatment groups without dropping a loser, or/and to retain the control group with a certain randomization rate for the purpose of statistical comparisons between the active groups and the control (dose level 1).

Step 7: Sample-Size Adjustment Sample-size determination requires anticipation of the expected treatment effect size, defined as the expected treatment difference divided by its standard deviation. It is not uncommon that the initial estimation of the effect size turns out to be too large or small, which leads to an underpowered or overpowered trial. Therefore, it is desirable to adjust the sample size according to the effect size for an ongoing trial. The sample-size adjustment is determined by a power function of the treatment effect size. Users can choose different power values to meet their particular requirements.

Step 8: Bayesian Prior If the response or utility is modeled using the Bayesian approach, you can choose one of three prior probability distributions for the Bayesian parameter in the response model: nonformative (uniform), truncated-normal, and truncated-gamma distributions. The priors should be based on information available during trial design.

Utility-Offset Model To have a high probability of achieving target patient distribution among the treatment groups, the probability of assigning a patient to a group should be proportional to the corresponding predicted or observed response rate minus the proportion of patients that have been assigned to the group. This is called the utility-offset model (Chang and Chow, 2005).

Maximum Utility Model The maximum utility model for adaptive randomization always assigns the next patient to the group that has the highest response rate based on a current estimation of either the observed or model-based predicted response rate.

8.2 CLASSICAL DESIGN WITH TWO PARALLEL TREATMENT GROUPS

Suppose that we are performing a phase II oncology trial with treatment groups and the primary endpoint of tumor response (PR and CR). The estimated response rates for the two groups are 0.2 and 0.3, respectively. We use

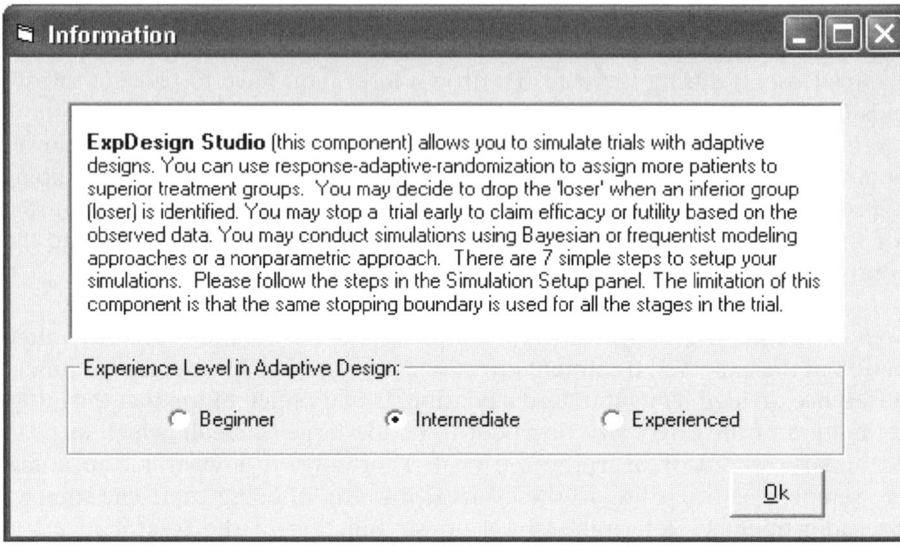

Figure 8.1 Selection of experience level with adaptive design.

simulation to calculate the sample size required given that $\alpha = 0.05$ and power = 80%.

Following are the steps in the simulation (⇒ indicates the next step):

1. Launch ExpDesign Studio ⇒ Click 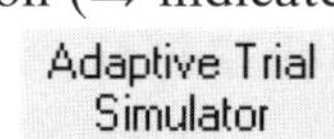

⇒ the **Intermediate** option on the panel for **Experience Level in Adaptive Design** (Figure 8.1). In what follows, we follow the steps in the **Simulation Setup** panel (Figure 8.2) to set up and run the simulations.
2. In the **Trial Objective** panel, choose the option for **To maximize the response rate** (Figure 8.2). Next, click on the option for **Step 2: Global Settings** in the **Simulation Setup** panel, and enter "10000" for **Number of simulations**, "600" for **Number of subjects**, "2" for **Number of dose levels**, "0.2" and "0.3" for **Response rate** corresponding to dose levels 1 and 2, respectively. You can click the arrow to navigate among dose levels (Figure 8.3).
3. Click the option for **Step 3: Response Model**, and select the **Null-model** option (Figure 8.4).
4. Click the option for **Step 4: Randomization Rule** and enter "600" for **Cluster size**, "100" for **Initial Balls**, and "0" for **balls for each response** (Figure 8.5). What we just specified is simple randomization, not an adaptive randomization.
5. Click the option for **Step 5: Early Stopping** and enter "1000" for **Total number of subjects randomized**. This implies that early stopping is not

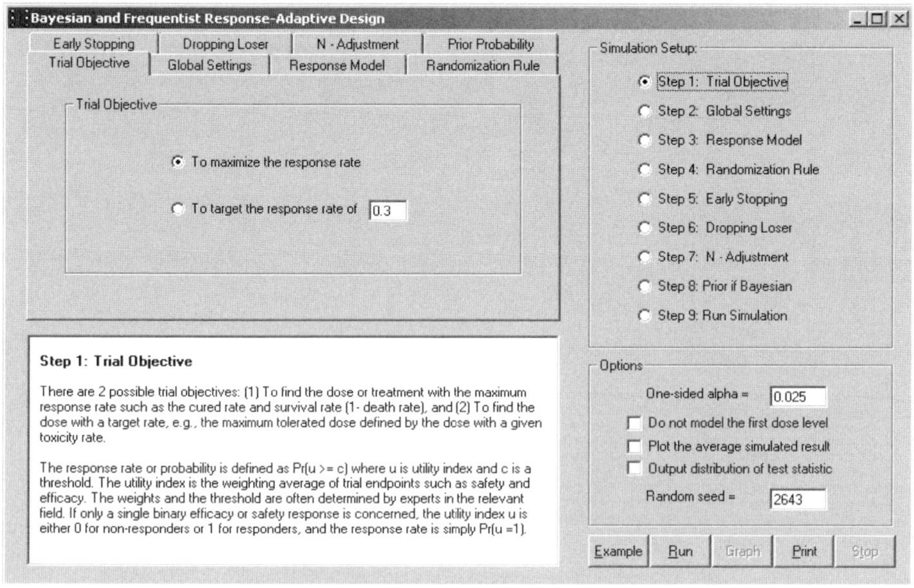

Figure 8.2 Step 1: trial objective.

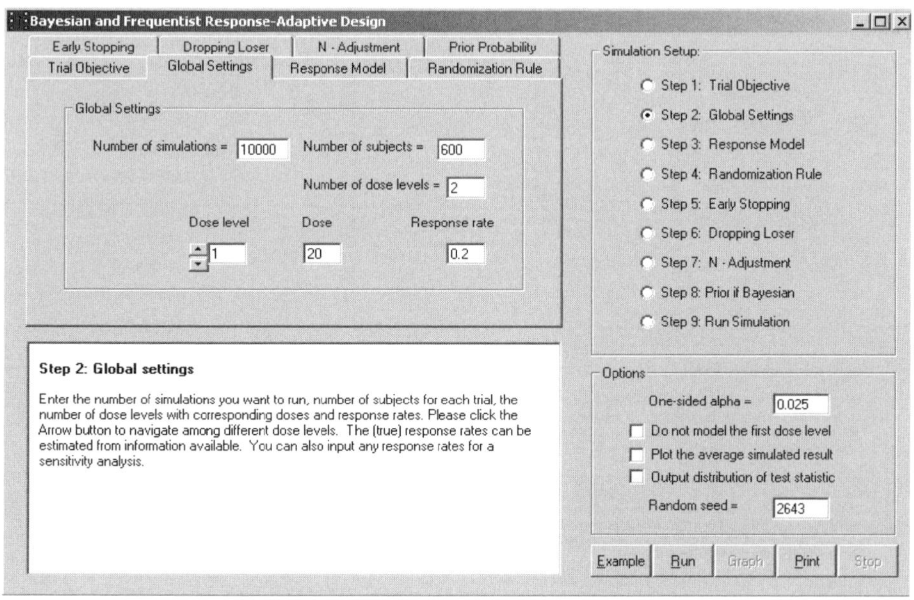

Figure 8.3 Step 2: global settings.

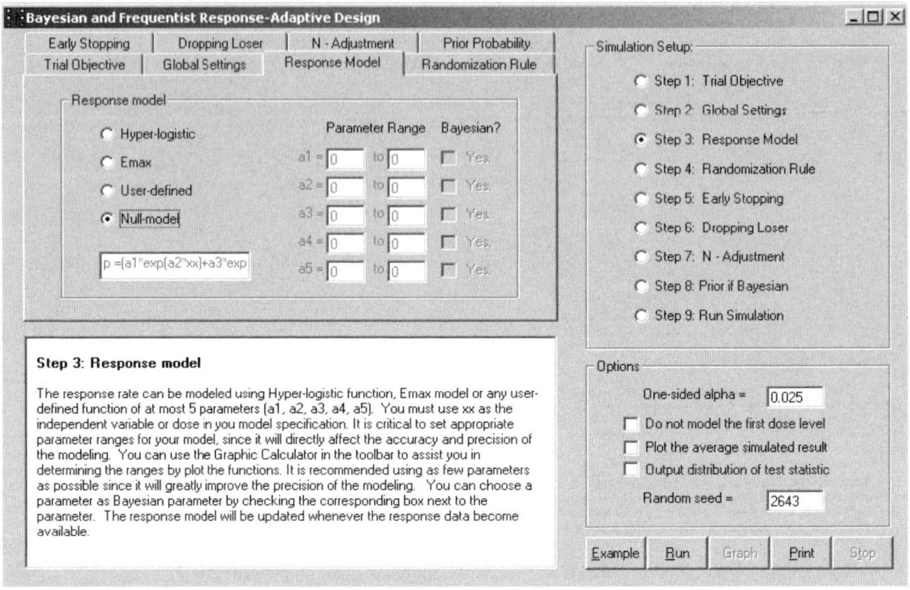

Figure 8.4 Step 3: response model.

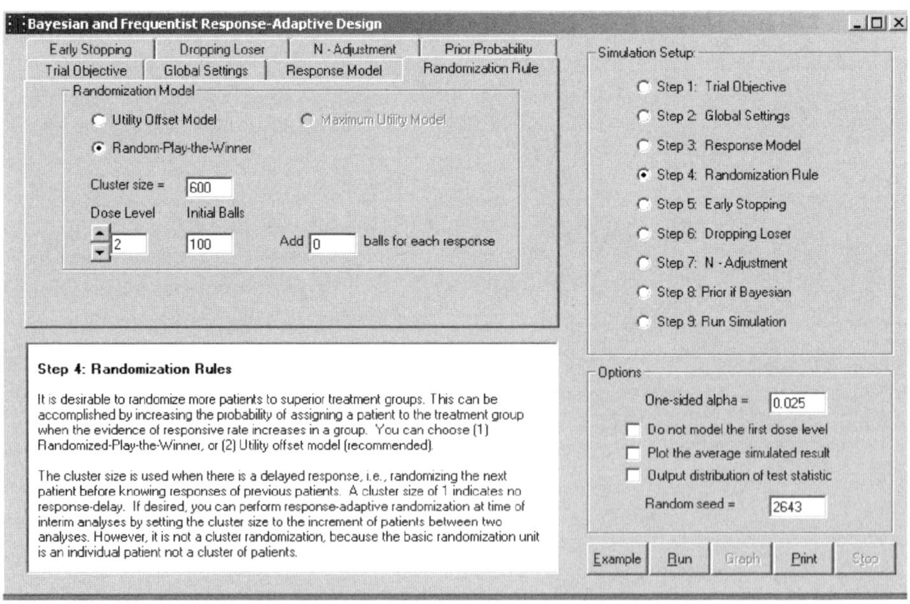

Figure 8.5 Step 4: randomization rule.

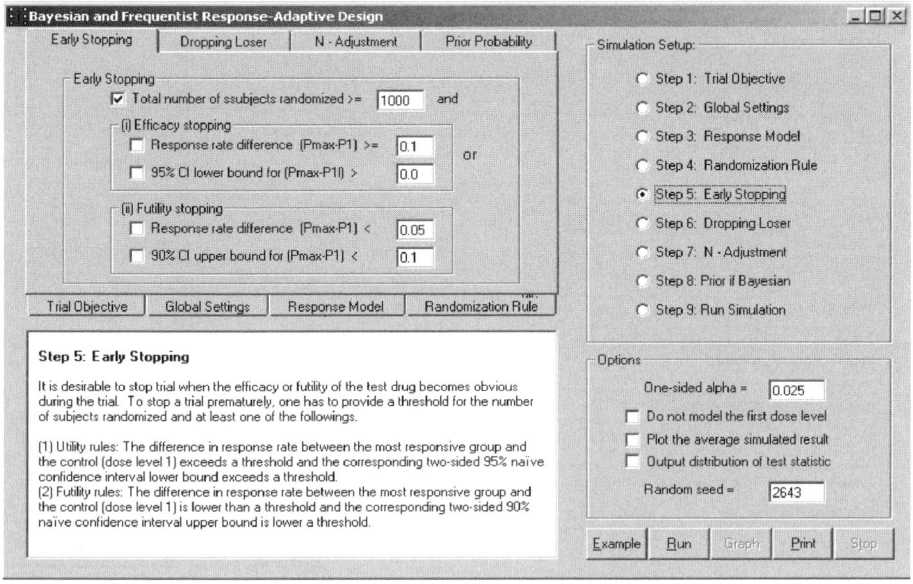

Figure 8.6 Step 5: early stopping.

allowed because the value of 1000 exceeds the planned number of subjects in the trial (i.e., 600) (Figure 8.6).

6. Click the option for **Step 6: Dropping Loser** ⇒ Check the box for **Retain all dose levels** (Figure 8.7).
7. Click the option for **Step 7: N - Adjustment** and enter "1000" for **Adjusted total sample size at information time, n**. This implies that there is no sample-size adjustment because the value of 1000 exceeds the total sample size in the trial (Figure 8.8).
8. Click the option for **Step 8: Prior if Bayesian** and leave as it is because we are not using the Bayesian approach (Figure 8.9).
9. Click the option for **Step 9: Run Simulations** and click 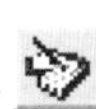 on the toolbar when it finished to view the simulation results, shown below.

Simulation Input The trial objective is to maximize the response rate. There are 10,000 simulations performed for the trial of two dose levels and 600 planned subjects in each simulation.

Simulation Results See Table 8.1. The average total number of subjects for each trial is 600. The total number of responses per trial is 150.1. The probability of predicting the most responsive dose level correctly is 0.998 based on

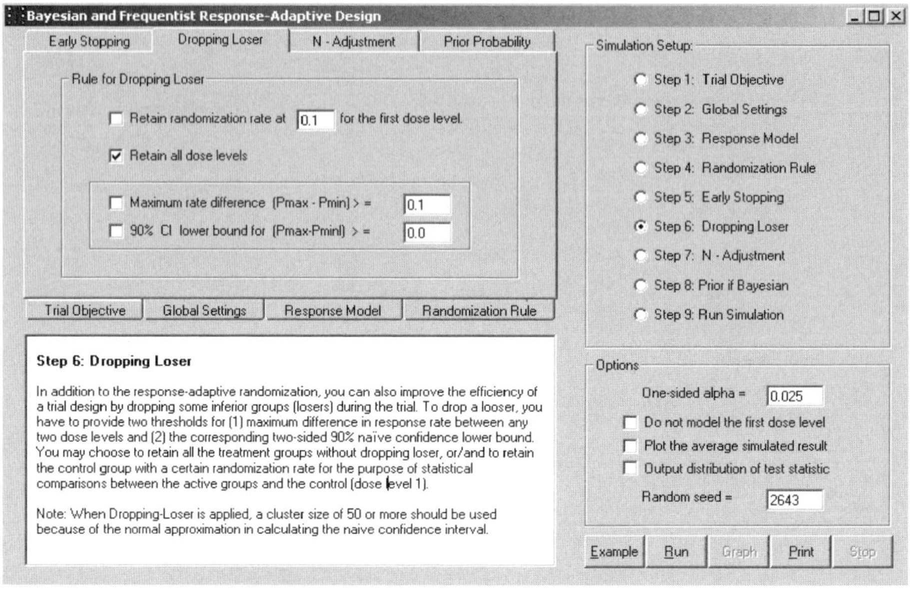

Figure 8.7 Step 6: dropping a loser.

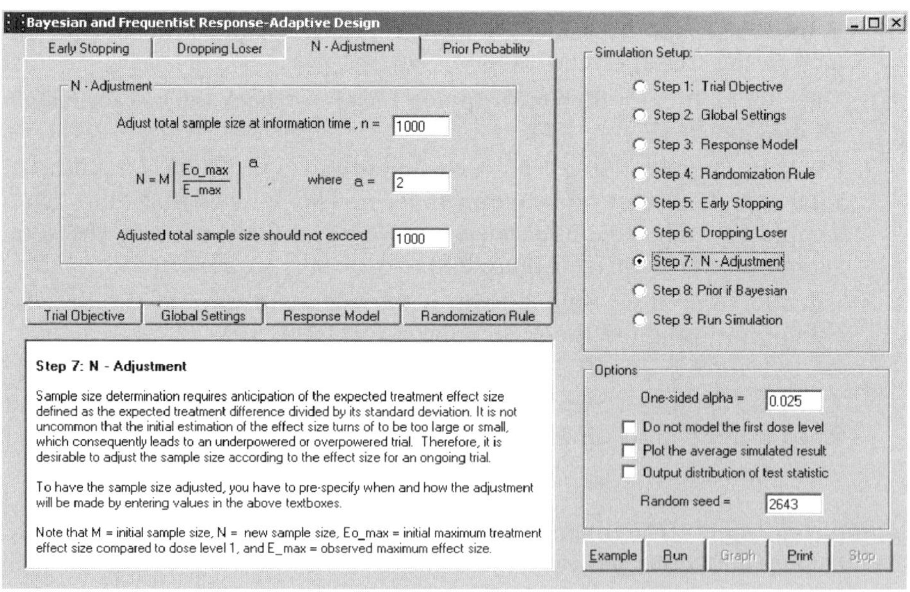

Figure 8.8 Step 7: sample-size adjustment.

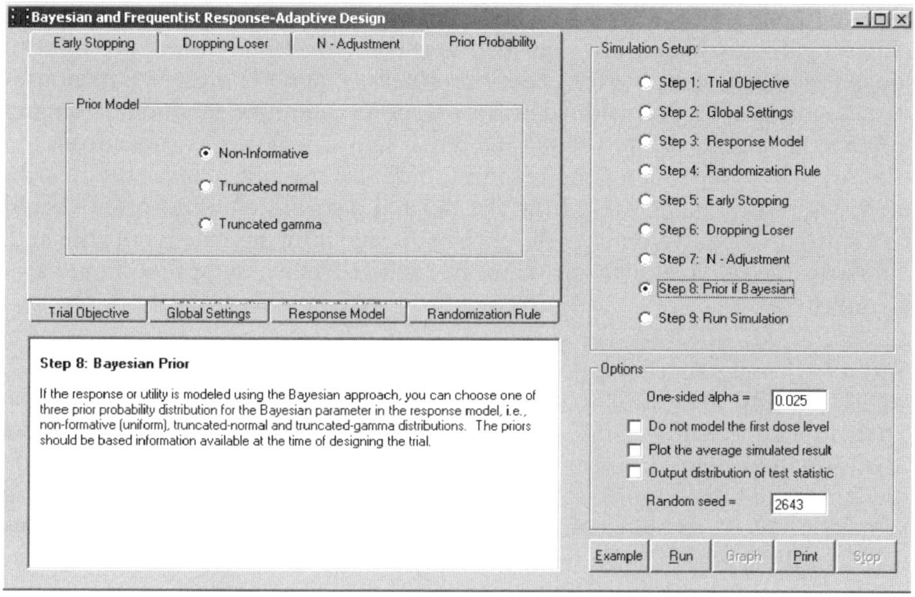

Figure 8.9 Step 8: prior for Bayesian approach.

TABLE 8.1

	Dose Level	
	1	2
Number of patients	299.648	300.351
Response rate	0.2	0.3
Mean rate observed	0.2	0.3
Std. dev. of rate observed	0.023	0.026

rates observed. The power for testing the treatment difference is 0.814 at a one-sided significant level (α) of 0.025.

8.3 FLEXIBLE DESIGN WITH SAMPLE-SIZE REESTIMATION

The power of a trial is heavily dependent on the estimated effect size; therefore, it is desirable to design a trial that allows modification of sample size at some point during the trial. Let us redesign the trial in section 8.2 and allow a sample-size reestimation and then study the robustness of the design.

The simulation can be classified in two stages. In the first stage you find the adjusted α. In the second stage you use the adjusted α and sample size to determine the power. The α adjustment is required when (1) there are multiple comparisons with more than two groups involved, (2) there are interim looks (i.e., early stopping for futility or efficacy), and (3) there is a response-dependent sampling procedure such as response-adaptive randomization and unblended sample-size reestimation. When samples or observations from the trial are not independent, the response data are no longer normally distributed. Therefore, the p-value from the normal distribution assumption should be adjusted, or equivalently, α should be adjusted if the p-value is not adjusted. Similarly, the other statistic estimates from the normal assumption should also be adjusted.

Stage 1 Keep everything the same as in the earlier example, but in step 2, create the null hypothesis condition by entering "0.2" for both dose levels. Then in step 7, enter "100" in the textbox for **Adjusted total sample size at information time, n**, "0.163" for Eo_max, "2" for parameter, **a**, and "1000" for the maximum sample size to be adjusted. Enter "100" for **Cluster size** in step 5. Now try different values for **One-sided alpha** in the **Options** panel until the power for the maximum effect (the family-wise error) becomes 0.025. The adjusted α is 0.023 in the present case. The average sample size is 960 under the null hypothesis. The value of 0.1633 for Eo_max is obtained from $(p_2 - p_1)/[p(1 - p)]$, where $p_1 = 0.2$ and $p_2 = 0.3$, $p = (p_1 + p_2)/2$ (Figure 8.10).

Stage 2 Change the response rate to the alternative hypothesis condition in step 2 (i.e., enter "0.2" for dose level 1 and "0.3" for dose level 2) (Figure 8.11). Run the simulation again by clicking 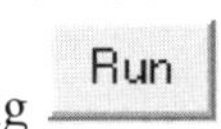

. When the simulation is finished, click 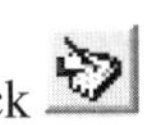 to view the simulation results. The design has 92.1% power with an average sample size of 821.5.

Now assume that the true effect sizes are not 0.2 versus 0.3 for the two treatment groups; instead, they are 0.2 and 0.28, respectively. We want to know to what the power of the flexible design pertains. Keep everything the same (also keep Eo_max = 0.1633), but change the response rates to 0.2 and 0.28 for the two dose levels and run the simulation again. The key results are shown below. The design has 79.4% power with an average sample size of 855.

Given the two response rates 0.2 and 0.28, a design with a fixed sample size of 880 has a power of 79.4%. We can see that there is a saving of 25 patients using the flexible design. If the response rates are 0.2 and 0.3 for 92.1% power, the sample size required is 828 with the fixed-sample-size design. The flexible design saves six or seven subjects. Flexible design increases sample size when the effect size observed is less than expected. Therefore, the power is protected.

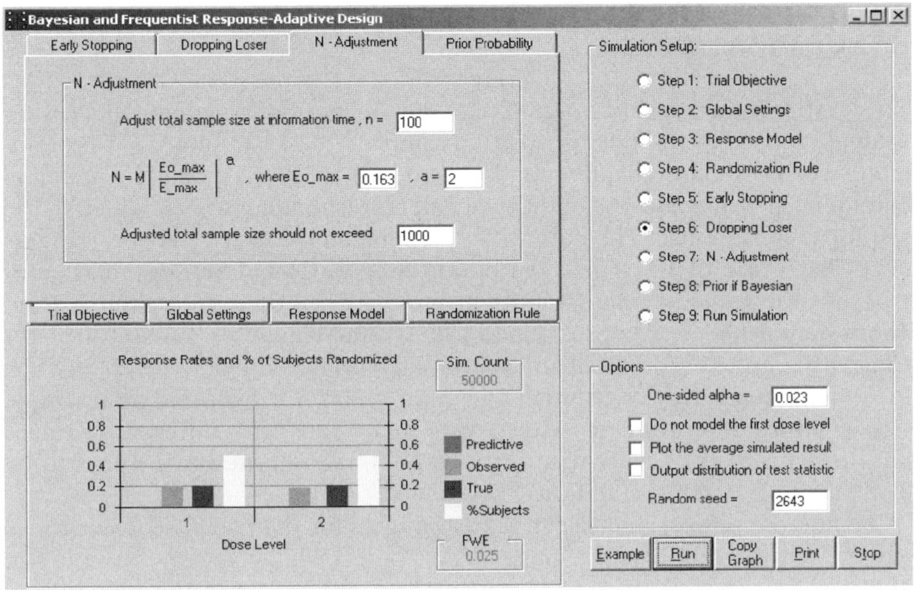

Figure 8.10 Finding the adjusted α in a sample-size reestimation.

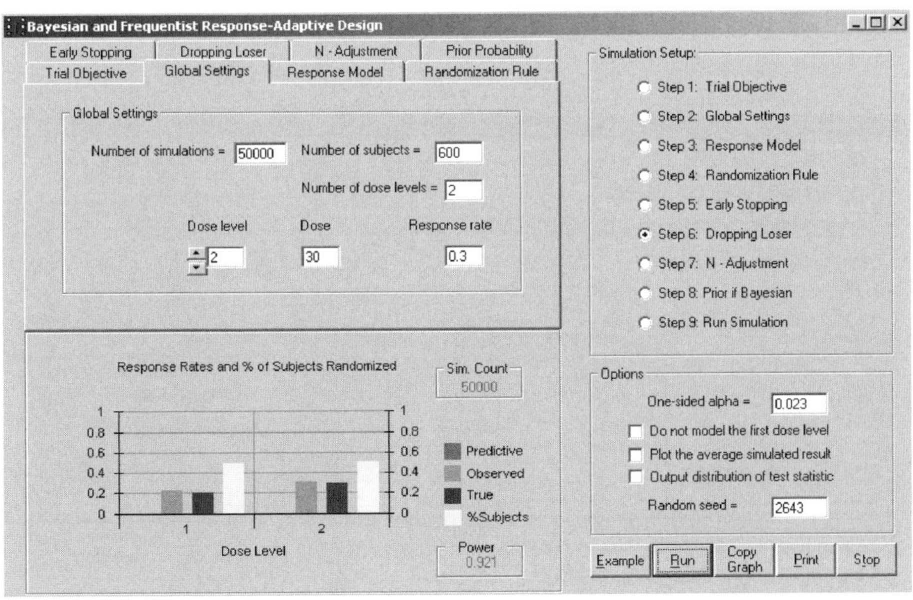

Figure 8.11 Finding the power in a sample-size reestimation.

8.4 DESIGN WITH RANDOM-PLAY-THE-WINNER RANDOMIZATION

To investigate the effect of random-play-the-winner randomization, the earlier example is used again, this time with a sample size of 600 subjects. The commonly used response-adaptive randomization is RPW(1,1); that is, one initial ball for each group and one additional ball corresponding will be added to the urn for each response. The data will be unblinded for every 100 new patients or a cluster size of 100. Click the option **Step 2: Global Settings**, and enter "0.2" for the response rate for both groups ⇒ Click the option **Step 4: Randomization Rule** ⇒ Choose **Random-Play-the-Winner** ⇒ Enter "100" for **Cluster size** and "1" for initial and additional balls for both dose levels ⇒ Click the option **Step 7: N - Adjustment** and enter "1000" for **Adjusted total sample size at information time, n**. After trying many runs with different α values until α matches the family-wise error (FWE), the adjusted α is found to be 0.02 based on 30,000 simulations (Figure 8.12).

To find the power, change the response rates for the two dose levels to 0.2 and 0.3, respectively. The design has 77.3% power with an average sample size of 600. On average, there are 223 subjects in dose level 1 and 377 in dose level 2 (Table 8.2).

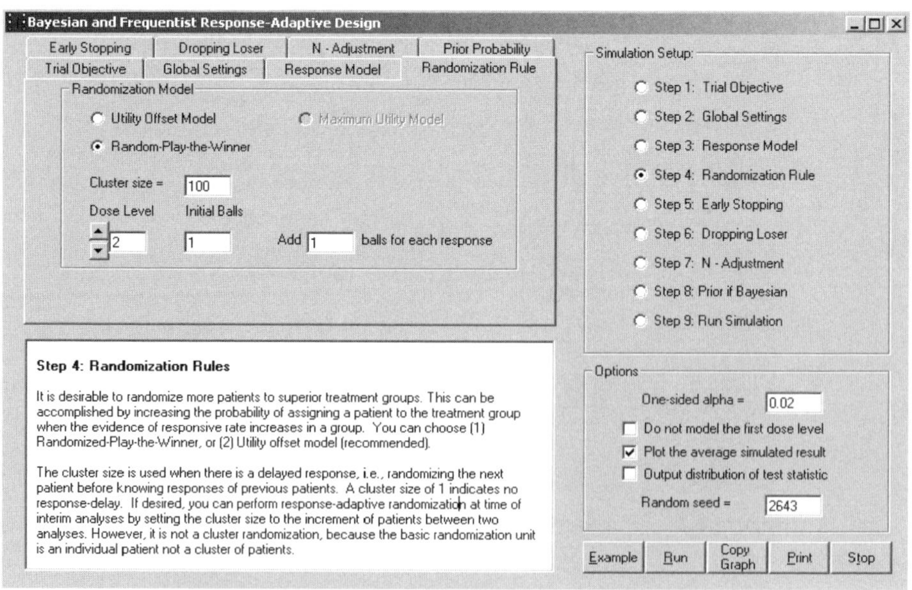

Figure 8.12 Effect of random-play-the-winner.

TABLE 8.2

	Dose level	
	1	2
Number of patients	222.972	377.028
Response rate	0.2	0.3
Mean rate observed	0.197	0.299
Std. dev. of rate observed	0.028	0.024

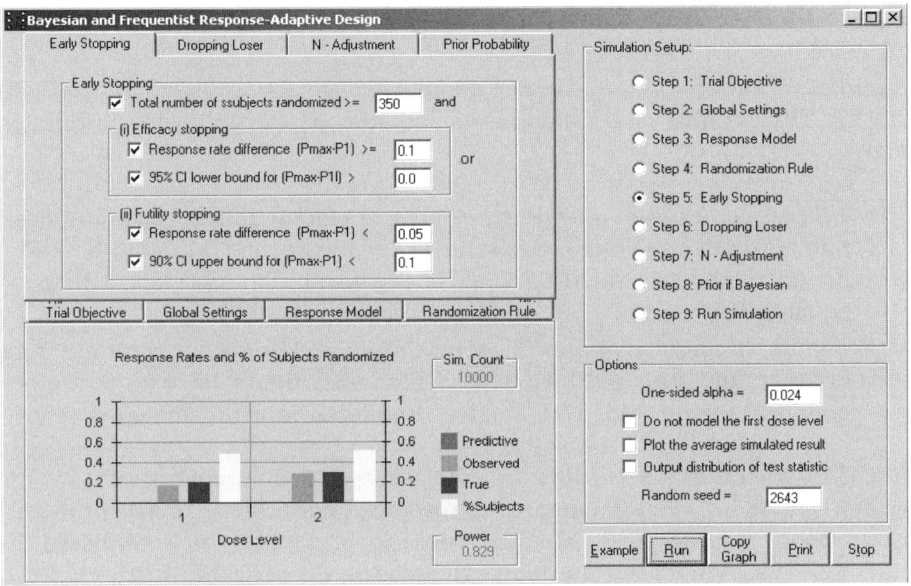

Figure 8.13 Group sequential design with one interim analysis.

8.5 GROUP SEQUENTIAL DESIGN WITH ONE INTERIM ANALYSIS

Similar to the example in Section 8.3 there two stages in the simulation. The first stage is used to find the adjusted α value, and the second stage, to find the power. Keep everything the same as in the earlier example, but click the option **Step 2: Global Settings**, and enter "700" for **Number of subjects** and "0.2" for both dose levels, then click the option **Step 5: Early Stopping**, and enter "350, 0.1, 0.0, 0.05, 0.1" for the five textboxes, in that order. Try different α values until the one-sided FWE = 0.025. The adjusted α is 0.024 for the current design. Now click the option **Step 2: Global Settings** in the **Simulation Setup** panel and enter "0.2" and "0.3" for the response rates of the two dose levels, respectively (Figure 8.13). The simulation results are presented below.

TABLE 8.3

	Dose Level	
	1	2
Number of patients	243.587	244.152
Response rate	0.2	0.3
Mean rate observed	0.198	0.303
Std. dev. of rate observed	0.028	0.033

Simulation Input The maximum number of subjects is 700. The trial will stop if 350 or more are randomized and one of the following criteria is met:

- *Efficacy (utility) stopping criterion.* The maximum difference in response rate between any dose and dose level 1 is larger than 0.1, with the lower bound of the two-sided 95% naive confidence interval larger than or equal to 0.0.
- *Futility stopping criterion.* The maximum difference in response rate between any dose and dose level 1 is smaller than 0.05, with the upper bound of the one-sided 95% naive confidence interval smaller than 0.1.

Simulation Results See Table 8.3. The average total number of subjects for each trial is 487.7. The total number of responses per trial is 122. The probability of predicting the most responsive dose level correctly is 0.988 based on rates observed. Under the alternative hypothesis, the probability of early stopping for efficacy is 0.5047 and the probability of early stopping for futility is 0.1035. The power for testing the treatment difference is 0.825.

8.6 DESIGN PERMITTING EARLY STOPPING AND SAMPLE-SIZE REESTIMATION

It is often desirable to have a design that permits both early stopping and sample-size modification. Keep everything the same as earlier, but enter "700" for **Number of subjects** in **Step 2: Global Settings** and "350" for **Cluster size** in **Step 4: Randomization Rule**. In step 7, enter "350" for **Adjusted total sample size at information time, n**, "1" for Eo_max, "2" for parameter a, and "1000" for **Adjusted total sample size should not exceed** (Figure 8.14). Similarly, the one-sided adjusted α value is found to be 0.05. The simulation results are presented below.

The maximum sample size is 700. The trial will stop if 350 or more are randomized and one of the following criteria is met:

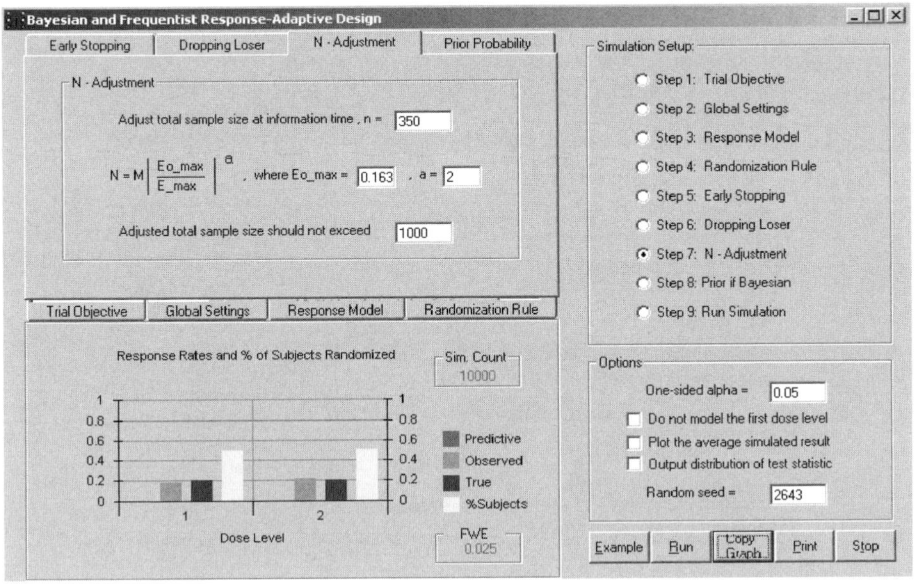

Figure 8.14 Early stopping and sample-size reestimation.

- *Efficacy (utility) stopping criterion.* The maximum difference in response rate between any dose and dose level 1 is larger than 0.1 with the lower bound of the two-sided 95% naive confidence interval larger than or equal to 0.0.
- *Futility stopping criterion.* The maximum difference in response rate between any dose and dose level 1 is smaller than 0.05 with the upper bound of the one-sided 95% naive confidence interval smaller than 0.1.

The sample size will be reestimated at the time when there 350 subjects are randomized. The new sample size will be N(Eo_max/E_max)^2, where Eo_max = 0.1633 and the initial sample size N = 1000 (Figure 8.15).

Simulation Results See Table 8.4. The average total number of subjects for each trial is 398.8. The probability of early stopping for efficacy is 0.0096. The probability of early stopping for futility is 0.9638.

To find the power of this design, you can change the response rates to 0.2 and 0.3 for the two dose levels, respectively (Table 8.5). The average total number of subjects for each trial is 543.5. The total number of responses per trial is 136. The probability of predicting the most responsive dose level correctly is 0.985 based on rates observed. The probability of early stopping for efficacy is 0.6225. The probability of early stopping for futility is 0.1546. The power is 0.842.

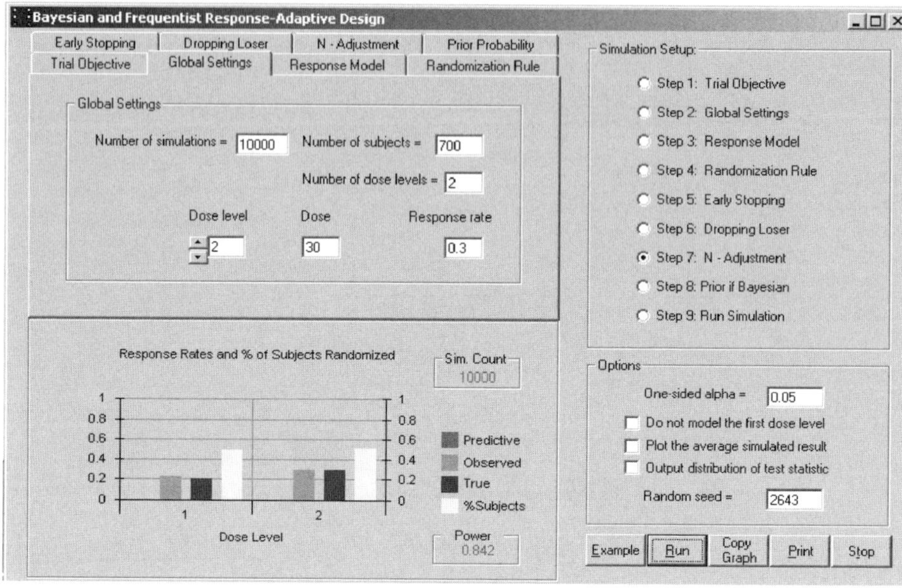

Figure 8.15 Power for group sequential trial with sample-size reestimation.

TABLE 8.4

	Dose Level	
	1	2
Response rate	0.2	0.2
Mean rate observed	0.202	0.198
Std. dev. of rate observed	0.028	0.028

TABLE 8.5

	Dose Level	
	1	2
Number of patients	271.463	272.029
Response rate	0.2	0.3
Mean rate observed	0.198	0.303
Std. dev. of rate observed	0.028	0.032

TABLE 8.6 Simulation Results Under the Alternative Hypothesis

	Dose Level					
	1	2	3	4	5	6
Number of patients	133	133	133	134	133	133
Response rate	0.5	0.4	0.5	0.6	0.7	0.55
Mean rate observed	0.499	0.4	0.5	0.6	0.7	0.55
Std. dev. of rate observed	0.043	0.043	0.044	0.043	0.04	0.043

The next set of examples is based on the same scenario in a six-arm study with response rates 0.5, 0.4, 0.5, 0.6, 0.7, and 0.55 for the six dose levels from 1 to 6, respectively.

8.7 CLASSICAL DESIGN WITH MULTIPLE TREATMENT GROUPS

Enter "800" for the number of subjects, "0.5" (assuming a response rate of 0.5 under H_o) for the response rate for all dose levels (the null hypothesis condition); enter "1" for initial balls and "0" for additional balls corresponding to each response in step 4. By altering α until the FEW becomes 0.025, we found that the final α is 0.0055. Next, we enter "0.5, 0.4, 0.5, 0.6, 0.7, and 0.55" for the six dose levels from 1 to 6, respectively. Enter "100" for the cluster in step 4 and "1000" for the number of subjects randomized in step 7. The simulation results are presented in Table 8.6.

The average total number of subjects for each trial is 800. The total number of responses per trial is 433.3. The probability of predicting the most responsive dose level correctly is 0.951 based on rates observed. The power for testing the maximum effect comparing any dose level to the control (dose level 1) is 0.803 at a one-sided significant level (α) of 0.0055. The powers for comparing each of the five dose levels to the control (dose level 1) at a one-sided significant level (α) of 0.0055 are 0, 0.008, 0.2, 0.796, and 0.048, respectively.

8.8 MULTIGROUP TRIAL WITH RESPONSE-ADAPTIVE RANDOMIZATION

It is desirable to randomize more patients to the superior treatment group, which can be accomplished by using response-adaptive randomization, such as RPW(1,1). Specify 800 for the number of subjets in step 1 and the number of balls based on RPW(1,1) with a cluster size of 100 in step 4, but retain the response rate for dose level 1 at 0.25 in step 6. Simulations under the null hypothesis result in a one-sided adjusted α value of 0.016 using this adjusted α and response rates 0.5, 0.4, 0.5, 0.6, 0.7, and 0.55 for dose levels 1 to 7, respectively. The simulation results shown below indicate that there are biases

TABLE 8.7 Simulation Results Under the Null Hypothesis

	Dose Level					
	1	2	3	4	5	6
Number of patients	200	120	120	119	120	121
Response rate	0.5	0.5	0.5	0.5	0.5	0.5
Mean rate observed	0.499	0.493	0.493	0.493	0.493	0.494

TABLE 8.8 Simulation Results Under the Alternative Hypothesis

	Dose Level					
	1	2	3	4	5	6
Number of patients	200	74	100	133	176	116
Response rate	0.5	0.4	0.5	0.6	0.7	0.55
Mean rate observed	0.499	0.388	0.493	0.595	0.697	0.544

in the estimated mean response rates in all dose levels except dose level 1, which has a fixed randomization rate. The design trial has 86% power and 447 responders per trial on average. Compared to 80% power and 433 responders for the simple randomization RPW(1,0), the adaptive randomization is superior in both power and number of responders. The simulation results are given in Tables 8.7 and 8.8.

The average total number of subjects for each trial is 800. The total number of responses per trial is 446.8. The probability of predicting the most responsive dose level correctly is 0.957 based on rates observed. The power for testing the maximum effect comparing any dose level to the control (dose level 1) is 0.861 at a one-sided significant level (α) of 0.016. The powers for comparing each of the five dose levels to the control (dose level 1) at a one-sided significant level (α) of 0.016 are 0, 0.008, 0.201, 0.853, and 0.051, respectively.

8.9 ADAPTIVE DESIGN FEATURING DROPPING LOSERS

Implementing the mechanism of dropping a loser can also improve the efficiency of a design. Enter "800" for the number of subjects in step 2, and enter "100" for the cluster in step 4 (meaning that for every 100 patients randomized, the data will be unblended, and a review and a decision will be make as to whether or not to drop a loser). Retain the randomization rate in dose level 1 at 0.25. An inferior group (loser) will be dropped if the maximum difference in response between the most effective group and the least effective group (loser) is larger than zero with the lower bound of the one-sided 95% naive

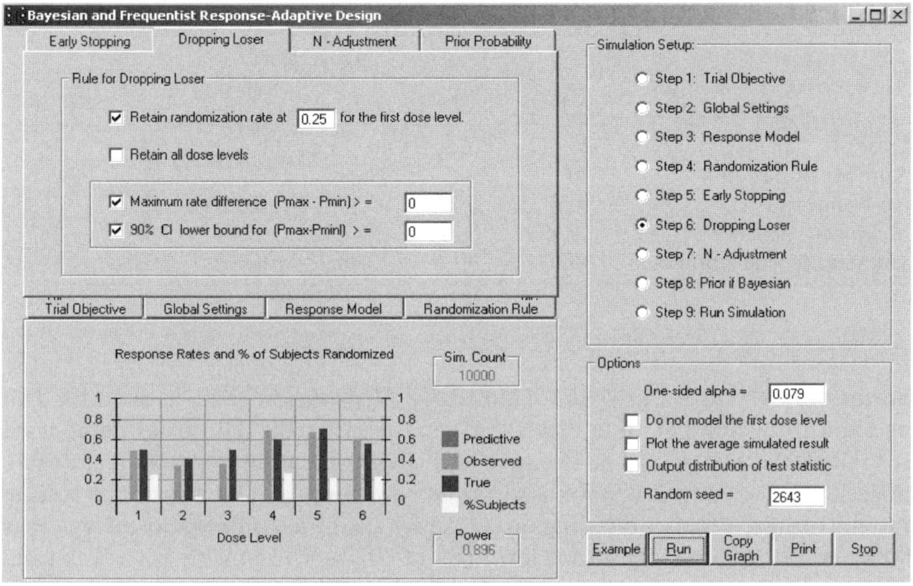

Figure 8.16 Dropping a loser.

TABLE 8.9

	Dose Level					
	1	2	3	4	5	6
Number of patients	200	114	121	122	122	122
Response rate	0.5	0.5	0.5	0.5	0.5	0.5
Mean rate observed	0.499	0.460	0.461	0.462	0.461	0.462
Std. dev. of rate observed	0.035	0.085	0.084	0.084	0.085	0.084

confidence interval larger than or equal to zero (Figure 8.16). Through the simulation, the adjusted α is found to be 0.079. From the simulation results below, some biases in mean rate can be observed with this design. The design has 90% power with 467 responders. The probability of predicting the most responsive dose level correctly is 0.965 based on rates observed. The design is superior to both RPW(1,0) and RPW(1,1).

Simulation Results Under the Null Hypothesis See Table 8.9. The power for testing the maximum effect comparing any dose level to the control (dose level 1) is 0.025 at a one-sided significant level (α) of 0.079. The powers for comparing each of the five dose levels to the control (dose level 1) at a one-sided significant level (α) of 0.079 are 0.007, 0.007, 0.005, 0.006, and 0.006, respectively.

TABLE 8.10

	Dose Level					
	1	2	3	4	5	6
Dose	20	30	40	50	60	70
Number of patients	200	26	68	172	240	95
Response rate	0.5	0.4	0.5	0.6	0.7	0.55
Mean rate observed	0.499	0.371	0.463	0.574	0.692	0.512
Std. dev. of rate observed	0.035	0.1	0.085	0.072	0.047	0.081

Simulation Results Under the Alternative Hypothesis See Table 8.10. The average total number of subjects for each trial is 800. The total number of responses per trial is 467.3. The probability of predicting the most responsive dose level correctly is 0.965 based on observed rates. The power for testing the maximum effect comparing any dose level to the control (dose level 1) is 0.896 at a one-sided significant level (α) of 0.079. The powers for comparing each of the five dose levels to the control (dose level 1) at a one-sided significant level (α) of 0.079 are 0.001, 0.007, 0.205, 0.889, and 0.045, respectively.

8.10 DOSE–RESPONSE TRIAL DESIGN

The trial objective is to find the optimal dose with the best response rate. There are five dose levels and 30 planned subjects in each simulation. The hyperlogistic model defined by the probability of response $p = 1/[0.1\exp(0.05x) + a_1\exp(-a_2x)]$, where $a_3 = [20,100]$ and $a_4 = [0,0.05]$. The RPW(1,1) is used for the randomization (Figure 8.17). The simulation results given in Table 8.11 show that the probability of predicting the most responsive dose level correctly is 0.992 by the model and only 0.505 based on rates observed.

8.11 DOSE-ESCALATION DESIGN FOR AN ONCOLOGY TRIAL

The trial objective is to find the MTD with a response rate (toxicity rate) of 0.3. The Bayesian continual reassessment method is used. The two-parameter logistic model is used to model the dose response. $p = 1/[1 + a_3\exp(-a_4x)]$, where $a_3 = [50,150]$, and Bayesian parameter a_4 with noninformative distribution over the range [0,0.3]. The maximum utility model is used for the randomization (i.e., the next patient is assigned to the dose level that has the highest predicted response rate). To consider the potential response delay, a cluster size of 3 is used. Due to safety concerns, dose escalation must proceed gradually (i.e., there must be no jump in dosage). See Figures 8.18 and 8.19 for the key parameter specifications to run the simulations.

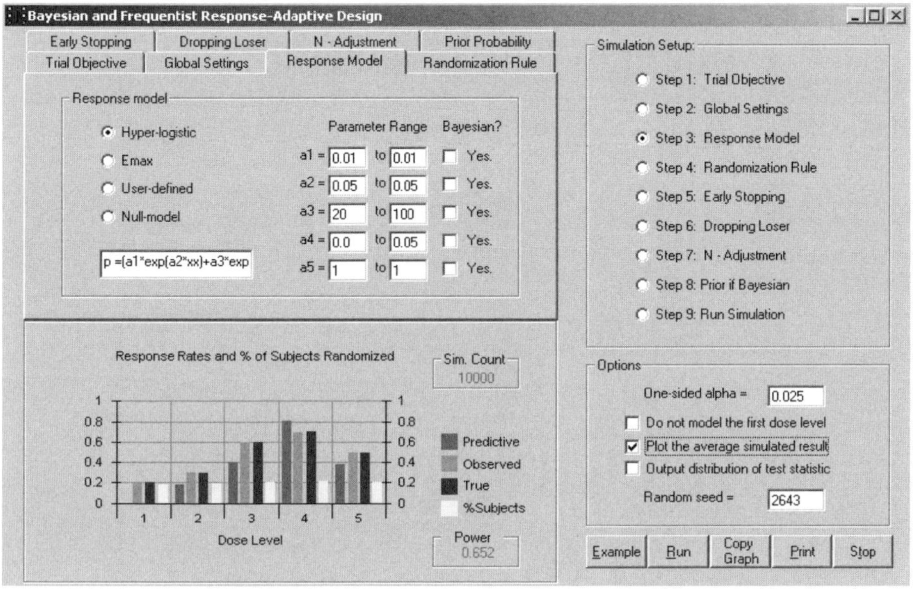

Figure 8.17 Hyperlogistic model for dose–response trial.

TABLE 8.11

	Dose Level				
	1	2	3	4	5
Dose	15	30	50	85	110
Number of patients	5.528	5.699	6.278	6.438	6.057
Response rate	0.2	0.3	0.6	0.7	0.5
Mean rate observed	0.193	0.294	0.593	0.691	0.489
Mean rate predicted	0.098	0.181	0.406	0.802	0.379
Std. dev. of rate observed	0.185	0.209	0.221	0.204	0.226
Std. dev. of rate predicted	0.074	0.073	0.104	0.151	0.056

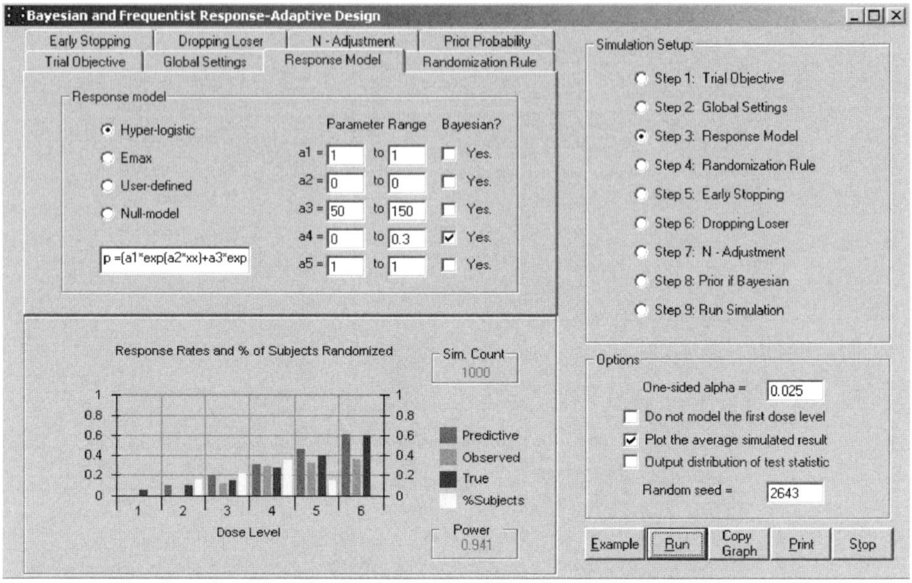

Figure 8.18 Hyperlogistic model with Bayesian parameter a_4.

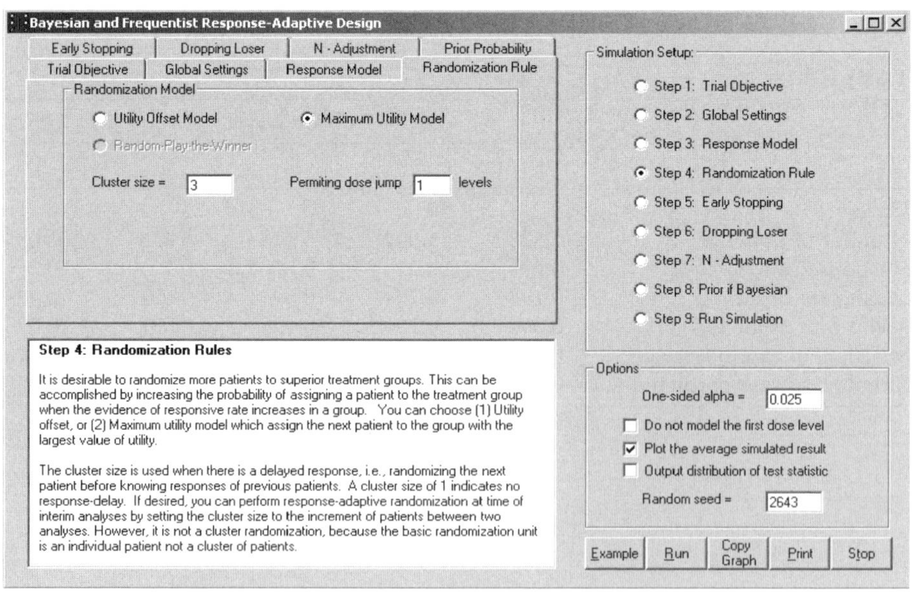

Figure 8.19 Maximum-utility model without a dose jump.

TABLE 8.12

	Dose Level					
	1	2	3	4	5	6
Dose	20	30	40	50	60	70
Number of patients	2.5	6.2	8.5	14.1	5.8	2.9
Response rate	0.05	0.1	0.15	0.28	0.4	0.6
Mean rate observed	0.012	0.048	0.108	0.281	0.324	0.353
Mean rate predicted	0.056	0.106	0.191	0.313	0.461	0.608
Std. dev. of rate observed	0.038	0.077	0.185	0.205	0.314	0.384
Std. dev. of rate predicted	0.02	0.041	0.073	0.104	0.124	0.127

The simulation results are given in Table 8.12. The average total number of subjects for each trial is 40. The total number of responses per trial is 10.2. The probability of predicting the most responsive dose level correctly is 1 by the model and 0.366 based on rates observed.

9 Further Assistance from ExpDesign Studio

9.1 EXPDESIGN PROBABILITY FUNCTIONS

Bernoulli Distribution This distribution best describes all situations where a "trial" is made resulting in either "success" or "failure," such as when tossing a coin or when modeling the success or failure of a surgical procedure. The Bernoulli distribution is defined as

$$f(x) = p^x(1-p)^{1-x}, \qquad x \in [0,1], \tag{9.1}$$

where p is the probability that a particular event (e.g., success) will occur.

Beta Distribution The beta distribution arising from a transformation of the F-distribution is typically used to model the distribution of order statistics. Because the beta distribution is bounded on both sides, it is often used to represent processes with natural lower and upper limits. The *beta distribution* is defined as

$$f(x) = \frac{\Gamma(v+w)}{\Gamma(v)\Gamma(w)} x^{v-1}(1-x)^{w-1}, \qquad 0 < x < 1, \quad v > 0, \quad \text{and} \quad w > 0, \tag{9.2}$$

where Γ is the gamma function and v and w are shape parameters.

Binomial Distribution The binomial distribution is useful for describing distributions of binomial events, such as the number of males and females in a random sample of companies, or the number of defective components in samples of 20 units taken from a production process. The binomial distribution is defined as

$$f(x) = \frac{n!}{x!(n-x)!} p^x(1-p)^{n-x} \qquad \text{for } x = 0, 1, \ldots, n, \tag{9.3}$$

Classical and Adaptive Clinical Trial Designs Using ExpDesign Studio™,
By Mark Chang

where p is the probability that the respective event will occur and n is the maximum number of independent trials.

Cauchy Distribution The Cauchy distribution is interesting for theoretical reasons. Although its mean can be taken as zero, since it is symmetrical about zero, the expectation, variance, higher moments, and moment generating function do not exist. The *Cauchy distribution* is defined as

$$f(x) = \frac{1}{\theta\pi(1+[(x-\eta)/\theta]^2)} \qquad \text{for } \theta > 0 \tag{9.4}$$

where η is the location parameter (median), θ is a scale parameter, and π is a constant (3.1415 . . .).

Chi-Square Distribution The sum of v independent squared random variables, each distributed following the standard normal distribution, is

$$f(x) = \frac{1}{2^{v/2}\Gamma(v/2)}(x^{v/2-1}e^{-x/2}) \qquad \text{for } v = 1, 2, \ldots \text{ and } x > 0, \tag{9.5}$$

where v represents the degrees of freedom, e is the base of the natural logarithm, sometimes called Euler's e (2.71 . . .), and Γ is the gamma function.

Exponential Distribution If T is the time between occurrences of rare events that happen on the average with a rate of l per unit of time, then T is distributed exponentially with parameter λ. Thus, the exponential distribution is frequently used to model the time interval between successive random events. Examples of variables distributed in this manner include the gap length between cars crossing an intersection, the lifetimes of electronic devices, or the arrivals of customers at a checkout counter in a grocery store. The *exponential distribution function* is defined as

$$f(x) = \lambda e^{-\lambda x} \qquad \text{for } \lambda > 0 \quad \text{and} \quad x \geq 0, \tag{9.6}$$

where λ is an exponential function parameter.

F-Distribution Snedecor's F-distribution is most commonly used in tests of variance (e.g., ANOVA). The ratio of two chi-squares divided by their respective degrees of freedom is said to follow an F-distribution. The F-distribution has the probability density function (for v = 1, 2, . . . ; w = 1, 2, . . .):

$$f(x) = \Gamma\left(\frac{v+w}{2}\right) \Big/ \Gamma\left(\frac{v}{2}\right) \Big/ \Gamma\left(\frac{w}{2}\right)\left(\frac{v}{w}\right)^{v/2} x^{v/2-1}\left(1+\frac{vx}{w}\right)^{-(v=w)/2}, \tag{9.7}$$

where $0 \leq x$, v and w (degrees of freedom) are positive integers, and Γ is the gamma function.

Gamma Distribution The probability density function of the exponential distribution has a mode of zero. In many instances it is known a priori that the mode of distribution of a particular random variable of interest is not equal to zero (e.g., when modeling the distribution of the lifetimes of a product such as an electric light bulb or the serving time taken at a ticket booth at a baseball game). In those cases, the gamma distribution is more appropriate for describing the underlying distribution. The *gamma distribution* is defined as

$$f(x) = \frac{1}{b\Gamma(c)}\left(\frac{x}{b}\right)^{c-1} e^{-x/b} \qquad \text{for } x \geq 0 \quad \text{and} \quad c > 0, \tag{9.8}$$

where c is a shape parameter and b is a scale parameter.

Geometric Distribution If independent Bernoulli trials are made until a "success" occurs, the total number of trials required is a geometric random variable. The *geometric distribution* is defined as

$$f(x) = p(1-p)^x \qquad \text{for } x = 1, 2, \ldots, \tag{9.9}$$

where p is the probability that a particular event (e.g., success) will occur.

Gompertz Distribution The Gompertz distribution is a theoretical distribution of survival times. Gompertz (1825) proposed a probability model for human mortality based on the assumption that the "average exhaustion of a man's power to avoid death to be such that at the end of equal infinitely small intervals of time he lost equal portions of his remaining power to oppose destruction which he had at the commencement of these intervals" (Johnson et al., 1995, p. 25). The resulting hazard function

$$r(x) = B\exp(x) \qquad \text{for } x \leq 0, \quad B > 0, \quad \text{and} \quad c \leq 1. \tag{9.10}$$

Laplace Distribution For interesting mathematical applications of the Laplace distribution, see Johnson et al. (1995). The *Laplace* (or *double exponential*) *distribution* is defined as

$$f(x) = \frac{1}{2b}\exp\left(\frac{|x-a|}{b}\right) \qquad \text{for } -\infty < x < \infty, \tag{9.11}$$

where a is the location parameter (mean) and b is the scale parameter.

Logistic Distribution The logistic distribution is used to model binary responses (e.g., gender) and is commonly used in logistic regression. The *logistic distribution* is defined as

$$f(x) = \frac{1}{b}\exp\left(-\frac{x-a}{b}\right)\left[1+\exp\left(-\frac{x-a}{b}\right)\right]^{-2} \quad \text{for } -\infty < x < \infty \text{ and } b > 0, \tag{9.12}$$

where a is a location parameter (mean) and b is a scale parameter.

Lognormal Distribution The lognormal distribution is often used in simulations of variables such as personal incomes, age at first marriage, or tolerance to poison in animals. In general, if x is a sample from a normal distribution, then $y = e^x$ is a sample from a lognormal distribution. Thus, the *lognormal distribution* is defined as

$$f(x) = \frac{1}{\sqrt{2}x\sigma}\exp\left[-\frac{(\ln x-\mu)^2}{2\sigma^2}\right] \quad \text{for } 0 < 0, \quad \mu \geq 0, \quad \text{and} \quad \sigma > 0, \tag{9.13}$$

where μ is a scale parameter and σ is a shape parameter.

Normal Distribution The normal distribution (the "bell-shaped curve" which is symmetrical about the mean) is a theoretical function commonly used in inferential statistics as an approximation to sampling distributions. In general, the normal distribution provides a good model for a random variable, when:

1. There is a strong tendency for the variable to take a central value.
2. Positive and negative deviations from the central value are equally likely.
3. The frequency of deviations falls off rapidly as the deviations become larger.

As an underlying mechanism that produces the normal distribution, one may think of an infinite number of independent random (binomial) events that bring about the values of a particular variable. For example, there are probably a nearly infinite number of factors that determine a person's height (i.e., thousands of genes, nutrition, diseases, etc.). Thus, height can be expected to be normally distributed in a population. The *normal distribution function* is determined by the formula

$$f(x) = \frac{1}{\sigma\sqrt{2\pi}}\exp\left(\frac{\mu-x}{2\sigma^2}\right) \quad \text{for } -\infty < x < \infty, \tag{9.14}$$

where μ is the mean and σ is the standard deviation.

Pareto Distribution The Pareto distribution is commonly used in a monitoring production processesor. The Pareto distribution can be used to model the length of wire between successive flaws. The *standard Pareto distribution* is defined as

$$f(x) = \frac{c}{x^{c+1}} \qquad \text{for } 1 \le x \quad \text{and} \quad c \ge 1, \tag{9.15}$$

where c is the shape parameter.

Poisson Distribution The Poisson distribution is also sometimes referred to as the *distribution of rare events*. Examples of Poisson-distributed variables are number of accidents per person, number of sweepstakes won per person, or the number of catastrophic defects found in a production process. The *Poisson distribution* is defined as

$$f(x) = \frac{\lambda^x e^{-\lambda}}{x!}, \qquad x = 0, 1, \ldots, \quad \text{and} \quad \lambda > 0, \tag{9.16}$$

where λ is the expected value of x (the mean).

Rayleigh Distribution If two independent variables y_1 and y_2 are independent of each other and normally distributed with equal variance, the variable $x = \sqrt{(y_1^2 + y_2^2)}$ will follow the Rayleigh distribution. Thus, an example (and appropriate metaphor) for such a variable would be the distance of darts from the target in a dart-throwing game, where the errors in the two dimensions of the target plane are independent and normally distributed. The *Rayleigh distribution* is defined as

$$f(x) = \frac{x}{b^2} \exp\left(-\frac{x^2}{2b^2}\right) \qquad \text{for } 0 \le x \quad \text{and} \quad b > 0, \tag{9.17}$$

where b is a scale parameter.

Rectangular Distribution The *rectangular distribution* is useful to describe random variables with a constant probability density over the defined range $a < b$:

$$f(x) = \frac{1}{b-a} \qquad \text{for } a < x < b; \text{ otherwise, } 0. \tag{9.18}$$

Student's t Distribution Student's t distribution is symmetric about zero, and its general shape is similar to that of the standard normal distribution. It is most commonly used in testing hypothesis about the mean of a particular population. *Student's t distribution* is defined as (for $n = 1, 2, \ldots$)

$$f(x) = \frac{\Gamma((v+1)/2)\sqrt{v\pi}}{\Gamma(v/2)}\left[1+\left(\frac{x^2}{v}\right)^{-(v+1)/2}\right] \tag{9.19}$$

where v is a shape parameter (degrees of freedom) and Γ is the gamma function.

Weibull Distribution As described earlier, the exponential distribution is often used as a model of time-to-failure measurements, when the failure (hazard) rate is constant over time. When the failure probability varies over time, the Weibull distribution is appropriate. Thus, the Weibull distribution is often used in reliability testing (e.g., of electronic relays, ball bearings, etc.; see Hahn and Shapiro, 1967). The *Weibull distribution* is defined as

$$f(x) = \frac{c}{b}\left(\frac{x}{b}\right)^{c-1} \exp\left(-\frac{x^c}{b^c}\right) \quad \text{for } 0 \geq x, \quad b > 0 \quad \text{and} \quad c > 0, \tag{9.20}$$

where b is a scale parameter and c is a shape parameter.

9.2 VIRTUAL TRIAL DATA GENERATION USING EXPDESIGN RANDOMIZOR

9.2.1 Random Number Generation Using ExpDesign

The randomizor in ExpDesign Studio can generate random numbers with the following distributions: Bernoulli, beta, binomial, Cauchy, chi-square, exponential, gamma, geometric, half-normal, hypergeometric, inverse Gaussian, laplace, lognormal, multinormal, negative binomial, Pareto, Pascal, Poisson, Rayleigh, Snedecor-F, standard normal, Student's-t, Uniform(0,1), Weibull.

To generate a uniformly distributed random number between 0 and 1, click 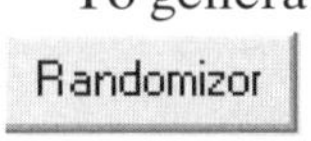

in the **ExpDesign Studio** window; then click 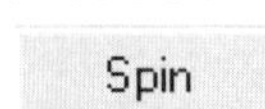

.

9.2.2 How to Generate a Random Univariate Using ExpDesign

To generate 40 random numbers with a standard normal distribution, enter "40" for **Number of random variables to be generated** and click 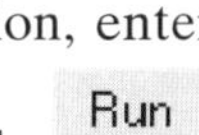

(Figure 9.1). The random numbers generated can be reviewed by clicking 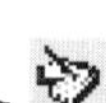 on the toolbar (Figure 9.2).

To generate five random numbers with the exponential distribution and sort them, select **Exp** in the **Distributions** box.

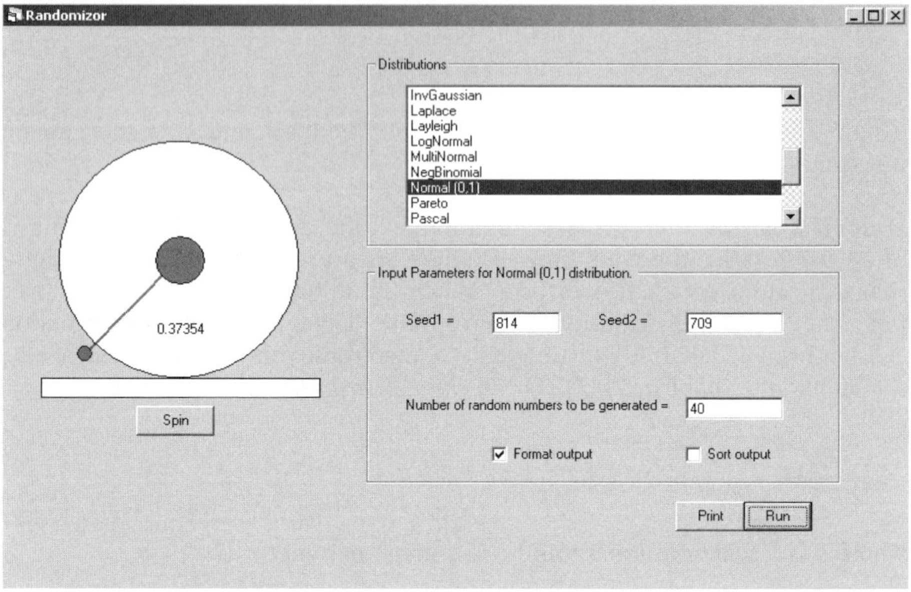

Figure 9.1 *N*(0,1) random number generation.

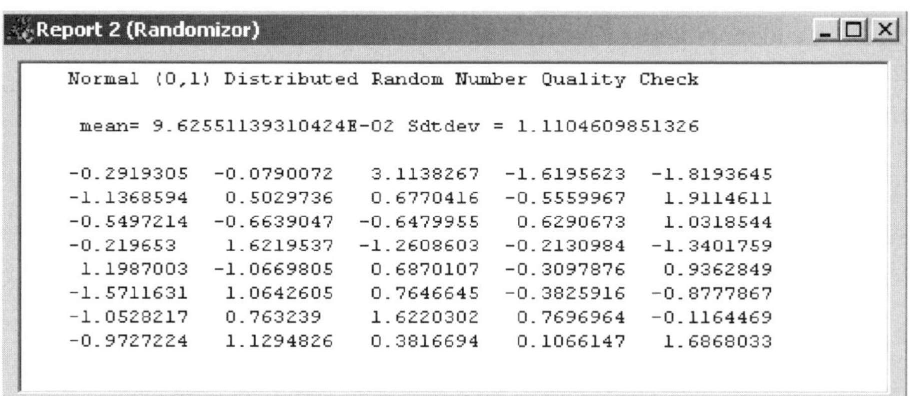

Figure 9.2 Random number generated using ExpDesign.

- Enter "5" for **Number of random variables to be generated**.
- Check the **Sort output** box.
- Click 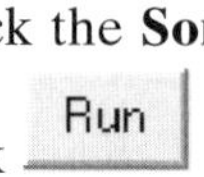

and the random numbers generated can be reviewed by clicking 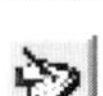 on the toolbar (Figures 9.3 and 9.4).

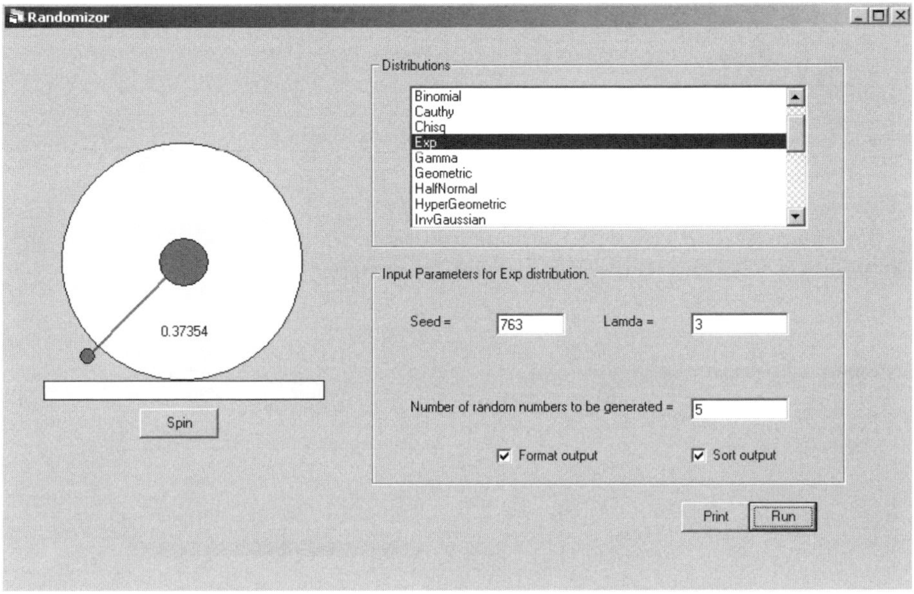

Figure 9.3 Exponential random number generation.

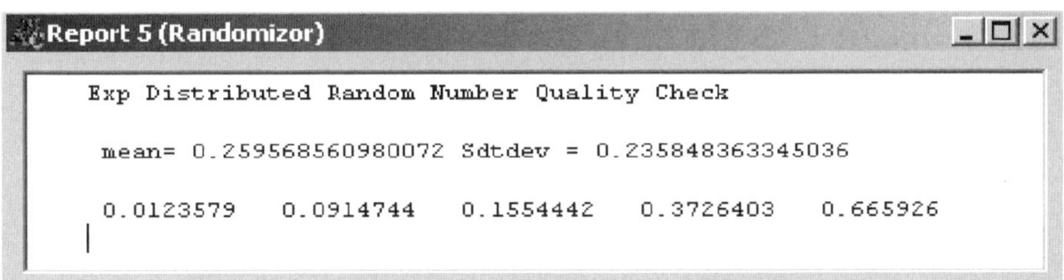

Figure 9.4 Exponential random number output.

9.2.3 How to Generate a Random Multivariate Using ExpDesign

To generate five rows of random numbers x_1, x_2, . . . of multivariate normal distribution with mean {0,0} and the following correlation matrix:

1	0.3
0.3	1

- Click 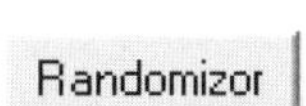

, then select **MultiNormal**.
- Enter “2” for **No. of Vars**.
- Enter “1, 0.3, 0.3, 1” for **Corr. Coef**.

- Enter "5" for **Number of random numbers to be generated**.
- Click Run.
- The random numbers generated can be reviewed by clicking 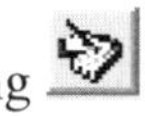 on the toolbar (Figures 9.5 and 9.6).

To generate five rows of random numbers x_1, x_2, . . . multivariate normal distribution with the following correlation matrix:

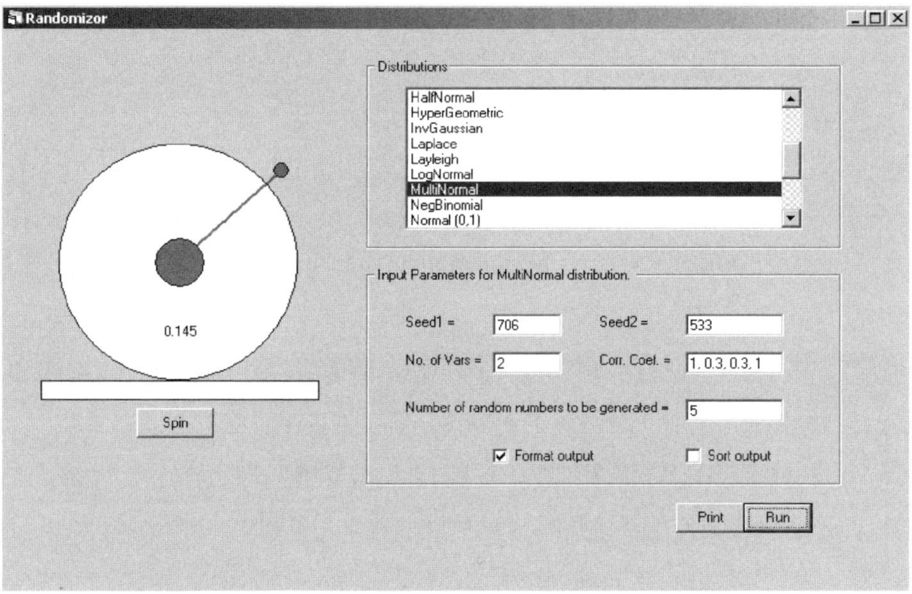

Figure 9.5 Multivariate random number generation.

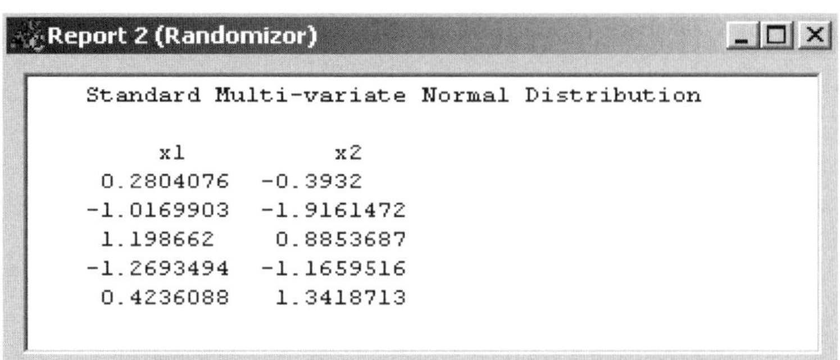

Figure 9.6 Multivariate normal random numbers.

1	0.5	0.5
0.5	1	0.5
0.5	0.5	1

- Select **MultiNormal** in the **Distributions** box.
- Enter "3" for **No. of Vars**.
- Enter "1, 0.5, 0.5, 0.5, 1, 0.5, 0.5, 0.5, 1" for **Corr. Coef**.
- Enter "5" for **Number of random variables to be generated**.
- Click 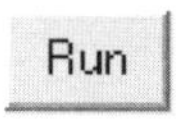.
- The random numbers generated can be reviewed by clicking  on the toolbar (Figures 9.6 and 9.7).

9.2.4 How to Generate a Random Multibinomial Using ExpDesign

To generate five rows of random numbers $x_1, x_2, \ldots,$ of multibinomial distribution with marginal proportion {0.4,0.5} and the following correlation matrix:

1	0.3
0.3	1

- Click 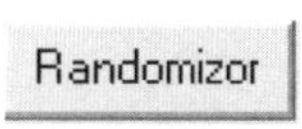 and the select **MultiBinomial**.
- Enter "2" for **No. of Vars**.
- Enter "0.4, 0.5" for the proportions.
- Enter "1, 0.3, 0.3, 1" for **Corr. Coef**.
- Enter "5" for **Number of random variables to be generated**.
- Click 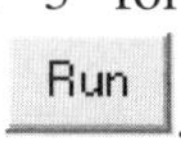.

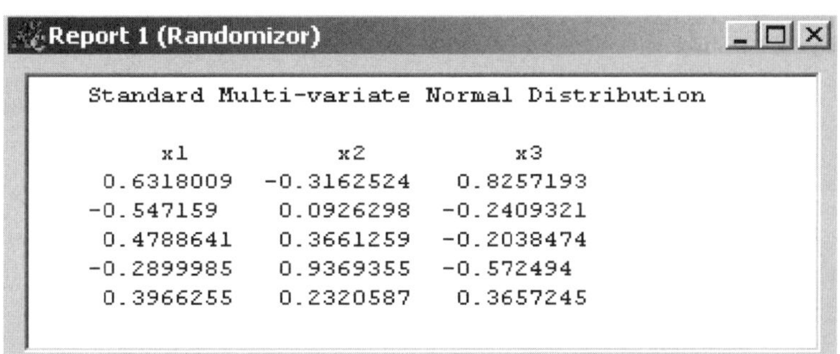

Figure 9.7 Three-variate normal distributions.

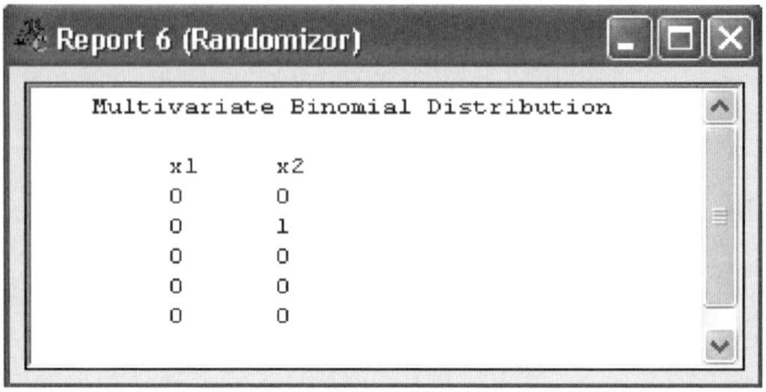

Figure 9.8 Two-variate binomial random numbers.

- The random numbers generated can be reviewed by clicking 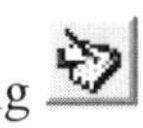 on the toolbar (Figures 9.8 and 9.9).

To generate five rows of random numbers $x_1, x_2, \ldots,$ of multibinomial distribution with marginal proportion {0.4, 0.5, 0.35} and the following correlation matrix:

1	0.3	0.3
0.3	1	0.3
0.3	0.3	1

- Click 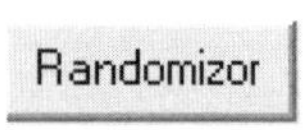 and then select **MultiBinomial**.
- Enter “3” for **No. of Vars**.
- Enter “0.4, 0.5, 0.35” for the **proportions**.
- Enter “1, 0.3, 0.3, 0.3, 1, 0.3, 0.3, 0.3, 1” for **Corr. Coef**.
- Enter “5” for **Number of random variables to be generated**.
- Click 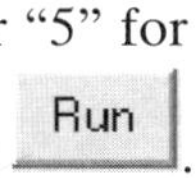.
- The random numbers generated can be reviewed by clicking  on the toolbar (Figure 9.9).

9.3 EXPDESIGN TOOLKITS

ExpDesign Studio toolkits include four tools: **Graphic calculator, statistical calculator, Confidence interval calculator,** and **show tip of day** (Figure 9.10). The toolkits can be accessed through the **Tools** menu or the icons on the

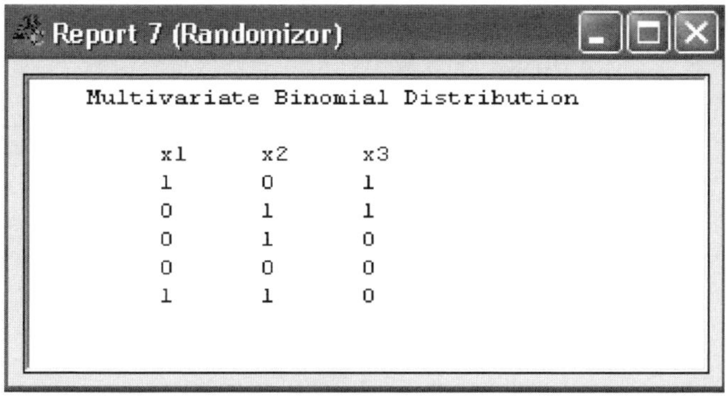

Figure 9.9 Three-variate binomial random numbers.

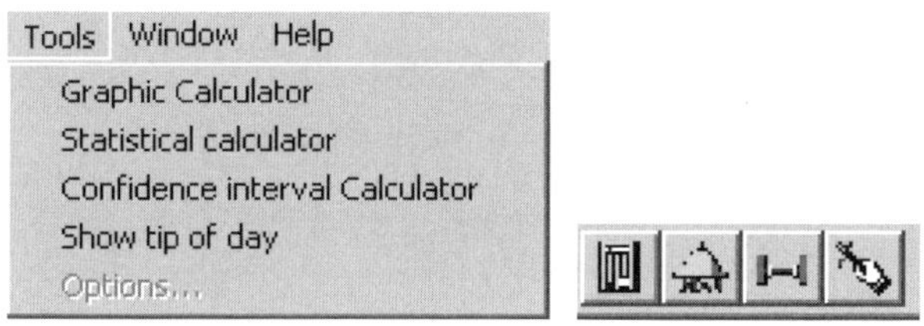

Figure 9.10 Menu and toolbar for expdesign toolkits.

toolbar. The tip text for each icon will indicate which icon is for which tool when you move the mouse over an icon (Figure 9.10).

9.3.1 Graphic Calculator

You can use the graphic calculator as a scientific calculator, a function plotter, or a data graphic tool.

To use as a scientific calculator:

- Click the icon for **Graphic Calculator** 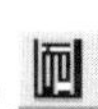.
- Enter functions and values to form a expression.
- Click **Compute** to obtain the desired output.

To use as function plotter:

- Click the icon for **Graphic Calculator** 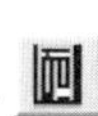.
- Choose **Function Plot** from the **Option** menu.
- Enter an expression in the textbox (the independent variable must be *x*).

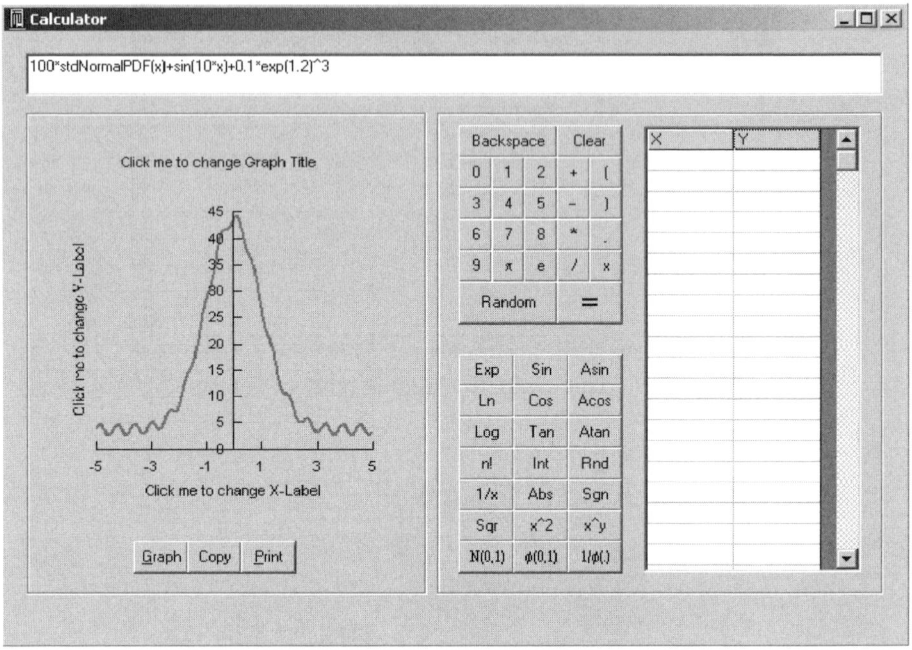

Figure 9.11 ExpDesign graphics calculator.

- Click **Graph** to plot the expression.
- Copy the graph by clicking the **Graph** button and paste into other application software such as MS Word using the **Paste** or **Paste-Special** method.
- Click Print to print the result (Figure 9.11).

To use as a data graphic tool:

- Choose the icon for **Graphic Calculator**.
- Enter data for x and y in the two columns in the spreadsheet. Click **Graph** to plot.
- You can change the title, axis labels, and ranges for the axis by clicking the corresponding area and entering the desired text in the textboxes that appear, then press the **Enter** key.
- Copy the graph by clicking the **Copy** button and paste into an application software such as MS Word using the **Paste** or **Paste-Special** method.
- Click Print to print the result.

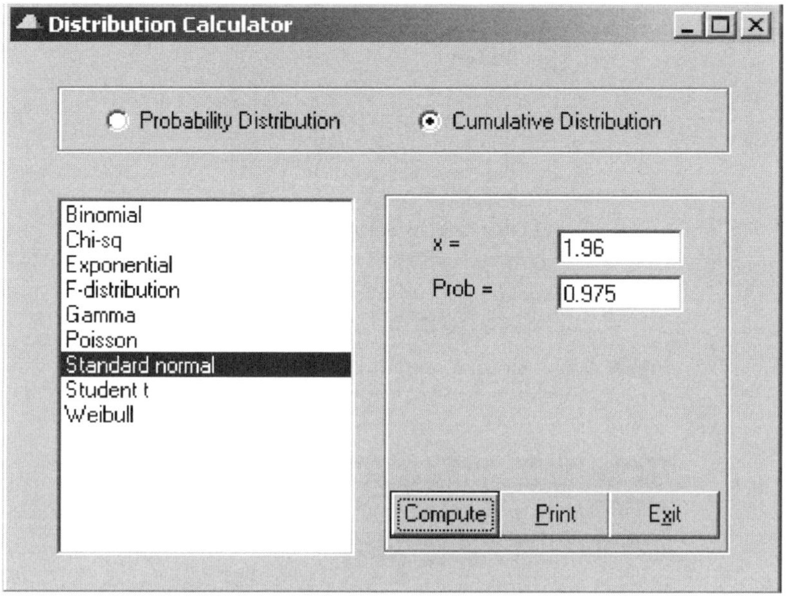

Figure 9.12 ExpDesign distribution calculator.

9.3.2 Statistical Calculator

The statistical calculator allows users to calculate the probability density, probabilities, and inverse probability functions for the following probability distributions: binomial, chi-square, exponential, gamma, Poisson, Suedecor-*F*, standard normal, Student's-t, and Weibull.

- Select the option for **Probability distribution** or **Cumulative distribution**.
- Select a probability distribution from the list.
- Enter appropriate values for the model parameters.
- Click 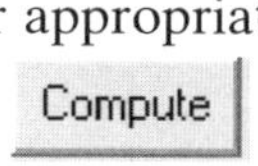 to obtain the desired output.
- Print the output by clicking 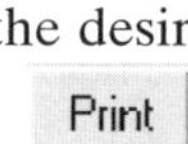 (Figure 9.12).

9.3.3 Confidence Interval Calculator

The confidence interval (CI) calculator allows users to calculate the following confidence intervals: one proportion exact CI, one proportion CI using normal approximation, one mean CI using the *t*-distribution, one mean CI using the normal approximation, two-proportion CI using the *t*-distribution, two-mean CI using the *t*-distribution, two-mean CI using the normal distribution, and CI for a one- or two-variance ratio using the *F*-distribution (Figure 9.13).

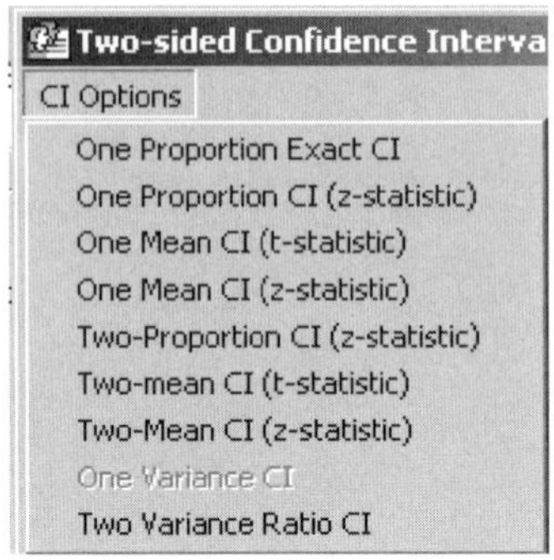

Figure 9.13 Confidence interval calculator options.

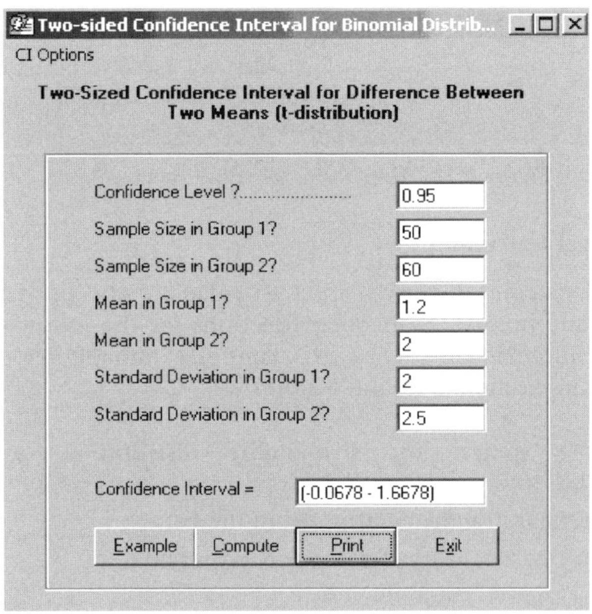

Figure 9.14 ExpDesign confidence interval calculator.

- Click the CI icon 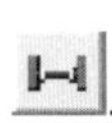.
- Choose the method desired for **CI Options.**
- Enter appropriate values for the model parameters.
- Click Compute to obtain the confidence interval.
- Click Print to print the result (Figure 9.14).

10 Classical Design Method Reference

10.1 SINGLE-GROUP DESIGN

10.1.1 One/Paired-Sample Hypothesis Test for the Mean

Sign Test for Median Difference for a Paired Sample
Objective: To calculate sample size based on the sign test for the difference between the medians of two distributions.

Technical Notes This formula for sample-size calculation is given by Noether (1987) under the assumption of a large sample. The sign test requires that observations in the two samples be taken in pairs, one from each distribution. Each observation should be taken under the same conditions, but it is not necessary for different pairs to be taken under similar conditions.

Wilcoxon Signed-Rank Test for One or a Paired Sample
Objective: To calculate sample size based on the Wilcoxon signed-rank test for the mean or median of a population, without requiring normality.

Technical Notes This formula for sample-size calculation is given by Noether (1987) under the assumption of a large sample. The Wilcoxon signed-rank test is a distribution-free test and requires a symmetrical population. The observations must be obtained randomly and independently.

Test for H_0: (u_0, σ_0) Versus H_a: (u_a, σ_a)—Large Sample
Objective: To calculate sample size based on a z-test for one sample mean with H_0: u_0 versus H_a: u_a, where u_a is a value that the research is interested in and u_0 is a value that the research is not interested in.

Technical Notes The formula is accurate if the population is normally distributed; otherwise, the sample size must be large (e.g., $n > 30$) (Lachin, 1981).

Classical and Adaptive Clinical Trial Designs Using ExpDesign Studio™,
By Mark Chang

One-Sample t-Test

Objective: To calculate sample size based on a one-sample *t*-test for the difference between an assumed population mean u_0 and a sample mean u_a.

Technical Notes This method for calculating the sample size is an exact method for a one-sample *t*-test. It is computed using a noncentral *t*-distribution with $n - 1$ degrees of freedom, and the noncentrality parameter is the square root of n times $(u_0 - u_a)/s$, where s is the standard deviation and n is the sample size (Devore, 1991).

One-Sample t-Test: Finite Population

Objective: To calculate sample size based on a one-sample *t*-test for the difference between an assumed population mean u_0 and a sample mean u_a. The population size is limited.

Technical Notes This method of calculating the sample size is an exact method for a one-sample *t*-test. It is first computed using a noncentral *t*-distribution with $n - 1$ degrees of freedom, and the noncentrality parameter is the square root of n times $(u_0 - u_a)/s/(1 - n/N)$, where s is the standard deviation, n is the sample size, and N is the population size. The resulting sample size is then adjusted for finite sample size (Devore, 1991).

Paired-Sample t-Test

Objective: To calculate sample size based on the paired-sample *t*-test for the difference between an assumed population mean u_0 and a sample mean u_a. A paired-sample *t*-test is often used to determine if a mean response changes under different experimental conditions using paired observations, such as pre- and post- study measurements.

Technical Notes This method for calculating the sample size is an exact method for a paired-sample *t*-test. It is computed using a noncentral *t*-distribution with $n - 1$ degrees of freedom and the noncentrality parameter square root of n times $(u_0 - u_a)/s$, where s is standard deviation and n is the sample size (Devore, 1991).

One-Way Repeated Measures ANOVA

Objective: To calculate sample size for testing constant correlation based on a one-way repeated measures ANOVA.

Technical Notes Sample size is computed using central and noncentral *F*. The numerator and denominator degrees of freedom are $(M - 1)$ and $(M - 1)(n - 1)$, and the noncentrality parameter is nM times the effect size, δ. $\delta = V/[S^2(1 - r)]$, where the variance of means $V = \Sigma\,(u_i - u)^2/k$, k is the number of levels, S is the common standard deviation at each level, and r is the correlation between levels.

One-Sample Multiple Test for Zero Means
Objective: To calculate sample size based on a one-sample multiple test for zero means.

Technical Notes The sample-size formula is given by Odeh and Fox (1991) for the three main effects based on a noncentral F-distribution. The numerator and denominator degrees of freedom are $m - 1$ and $N - m$, respectively.

10.1.2 One/Paired-Sample Hypothesis Test for Proportion

One-Sample Exact Test for Proportion Using Binomial Distribution
Objective: To calculate sample size based on a one-sample exact test for proportion using binomial distribution.

Technical Notes Sample size is calculated using cumulative binomial distribution (Devore, 1991). The critical point for rejecting the null hypothesis is calculated as the largest k for which the probability of observing k or fewer responses is less than α when $p = p_0$ for a one-sided test with H_0: $p_a < p_0$. For a one-sided test with H_0: $p_a > p_0$, the smallest k is chosen for which the probability of observing k or more successes is $\leq\alpha$. For a two-sided test, both probabilities are required to be less than or equal to $\alpha/2$. Because of the discrete nature of the binomial distribution, power is not a monotonic function of sample size. Therefore, a small sample-size increase may result in a decrease in power. The sample size provided by this software ensures that a sample size beyond this size will not reduce the power.

McNemar's Test for a Paired Sample
Objective: To calculate sample size based on McNemar's test for the equality of binary response rates from two populations, where the data consist of paired dependent responses, one from each population.

Technical Notes This sample-size formula is given by Miettinen (1968) based on McNemar's test, which is identical to the binomial test using a normal approximation. It should be used only when normality is met. That is, $C_{12}C_{12} \geq C_{21}(4 - C_{12})$ and $C_{21}C_{21} \geq C_{12}(4 - C_{21})$, where C_{ij} is the cell frequency in a 2×2 table.

Chi-Square Test for One Sample Proportion
Objective: To calculate sample size based on the chi-square test for one sample proportion.

Technical Notes This method is only applicable to a large sample due to the normality approximation. The sample size for the one-sided test is calculated using the following formula: $n = (z_{1-\alpha}d_0 + z_{1-\beta}d_1)^2/(p_0 - p_1)^2$, where

$d_i = [p_i\,(1 - p_i)]^{0.5}$ and p_i is the proportion. For a two-sided test, replace the α in the equation by $\alpha/2$ (Devore, 1991).

Chi-Square Test for One Sample Proportion: Finite Population

Objective: To calculate sample size based on the chi-square test for one-sample proportion with finite population adjustment.

Technical Notes This method is only applicable to a large sample due to the normality approximation. The unadjusted sample size for the one-sided test is calculated using the following formula: $n = (z_{1-\alpha}\,d_0 + z_{1-\beta}\,d_1)^2/(p_0 - p_1)^2$, where $d_i = [p_i\,(1 - p_i)]^{0.5}$ and p_i is the proportion. For a two-sided test, replace the α in the equation by $\alpha/2$. To adjust for finite population size N, use a factor of $n/(n + N)$. That is, the adjusted sample size will be $nN/(n + N)$ (see Devore, 1991).

10.1.3 One/Paired-Sample Hypothesis Test for Others

Test for Bloch–Kraemer Intraclass κ Coefficient

Objective: To calculate sample size based on the test for Bloch–Kraemer intraclass κ coefficient for binary outcomes.

Technical Notes The sample size is calculated based on the formula $n = [(z_{1-\alpha} + z_{1-\beta})/(Z_0 - Z)]^2\,V_z$, where Z is the z-transform of the κ coefficient, and V_z is the variance of Z. The κ coefficient = (variance of p)/[$p(1 - p)$], and p is the proportion of response (Bloch and Kraemer, 1989).

Test for Bloch–Kraemer Intraclass κ Using z-Transformation

Objective: To calculate sample size based on the test for the Bloch–Kraemer intraclass κ coefficient (binary outcome) with Kraemer's Z-transformation.

Technical Notes The sample size is calculated based on the formula $n = (z_{1-\alpha}/w)^2 V_k$, where the variance of the κ coefficient $V_k = (1 - \kappa)\{(1 - \kappa)(1 - 2\kappa) + \kappa(2 - \kappa)/[2p(1 - p)]\}$, the kappa coefficient = (variance of p)/[$p(1 - p)$], and p is the proportion of response. It is assumed that κ is normally distributed. This assumption may not hold in some situations; therefore, it is better to use the z-transform (Bloch and Kraemer, 1989).

Test H_0: Correlation = Zero Using Fisher's Arctan Transformation

Objective: To calculate sample size based on a test for single correlation.

Technical Notes The formula is developed using Fisher's arctanh transformation: $Z(r) = 0.5\ln[(1 + r)/(1 - r)]$, where r is the sample correlation. $Z(r)$ is normally distributed with mean $Z(r_0)$ and variance $1/(N - 3)$, where r_0 is the true correlation and N is the sample size (Lachin, 1981).

Test H_0: Regression Coefficient = Zero Using Arctan Transformation
Objective: To calculate sample size based on a test for the regression coefficient.

Technical Notes The formula is developed using Fisher's arctanh transformation: $Z(r) = 0.5 \ln[(1 + r)/(1 - r)]$, where r is a sample regression coefficient. $Z(r)$ is normally distributed with mean $Z(r_0)$ and variance $1/(N - 3)$, where r_0 is the true regression coefficient and N is the sample size (Lachin, 1981).

Logistic Regression on x for a Binary Outcome
Objective: To calculate sample size based on logistic regression on a single variable x for binary outcomes.

Technical Notes Logistic regression is commonly used in the analysis of epidemiologic data to examine the relationship between possible risk factors and a disease. In follow-up studies the proportion of persons with the disease (event) is usually low, but it is higher in case–control studies. The method was developed by Whitehead (1993) using the normal approximation. He has found the sample size required to be very sensitive to the distribution of covariates. The sample size is given by $N = [z_{1-\alpha} + \exp(-Q^2/4)z_{1-\beta}]^2(1 + 2P\delta)/(PQ^2)$, where P is the proportion at the mean of the covariate and $\delta = [1 + (1 + Q^2) \exp(5Q^2/4)]/[1 + \exp(-Q^2/4)]$ (see Hsieh, 1989).

Logistic Regression on x for a Binary Outcome with Covariates
Objective: To calculate sample size based on logistic regression on covariates for binary outcomes.

Technical Notes Similar to the preceding method, this method was also developed by Whitehead (1993) using the normal approximation. He has found the required sample size to be very sensitive to the distribution of covariates. The sample size is given by $N = [z_{1-\alpha} + \exp(-Q^2/4)z_{1-\beta}]^2(1 + 2P\delta)/(PQ^2)/(1 - r^2)$, where P is proportional to the mean of the covariate, Q is the log odds ratio, $\delta = [1 + (1 + Q^2) \exp(5Q^2/4)]/[1 + \exp(-Q^2/4)]$, and r is the correlation of x with the covariates included (Hsieh, 1989).

Linear Regression; Test for H_0: Correlation Coefficient = 0
Objective: To calculate sample size based on linear regression (test for null hypothesis H_0: correlation coefficient = 0).

Technical Notes The sample size is computed using the noncentral F-distribution with numerator and denominator degrees of freedom 1 and $n - 2$. The noncentrality parameter is $nr^2/(1 - r^2)$, where r is a correlation coefficient (Cohen, 1988).

Multiple Linear Regression; Test for H_0: Multiple Correlation $R = 0$

Objective: To calculate sample size based on multiple linear regression (test for H_0: multiple correlation $R = 0$).

Technical Notes The sample size is computed using noncentral F-distribution with numerator and denominator degrees of freedom k and $n - k - 1$. The noncentrality parameter is $nr^2/(1 - r^2)$, where r is a correlation coefficient (Cohen, 1988).

Multiple Regression; Test, Zero Increase in R^2 Due to Extra b Covariates

Objective: To calculate sample size based on multiple regression to test for the significance of the effect of additional covariates.

Technical Notes The sample size is computed using the noncentral F-distribution with numerator and denominator degrees of freedom b and $n - a - b - 1$, where a is the number of covariantes for the prior model. The noncentrality parameter is $n(R_{ab}^2 - R_a)/(1 - R_{ab}^2)$, where R_a and R_{ab} are the correlation coefficients for the prior and the larger models (Cohen, 1988).

Linear Regression $y = a + bx$; Test H_0: $b = b_0$

Objective: To calculate sample size based on linear regression: $y = a + bx$ (test H_0: $b = b_0$, vs. H_a: $b \neq b_0$).

Technical Notes The sample size is calculated based on noncentral t, with $n - 2$ degrees of freedom. The noncentrality parameter is $\sqrt{n}\ |b - b_0|\ S/S_e$, where S is the standard deviation of x and S_e is the standard deviation of error.

Kendall's Test of Independence

Objective: To calculate sample size based on Kendall's test for independence between two series of observations obtained in pairs.

Technical Notes This formula was introduced by Noether (1987) under the assumption of a large sample. Kendall's test requires the two population distributions to be continuous and the observations x_i and y_i to have been obtained in pairs (Noether, 1987).

10.1.4 Paired-Sample Equivalence Test for the Mean

Paired t-Test for Equivalence of Means

Objective: To calculate sample size based on the paired t-test for equivalence of means.

Technical Notes This is an exact method. The sample size is computed using noncentral t-distribution with the degree of freedom and the noncentrality parameter the square root of n times $(u_0 - u_a)/s$, where s is the standard deviation and n is the sample size (Chow and Liu, 1998).

10.1.5 Paired-Sample Equivalence Test for Proportion

Paired Response: Equivalence of p_1 and p_2 (Large Sample)
Objective: To calculate sample size based on the equivalence of the paired proportion.

Technical Notes The sample size (number of pairs) is calculated using the formula $n = v\,(z_{1-\alpha} - z_{1-\beta})^2/(\delta_0 - \delta_1)^2$, where $v = \max[p_0(1 - p_0), p_1(1 - p_1)]$; δ_0 and δ_1 are the allowable difference in proportion and the expected difference in proportion, respectively. This formula can be derived from the Mukuch–Simon method for a two-sample equivalence problem, noting that variance for a one-sample problem is half of the variance for the two-sample problem. This method is only applicable for a large sample, due to the normal approximation (Makuch and Simon, 1978).

10.1.6 One-Sample Confidence Interval for the Mean

One-Sample Mean Confidence Interval Method
Objective: To calculate sample size based on precision analysis of a one-sample problem.

Technical Notes Precision analysis for the sample size is based on a confidence interval. The maximum half-width of the $(1 - \alpha)100\%$ confidence interval is usually referred to as the maximum error of an estimate of unknown parameter. The precision method requires one to specify the maximum error allowed. The formula to calculate sample size is $n = (z_{\alpha/2})^2V/E^2$, where V is the sample variance and E is the maximum error that we are willing to accept. Note that the precision method is based on the confidence interval corresponding to the hypothesis method with 50% power. Hence, the sample-size formula does not include the term power (Chow and Liu, 1998).

One-Sample Mean Confidence Interval Method: Finite Population
Objective: To calculate sample size based on precision analysis for a one-sample problem adjusted for finite population size.

Technical Notes The sample-size calculation is similar to preceding one, but adjusted for the finite population. The precision method requires one to specify the maximum error allowed. The formula to calculate sample size is $n = z_{1-\alpha/2}^2 V(1 - n/N)/E^2$, where N is the population size, V is the sample variance, and E is the maximum error that we are willing to accept (Chow and Liu, 1998).

Paired-Sample Mean Confidence Interval Method: Large Sample
Objective: To calculate sample size based on precision analysis for a paired-sample problem.

Technical Notes The formula to calculate sample size is $n = z_{1-\alpha/2}^2 V/E^2$, where V is the sample variance and E is the maximum error that we are willing to accept (Chow and Liu, 1998).

Paired-Sample Mean Confidence Interval Method: Finite Population
Objective: To calculate sample size based on precision analysis for a one-sample problem adjusted for finite population size N.

Technical Notes The sample-size determination is based on the confidence interval width. It requires that the maximum error rate available be specified. The formula to calculate the sample size is $n = z_{1-\alpha/2}^2 V(1-n/N)/E^2$, where N is the population size, V is the sample variance, and E is the maximum error that we are willing to accept (Chow and Liu, 1998).

Confidence Interval for Repeated Measures Contrast
Objective: To calculate sample size based on the confidence interval for repeated measures contrast.

Technical Notes Normality assumption is used in the sample-size calculation. The sample size is given by $N = z_{1-\alpha}^2 S^2(1-r)D^2/w^2$, where S is the standard deviation, r is the correlation coefficient, w is the 0.5 interval width (Devore, 1991).

One-Sample Confidence Interval for a Mean Based on the t-Statistic
Objective: To calculate sample size based on precision analysis for a one-sample problem adjusted for finite sample size N.

Technical Notes The method allows one to specify the coverage probability for the confidence interval. When the coverage probability = 0.5, the resulting sample size is consistent with that obtained from the common precision method (Chow and Liu, 1998).

Paired Mean Confidence Interval Based on the t-Statistic
Objective: To calculate sample size based on precision analysis for a paired-sample problem adjusted for finite sample size N.

Technical Notes The method allows one to specify the coverage probability for the confidence interval. When specifying the coverage probability as 0.5, the resulting sample size is consistent with that obtained from the common precision method (Chow and Liu, 1998).

10.1.7 One-Sample Confidence Interval for Proportion

Confidence Interval for a Proportion: Large n
Objective: To calculate sample size based on the confidence interval for a one-sample proportion.

Technical Notes The sample-size formula is developed using the normal approximation to the binomial distribution [i.e., the sample size $n = p(1 - p)(z_{1-\alpha}/w)^2$ for the one-sided confidence interval]. For the two-sided test, replace α in the formula by $\alpha/2$. Note that the confidence interval method has only 50% coverage probability or power (Devore, 1991).

Confidence Interval for an Odds Ratio for Paired Proportions: Large n
Objective: To calculate sample size based on the confidence interval for the odds ratio in a matched case–control study.

Technical Notes O'Neill (1984) proposed confidence estimation of the odds ratio as a basis for sample-size determination in unmatched design. Using findings of Breslow (1981) and Smith et al. (1985, Eq. 8) developed a sample-size calculation based on the confidence interval odds ratio in a matched case–control study as follows: The sample size in number of pairs for a one-sided test is given by $n = (z_{1-\alpha}/w)^2(1 + 1/\mathrm{OR})/p_{01}$, where OR is the expected odds ratio (the proportion expected in an experimental group divided by the proportion expected in the control group), and p_{01} is the proportion in the control group. Note that the sample size obtained from this formula is very sensitive to the estimation of the proportion in the control group; therefore, a trial designer should make a great effort to get the best estimate of the proportion.

Confidence Interval for Proportion: Finite Population
Objective: To calculate sample size based on the confidence interval for one sample, with adjustment for finite sample size.

Technical Notes The sample-size formula is applicable to a large sample only because it is developed using the normal approximation to the binomial distribution. The unadjusted sample size is given by $n = p(1-p)(z_{1-\alpha/2}^2/w)^2$ for a one-sided confidence interval. The adjusted sample size $n_{\text{adjusted}} = nN/(n + N)$, where N is the population size. For the two-sided test, replace α in the formula by $\alpha/2$ (Devore, 1991).

Confidence Interval for the Probability of Observing a Rare Event
Objective: To calculate sample size based on the probability of observing a rare event.

Technical Notes The sample is calculated using the formula $n = \ln(1 - p)/\ln(1 - p_0)$, where p is the probability of observing one or more events and p_0

is the actual or expected probability of the event. The formula is the direct result of the fact that the probability of observing one or more events, p, is $p = 1 - (1 - p_0)^n$ (see Kanji, 1999).

10.1.8 One-Sample Confidence Interval for Others

Confidence Interval for a Correlation Coefficient

Objective: To calculate sample size based on the confidence interval for a correlation coefficient.

Technical Notes The sample size is computed based on the large-sample normal approximation using Fisher's z-transformation. The sample size is given by $n = (z_{1-\alpha/2} + z_{1-\beta})^2/[\mathrm{FZ}(r_1 - FZ(r_0)]^2 + 3$, where FZ(·) denotes Fisher's z-transform (Fisher and Belle, 1993, p. 379), $\mathrm{FZ}(r) = 1/2 \ln[(1 + r)/(1 - r)]$ (see Fisher and Belle, 1993).

Linear Regression y = a + bx, Confidence Interval for b

Objective: To calculate sample size based on the confidence interval for b where b is the coefficient from the linear regression: $y = a + bx$.

Technical Notes The sample size is calculated based on the large-sample normal approximation and given by $n = (z_{1-\alpha/2}S_e/L/S)^2$, where S_e is the standard error, S is the standard deviation of x, and L is the tolerable limit for the confidence interval width.

10.2 TWO-GROUP DESIGN

10.2.1 Two-Sample Hypothesis Test for the Mean

Two-Sample t-Test

Objective: To calculate sample size based on the two-sample t-test for the difference between the means of two independent populations.

Technical Notes The sample size is calculated using noncentral t-distribution with the degree of freedom = $2n - 2$ and the noncentral parameter = $\sqrt{n/2}$ (d/s), where n is the sample size, d is the absolute value of mean difference, and s is the standard deviation (Graybill, 1976).

Mann–Whitney U/Wilcoxon Rank-Sum Test for Two Samples

Objective: To calculate sample size based on the Wilcoxon–Mann–Whitney or Wilcoxon rank-sum test for median difference between two independent samples.

Technical Notes This formula is given by Noether (1987) under the assumption of a large sample. The Wilcoxon–Mann–Whitney test requires that two distributions have the same general shape, but with one shifted relative to the other by a constant amount under the alternative hypothesis: shift alternatives. If one is interested primarily in differences in location between the two distributions, the Wilcoxon test also has the disadvantage of reacting to other differences between the distributions, such as differences in shape. When the assumptions of the two-sample t-test hold, the Wilcoxon test will be slightly less powerful than the two-sample t-test (Noether, 1987).

Two-Sample z-Test: Large Sample or Population Variance Known

Objective: To calculate sample size based on the z-test for mean difference between two treatment groups.

Technical Notes The formula is accurate if the population is normally distributed; otherwise, the sample size must be large (e.g., $n > 30$) (Lachin, 1981).

2 × 2 Crossover Study

Objective: To calculate sample size for a two-treatment, two-sequence, and two-period crossover design.

Technical Notes A crossover design is considered efficient in terms of sample size because each patient receives multiple treatments in sequence (Fleiss, 1986). It also controls intrasubject variability. However, some disadvantages exist. For example, it may require a longer study duration and there may be confounding issues (e.g., you may not be able to differentiate carryover effect and treatment by period effect). The sample size from the 2 × 2 crossover design relates the sample size from the two-group parallel design by the intraclass correlation coefficient R = intersubject variance/total variance. The sample size will decrease by a factor of $1 - R$.

One-Way Repeated Measures ANOVA for Two Groups

Objective: To calculate sample size based on one-way repeated-measures ANOVA for two groups.

Technical Notes Chow and Liu (1998, p. 453) propose this method to compute sample size and power for correlated observations. The sample size is given by the formula $n = (z_{\alpha/2} + z_{\beta})^2 s^2 [1 + (m - 1)r]/[p(1 - p)md^2]$, where r is the within-subject correlation, p is the proportion of subjects in the treatment group, and d is the difference in practical importance (Chow and Liu, 1998).

Test for a Treatment Mean Difference with a 2 × 2 Crossover Design

Objective: To calculate sample size based on a test for treatment mean difference for the 2 × 2 crossover design.

Technical Notes This method is applied to the 2×2 crossover study without consideration of unequal carryover effects (Chow and Liu, 1998).

Two-Sample Multiple Test for Mean Differences
Objective: To calculate sample size based on the two-sample multiple test for zero means.

Technical Notes This sample-size formula is developed by Odeh and Fox (1991) for the three main effects based on a noncentral F-distribution. The numerator and denominator degrees of freedom are $m - 1$ and $N - m$, respectively, where m is the number of tests and N is the sample size (Odeh and Fox, 1991).

Comparing DNA Expression Profiles Among Predefined Classes
Objective: To calculate sample size for comparison of expression profiles among predefined classes using DNA microarrays.

Technical Notes DNA microarrays are arrays that provide information about expression levels of thousands of genes simultaneously and are consequently finding wide use in biomedical research. Simon et al. (2002) proposed this method for planning a sample size for testing whether a particular gene is expressed differentially between two predefined classes. This method may be used for two-color arrays using reference designs or for single-label oligonucleotide arrays. Suppose that some function of the expression levels (e.g., log ratios for cDNA arrays) is approximately normally distributed in the two classes. Let σ denote the standard deviation of the expression level among samples within the same classes and suppose that the means of the two classes differ by δ. For example, with base 2 log ratio or log intensities, a value of $\delta = 1$ corresponds to a twofold difference between classes. The total sample size is given by $N = (k + 1)^2/k(z_{\alpha/2} + z_\beta)^2\sigma^2/\delta$. To control the number of false positives, it is suggested that α be $1/n$, where n is the number of genes expressed equally in the two classes. Similarly, the expected number of false-negative conclusions for genes that are actually differentially expressed between the two classes by δ-fold is βm, where m is the number of such genes. If we want the number of false negatives to be F, then $\beta = F/m$. In general, α and β should not exceed 0.001 and 0.05, respectively (Simon et al., 2002).

Donner's Method for Mean Difference Using Cluster Randomization
Objective: To calculate sample size for a trial with cluster randomization.

Technical Notes This method is proposed by Donner et al. (1981) for a cluster randomization trial with normally distributed response.

10.2.2 Two-Sample Hypothesis Test for Proportion

Asymptotic z-Method Considering Variance Difference

Objective: To calculate sample size based on Pearson's chi-square test (without Yates's continuity correction) for the proportion difference in two independent groups.

Technical Notes This formula is developed by Halperin et al. (1968) based on the asymptotic normality of the untransformed binomial proportion. Halperin's method takes into account the different variances associated with two sample proportions. However, it can only be applied in a situation with large sample size, due to the normality assumption. This is not a conservative approach compared to Fisher's exact formula (Sahai and Khurshid, 1996).

Fisher's Exact Test

Objective: To calculate sample size based on Fisher's exact test for the proportion difference between two independent samples.

Technical Notes The p-value for a one-sided test for the null hypothesis H_0: $P_2 - P_1 \le 0$ is given by (Thomas and Conlon, 1992)

$$p = \sum_{i=\max\{0, m_1+m_2-n_2\}}^{m_1} \frac{\binom{n_1}{i}\binom{n_2}{m_1+m_2-i}}{\binom{n_1+n_2}{m_1+m_2}},$$

where m_1 and m_2 are numbers of responders from the groups with sample sizes n_1 and n_2, respectively. Because m_1 and m_2 follow binomial distributions, the power for the Fisher exact test is given by

$$\text{power} = \sum_{m_1=0}^{n_1} \sum_{m_2=0}^{n_2} p\delta_\alpha(p)\text{bn}(n_1, m_1, p_1)\text{bn}(n_2, m_2, p_2),$$

where bn(., .) is a binomial p.d.f.:

$$\delta_\alpha(p) = \begin{cases} 1, & \text{if } p \le \alpha \\ 0, & p > \alpha. \end{cases}$$

Pearson's Chi-Square Test: Kramer–Greenhouse

Objective: To calculate sample size based on Pearson's chi-square test for the proportional difference between two independent samples.

Technical Notes This formula was developed by Casagrande et al. (1978). It provides an excellent approximation to values obtained via Fisher's exact formula (Sahai and Khurshid, 1996).

Whitehead Logistic Model for Two Groups with k Categories

Objective: To calculate sample size based on the proportional odds ratio model with k categories and two treatments.

Technical Notes Many clinical trials yield data on an ordered categorical scale such as *very good, good, moderate*, or *poor*. Under the assumption of proportional odds, such data can be analyzed using techniques of logistic regression. In simple comparisons of two treatments, this approach becomes equivalent to the Mann–Whitney test. Whitehead (1993) derived this method of sample-size calculation for ordered categorical data consistent with an eventual logistic regression analysis. The method is accurate only when it generates moderate to large sample size. The proportional odds model (McCullagh, 1980) is also assumed. That is, the odds ratio between the two treatment groups is constant over all the categories and the common odds ratio. McCullagh studied the effect of the number of categories on sample size and power using computer simulations, and concluded that for $k > 5$, an increased number of categories will not increase the efficiency or reduce the sample size required. The limiting case is approached in a large sample in which a full ranking of patient outcomes is achieved, as envisaged in the Mann–Whitney test. A full ranking is equivalent to a categorization with only one patient in each category. When data are normally distributed, the full Mann–Whitney test is in turn 94% efficient relative to a t-test (Lehmann, 1975). The design based on five equally probable categories is 90% efficient relative to the t-test when data are normally distributed.

The author also studied the influence of prognostic factors. It is well know that adjustment for prognostic factors improves the power of analyses of normally distributed data. For survival data, adjustment has little effect on power (Schoenfeld, 1983). Robinson and Jewell (1991) have pointed out that covariate adjustment in the logistic regression analysis of binary data can lead to an apparent loss of power. Whitehead (1993) further stated that the same is true in the case of ordered categorical data. To preserve power, it will be necessary to increase sample size (Whitehead, 1993).

Lachin's Test for Two Treatments by Three Time-Point Interactions

Objective: To calculate sample size based on a test for treatment by time interaction.

Technical Notes This method was developed by Lachin (1977) for the case of two treatment groups and two time-point repeated measures. For a more general method for an $r \times c$ comparative trial, see Lachin's paper.

Mantel–Haenszel Test for an Odds Ratio with k Strata: Large Sample

Objective: To calculate sample size based on the Mantel–Haenszel test for an odds ratio with k strata.

Technical Notes This formula assumes a constant odds ratio (rather than relative risk) over strata and the random treatment assignment with each stratum. One wishes to compare event rates within each of the resulting 2×2 tables and to obtain an overall comparison to test whether the (assumed) common odds ratio equals unity. The large-sample assumption is used in the formula (Lachin, 1977).

Mantel–Haenszel Test for an Odds Ratio with k Strata: Continuity Correction

Objective: To calculate sample size based on Cochran's test (1954) with the continuity correction and the overall type I error controlled.

Technical Notes Information on a possible confounding effect is important in choosing correctly between a strata-matched or strata-nonmatched design in a case–control study. The Mantel–Haenszel test and Cochran's test are asymptotically equivalent, but the former uses a hypergeometric distribution conditioned on all marginal total fixed, whereas the latter uses a pair of binomials in each stratum. Woolson et al. (1986) present a simple approximation of sample size for Cochran's test for detecting association between exposure and disease. Nam (1992) derives this sample-size formula for Cochran's statistic with continuity correction, which guarantees that the actual type I error rate of the test does not exceed the nominal level. The corrected sample size is necessarily larger than the uncorrected size given by Woolson et al. (1986), and the relative difference between the two sample sizes is considerable. When any effect of stratification is absent, Cochran's stratified test, although valid, is less efficient than the unstratified test, except for the important case of a balanced design (Nam, 1992).

Chi-Square Test for a Two-Sample Proportion with k Categories

Objective: To calculate sample size based on a chi-square test for two-sample proportions with k categories.

Technical Notes This method is only applicable to a large sample. The sample size is calculated using a noncentral chi-square distribution with $k - 1$ degrees of freedom, and Patnaik's parameter of noncentrality $= n \sum (p_{1j} - p_{0j})^2/(p_{1j} + p_{0j})$, where p_{1j} and p_{0j} are the expected proportions in the jth category of the two treatment groups, and the sum is performed over all k categories. Patnaik (1949) developed a method for the asymptotic Pearson chi-square test for goodness of fit with k classes. Before Patnaik, Eisenhart (1938) had presented a more general result for the test with $k - s$ degrees of freedom, where s is the number of parameters of the assumed distribution (Kendall and Stuart, 1967; Lachin, 1977).

Repeated Measures for Two Proportions
Objective: To calculate sample size based on one-way repeated measures ANOVA for two groups.

Technical Notes Chow and Liu (1998) proposed this method to compute sample size and power with correlated observations. The sample size given by $n = (z_{\alpha/2} + z_{\beta})^2 s^2[1 + (m - 1)r]/[p(1 - p)md^2]$, where r is the within-subject correlation, p is the proportion of subjects in the treatment group, s is the standard deviation, and d is the difference of practical importance in the mean. This formula can be applied to the case where two treatments are compared with binary responses, with the following modification (Chow and Liu, 1998):

$$n = \frac{(z_{1-\alpha/2} + z_{1-\beta}^2)^2 s^2[1+(m-1)r][pp_0(1-p_0)+(1-p)p_1(p_1-p_1)]}{p(1-p)m(p_1-p_2)^2}$$

10.2.3 Two-Sample Hypothesis Test for Others

Exponential Survival Distribution with Uniform Patient Enrollment
Objective: To calculate sample size based on a test for the difference in median survival time.

Technical Notes It is not realistic in clinical trials that all patients will be followed to the terminal event no matter how long is required for the last patient to reach that event. A more realistic approach is to follow the trial to termination at time T. This method assumes that patients enter the trial at a uniform rate over the time interval 0 to T and that exponential survival applies. The formula is derived based on exponential survival distribution. If this assumption is seriously violated, the sample size obtained from this formula will not be appropriate. The model may not be very realistic, because as soon as the last patient enters the study, the trial will stop. Also, the assumption of uniform patient enrollment should be checked before the formula is used (Lachin, 1981).

Exponential Survival Distribution with Uniform Enrollment and Follow-up
Objective: To calculate sample size based on a test for the difference in median survival time.

Technical Notes It is desired in a clinical trial to recruit patients for study over the time interval 0 to T_0 and then to follow all recruited patients to the time of the terminal event or to the end of the trial, whichever is shorter. This method assumes that patients enter the trial at a uniform rate over the interval 0 to T_0 and that exponential survival applies. In the event that all patients enter the trial at the same time, T_0 should be set to a very small value (Lachin, 1981).

Test Interaction in a Model with an Exponential Survival Function: Two Strata

Objective: To calculate sample size (number of events) based on a test for the interaction in a model with an exponential survival function.

Technical Notes This formula is applicable to the case with two treatments, two strata, and equal size in each cell of a 2×2 table. The method was developed by Peterson and George (1993). The authors show via simulations that the formula gives valid powers for the test score of the interaction effect available from fitting the proportional hazards model, as long as the proportional hazards model holds. The authors also point out that even moderate interaction effects can have a profound impact on the power of the standard statistical procedure. The assumption of an equal number of failures per cell can be used as long as the sample-size ratio between any two cells does not exceed 2. The authors also give a formula for calculating the sample size for a situation with k strata (Peterson and George, 1993).

Test Interaction in a Model with an Exponential Survival Function: k Strata

Objective: To calculate sample size (number of events) based on a test for interaction in a model with an exponential survival function.

Technical Notes A formula developed by Peterson and George (1993) is applicable to a case with two treatments, k strata, and equal size in each cell of a $2 \times k$ table. The authors show via simulations that the formula gives valid powers for the score test of the interaction effect available from a fitting of the proportional hazards model, as long as the proportional hazards model holds. The authors also point out that even moderate interaction effects can have a profound impact on the power of the standard statistical procedure. Even with the assumption of an equal number of failures per cell, the formulation can still be used as long as the sample-size ratio between any two cells does not exceed 2 (Peterson and George, 1993).

Log-rank Test for Survival Analysis

Objective: To calculate sample size based on the log-rank test for survival analysis.

Technical Notes In practice, methods are sometimes applied even though assumptions are violated or theoretical justification is lacking. It is common to see binomial sample-size calculation when the intended analysis will be a comparison of two survival curves when the exponential or proportional hazards assumption is not realistic. The log-rank statistic can still be used for analysis when, as in many trials, the proportional hazards assumption is violated (Lakatos and Lan, 1992). Lakatos (1988) derives the sample size required for a log-rank statistic in this general case by using a discrete nonstationary Markov process that follows any pattern of survival, noncompliance, loss to follow-up, drop-in, and lag in the effectiveness of treatment during the course of a clinical trial. If the survival distributions are exponential, the proportional hazards assumption is satisfied. It can be shown that after an appropriate time transformation, the converse is true when there is no censoring. Since the log-rank statistic is no longer optimal when the hazards are nonproportional, hazard functions are really known precisely. There are definite risks involved with assuming that one knows a nonproportional hazards alternative and choosing the optimally weighted statistic for the final analysis (Lakatos and Lan, 1992).

Exponential Survival Distribution with a Uniform Patient Enrollment Rate over Time T_0, a Follow-up Period, and Dropouts

Objective: To calculate sample size based on a test for the difference in mean/median survival time for two independent samples with exponential survival distribution and exponential loss to follow-up distribution.

Technical Notes The assumption of exponential survival distribution and exponential loss to follow-up distribution must both be met. Otherwise, the resulting sample size will not be accurate (Lachin and Foulkes, 1986).

Exponential Survival Distribution with a Bernoulli Confounding Variable

Objective: To calculate sample size based on a test for the difference in median survival time between two treatment groups with exponential survival distribution and a dichotomous confounder.

Technical Notes This method was developed by Liu (1992) based on an exponential covariate model. In clinical trials, random assignment of treatments to individuals is generally used to eliminate the effects of confounding variables. When there is censorship in the data, however, confounding effects may not automatically be removed solely by the randomization procedure under the exponential model (Gail et al., 1984). Therefore, in this situation, sample-size calculation without consideration of the confounding effects is not appropriate (Feigl and Zelen, 1965). Unlike other papers describing studies of sample size with the presence of a confounder, in his paper Lui takes into account the distribution of response times and their possible censorship. In the presence of censorship and confounders under an exponential model, the MLE of the treatment effect is asymptotically biased in randomized trials when there is a difference between the two treatment effects under consideration (Feigl and Zelen, 1965).

Testing Two Correlation Coefficients Using Fisher's Arctan Transformation

Objective: To calculate sample size based on a test for two independent correlations.

Technical Notes This formula is developed by using Fisher's arctanh transformation: $Z(r) = 0.5\ln[(1 + r)/(1 - r)]$, where r is a sample correlation. $Z(r)$

is normally distributed with mean $Z(r_0)$ and variance $1/(N-3)$, where r_0 is the true correlation and N is the sample size (Lachin, 1981).

Linear Regression $y_1 = a_1 + b_1$x, $y_2 = a_2 + b_2$x; Test H_o: $b_1 = b_2$
Objective: To calculate sample size based on the hypothesis test H_o: $b_1 = b_2$ versus H_a: $b_1 \neq b_2$, where b_i is the coefficient from the linear regression $y_1 = a_1 + b_1x$, $y_2 = a_2 + b_2x$.

Technical Notes The sample size is calculated based on the noncentral t-distribution with $2n - 4$ degrees of freedom. The noncentrality parameter is $\sqrt{n/2}\,|b-b_0|S|S_e$, where S is the standard deviation of x and S_e is the standard deviation of error.

10.2.4 Two-Sample Equivalence/Noninferiority Test for the Mean

Noninferiority Test for Two Means Based on a One-Sided Two-Sample t-Test
Objective: To calculate sample size for a noninferiority test for mean difference based on a one-sided two-sample t-test.

Technical Notes This method may be used for noninferiority studies but is not appropriate for bioequivalence studies. Chow and Liu (1998) pointed out that the power approach to sample-size determination based on the hypothesis of equality is not statistically valid in assessing equivalence between treatments (refer to Schuirmann, 1987).

Two One-Sided t-Tests for Equivalence: Parallel Design (Bivariate t)
Objective: To calculate sample size based on two one-sided t-tests for an equivalence study with a parallel design.

Technical Notes The sample size is computed based on the bivariate noncentral t-distribution with degrees of freedom $2(n-1)$ and noncentrality parameters $(u_T - u_s - d_L)\sqrt{n/2}\,/\,S$ and $(u_T - u_s - d_U\sqrt{n/2}\,/\,S$, where d_L and d_U are the lower and upper limits for the mean difference between the two groups and S is the common standard deviation (Schuirmann, 1987).

Two One-Sided Tests for Equivalence Based on a Ratio of Means: Parallel Design (Bivariate t)
Objective: To calculate sample size for an equivalence test of two means based on Schuirmann's two one-sided t-tests (Schuirmann, 1987).

Technical Notes This is an exact method based on the bivariate noncentral t-distribution (Owen, 1965). The power approach described in the literature for sample-size determination based on a hypothesis of equality is not statistically valid in assessing equivalence between treatments (Chow and Liu, 1998; Schuirmann, 1987).

Two One-Sided t-Tests for Equivalence Based on a Ratio of Two Means: Crossover Design (Bivariate t)

Objective: To calculate sample size for an equivalence test based on a ratio of two means using Schuirmann's (1987) two one-sided t-tests for a 2×2 crossover study.

Technical Notes This is an exact method based on the bivariate noncentral t-distribution. For the assessment of equivalence between treatments under the standard two-sequence, two-period crossover design, it is suggested that the following interval hypotheses be tested (Owen, 1965; Schuirmann, 1987; Chow and Liu, 1998):

$$H_0: u_T - u_p < Q_L \text{ or } u_T - u_p \geq Q_U \text{ vs. } H_a Q_L < u_T - u_p < Q_U,$$

where u_T and u_p are the two means of the log-transformed data for the two treatment groups, and Q_L and Q_U are some clinically meaningful limits for equivalence. The hypotheses can be decomposed into two sets of one-sided hypotheses:

$$H_0: u_T - u_p \leq Q_L \text{ vs. } H_a: u_T - u_p > Q_L$$
$$H_0: u_T - u_p \geq Q_U \text{ vs. } H_a: u_T - u_p < Q_U.$$

Two One-Sided t-Tests for Equivalence Based on a Mean Ratio for Lognormal Data: Parallel Design (Bivariate t)

Objective: To calculate sample size for an equivalence test for the ratio of two means based on Schuirmann's (1987) two one-sided t-tests for a parallel design.

Technical Notes This is an exact method based on the bivariate noncentral t-distribution (Owen, 1965; Schuirmann, 1987; Chow and Liu, 1998).

Schuirmann–Chow's Two One-Sided t-Tests for Equivalence

Objective: To calculate sample size for an equivalence test for two means based on Chow's approximation to Schuirmann's (1987) two one-sided t-tests.

Technical Notes This sample size is an approximation method developed by Chow and Liu (1998). During the implementation of the method, normal distribution is used in place of a t-distribution in Chow's equation. For exact sample size for the same problem, sample-size calculation for equivalence test for difference of two means should be used based on two one-sided t-tests using bivariate noncentral t-distribution (Owen, 1965; Schuirmann, 1987, Chow and Liu, 1998).

10.2.5 Two-Sample Equivalence/Noninferiority Test for Proportion

Equivalence Test for Two Proportions: Large n

Objective: To calculate sample size based on an equivalent test for two independent proportions.

Technical Notes This method was originally proposed by Farrington and Manning (1990) using the asymptotic approximation. It is applicable only to the large-sample case. Sample size is calculated using the formula $n = (z_{1-\alpha} + z_{1-\beta})^2[p_1(1 - p_1) + p_2(1 - p_2)]/(\delta - \delta_0)^2$, where δ_0 is the allowable difference and δ is the expected difference of proportions p_1 and p_2. However, this method underestimates the sample size when $\delta_0 < \delta$, which is often the case in practice. A better method but a little conservative approach is given by (S. C. Lin, 1995; Chow, Shao and Wang, 2003)

$$n_1 = \frac{(z_{1-\alpha} + z_{1-\beta/2})^2}{(\delta - |\varepsilon|)^2}\left[\frac{p_1(1-p_1)}{r} + p_2(1-p_2)\right],$$

$$n_2 = rn_1.$$

Note that β, not α, is divided by 2 in the formulation (see Farrington and Manning, 1990; S. C. Lin, 1995; Chow et al., 2003).

One-Sided Noninferiority Test for Two Proportions *Objective:* To calculate sample size for a one-sided noninferiority test for two proportions based on a large-sample assumption.

Technical Notes Normal approximation is used in this formula and is applicable only to large sample-size. The sample-size formulation is given by (M. Chang, 2007e; Chow et al., 2003)

$$n_1 = \frac{(z_{1-\alpha} + z_{1-\beta})^2}{(\delta - \varepsilon)^2}\left[\frac{p_1(1-p_1)}{r} + p_2(1-p_2)\right].$$

$$n_2 = rn_1.$$

10.2.6 Two-Sample Equivalence/Noninferiority Test for Survival

Noninferiority Test for Survival with Uniform Accrual and Follow-up

Objective: To calculate sample size for a noninferiority test for survival difference based on normal approximation.

Technical Notes Normal approximation is used in this formula (Chow et al., 2003; M. Chang, 2007e).

Equivalence Test for Survival with Uniform Accrual and Follow-up
Objective: To calculate sample size for an equivalence test for two hazard rate differences based on two one-sided tests.

Technical Notes The sample size is calculated using two one-sided tests based on a large-sample assumption. Normal approximation is used and the equivalent standard deviation can be found (Chang, 2007a; Chow et al., 2003).

10.2.7 Two-Sample Confidence Interval for the Mean

Confidence Interval for Difference of Two Means: Large Sample
Objective: To calculate sample size based on a precision analysis for the mean difference between two independent samples.

Technical Notes A precision analysis for sample size is based on the maximum half-width of the confidence interval that one is willing to accept for the underlying parameter. Therefore, the sample size is independent of power. The sample size given by this formula can be expressed as $n = 2z_{1-\alpha/2}^2 V/E^2$, where V is the sample variance and E is the confidence interval width (Chow and Liu, 1998).

10.2.8 Two-Sample Confidence Interval for Proportion

Confidence Interval for the Difference in Two Proportions: Large n
Objective: To calculate sample size based on the confidence interval for difference in proportions between two samples.

Technical Notes This method is applicable only to large-sample cases, due to a normality approximation. The sample size per group is given by $n = (z_{1-\alpha}/w)^2[p_1(1-p_1) + p_2(1-p_2)]$, where p_i is the expected proportion in the ith treatment group and w is the allowable confidence interval width (Lachin, 1977).

Confidence Interval for Proportional Difference with Minimum Total Size
Objective: To calculate sample size based on the confidence interval for the proportional difference between two groups.

Technical Notes This formula is derived based on Makuch and Simon's method. The minimum sample size is obtained by taking the derivate of the quantity $n_1 + n_2$ with respect to r (Makuch and Simon, 1978).

Confidence Interval for ln(Odds Ratio): Unmatched Case–Control Study
Objective: To calculate sample size based on the confidence interval for a log odds ratio.

Technical Notes Gart and Thomas (1982) compared the performance of three approximate confidence limit methods for an odds ratio: the method proposed by Cornfield (1956), the logit method proposed by Woolf (1955), and the test-based method proposed by Miettinen (1976). Grat and Thomas concluded that Cornfield's method without a continuity correction is the preferred method in the unconditional sample space: that is, the sample space of two independent binomial distributions. Brown (1981) and Gart and Thomas (1972) have shown that Cornfield's method with continuity correction is the preferred method in the conditional space: that is, with all marginal totals fixed. This method was developed by O'Neill (1984) to calculate sample size based on a logit method using an allowable confidence width = $2d$ for the log odds ratio, which, because of symmetry on the log odds ratio scale, allows for an intuitively appealing way of approximating sample sizes needed to achieve a certain fixed level of precision for the log odds ratio. Confidence for the odds ratio is given by $w = \text{OR}[\exp(d) - \exp(-d)]$, where OR is the odds ratio. The sample size for the control is given by $n_0 = \{(1/r/[p_1(1 - p_1)] + 1/[p_0(1 - p_0)]\}(z_{1-\alpha/2}/d)^2$, where r is the sample size ratio n_0/n_1 (O'Neill, 1984).

10.3 MULTIGROUP TRIAL DESIGN

10.3.1 Multisample Hypothesis Test for the Mean

One-Way ANOVA for Parallel Groups
Objective: To calculate sample size based on one-way ANOVA with the null hypothesis H_0 that all means are equal. The alternative hypothesis is that H_0 is not true.

Technical Notes This is an exact method using a central F-distribution (Fleiss, 1986). The degree of freedoms are $g - 1$ for the numerator and $n - g$ for the denominator, where g is the number of treatment groups and n is the total sample size. The noncentral parameter $\delta = n$ times variance between treatments divided by the common variance (variance within treatment).

One-Way Contrast Between Means
Objective: To calculate sample size based on the null hypothesis H_0 with specific contrast.

Technical Notes A contrast test is often used for dose–response studies. M. Chang (2007e) developed a uniform sample-size formulation for superiority and noninferiority tests with mean, proportion, and survival endpoints and suggested the selection of contrasts with opposite signs between the control and test groups. He also proved that the Cochran–Armitage test for dose–reponse is a special case of the general formulation.

Two-Way ANOVA with an Interaction Term

Objective: To calculate sample size based on two-way ANOVA with an interaction term.

Technical Notes The sample-size formula is given by Odeh and Fox (1991) based on the noncentral F-distribution. The numerator degrees of freedom are $a - 1$, $b - 1$, and $(a - 1)(b - 1)$ for the two main effects and the interaction effects, respectively, and the denominator degrees of freedom are $ab(n - 1)$, where a and b are the number of levels for factors A and B, respectively, and n is the sample size. The noncentrality parameters are abn times the respective effect sizes for factors A and B and the interaction (Odeh and Fox, 1991, pp. 12–13, Case 1, Eq. 2.8).

Two-Way ANOVA Without Interaction

Objective: To calculate sample size based on two-way ANOVA without an interaction term.

Technical Notes The sample-size formula is given by Odeh and Fox (1991) based on the noncentral F-distribution. The numerator degrees of freedom are $a - 1$ and $b - 1$ for the two main effects, respectively, and the denominator degrees of freedom are $abn - a - b - 1$, where a and b are the number of levels for factors A and B, respectively, and n is the sample size. The noncentrality parameters are abn times the respective effect sizes for factors A and B and the interaction (Odeh and Fox, 1991, pp. 12–13).

One-Way Random Block Design

Objective: To calculate sample size based on one-way random block design.

Technical Notes The sample-size formula is given by Odeh and Fox (1991) based on the noncentral F-distribution. The numerator degrees of freedom are $a - 1$ and $n - 1$ for the main and block effects, respectively, and the denominator degrees of freedom are $(a - 1)(n - 1)$, where a and b are the number of levels for factors A and B, respectively, and n is the sample size. The noncentrality parameter is equal to na times the respective effect sizes for factors A and B and the interaction (Odeh and Fox, 1991, pp. 16–17).

ANOVA with Latin Square Design

Objective: To calculate sample size based on ANOVA with a Latin square design.

Technical Notes The sample-size formula is given by Odeh and Fox (1991) for the three main effects based on noncentral F-distribution. The numerator and denominator degrees of freedom are $m - 1$ and $N - 3m - 2$, respectively. The noncentranality parameter = N MS_A/MS_Error (Odeh and Fox, 1991).

William's Test for Minimum Effective Dose
Objective: To calculate sample size based on William's test for minimum effective dose.

Technical Notes This sample-size method is given by Chow and Liu (1998) based on William's test for dose–response (William 1971, 1972).

10.3.2 Multisample Hypothesis Test for Proportion

Cochran–Armitage Test for Linear/Monotonic Trend: Dose Response
Objective: To calculate sample size based on the Cochran–Armitage test for dose–response.

Technical Notes This approximate sample-size formula is given by Nam (1987) for detecting a linear trend in proportions. The author gives formulas for both uncorrected and corrected Cochran–Armitage tests. For two binomial proportions these reduce to those given by Casagrande et al. (1978). An asymptotic test of significance of a linear trend in proportions is given by Cochran (1954) and Armitage (1955). This test is known to be more powerful than the chi-square homogeneity test in identifying a trend (Chapman and Nam, 1968). A dose–response curve is not necessarily linear in proportion, and a logistic model may be more reasonable for some cases. Nam shows numerically that the sample size based on logistic dose–response alternative differs little from that of a linear alternative. As the nature of the dose–response curve is usually not known prior to the chronic bioassay study, it may be reasonable to use a linear model in determining a sample size since the model could grossly approximate many monotonically increasing curves (Nam, 1987; M. Chang, 2006).

Chi-Square Test for Equal Proportions in m Groups in k Categories
Objective: To calculate sample size based on a chi-square test for equal proportions in m groups.

Technical Notes The sample-size calculation is based on a noncentral chi-square distribution with the degrees of freedom $m - 1$ and the noncentral parameter $\delta = 1/[P_{\text{mean}}(1 - P_{\text{mean}})]\sum[R_i(P_i - P_{\text{mean}})^2]/\sum R_i$, where R_i is the sample size ratio N_i/N_1 (see Lachin, 1977).

Chi-Square Test for Equal Proportions in m Groups
Objective: To calculate sample size based on a chi-square test for equal proportions in m groups.

Technical Notes The sample-size calculation is based on a noncentral chi-square distribution with degrees of freedom $m - 1$ and the noncentral parameter $\delta = 1/[P_{\text{mean}}(1 - P_{\text{mean}})]\sum[R_i(P_i - P_{\text{mean}})^2]/\sum R_i$, where R_i is the sample-size ratio N_i/N_1 (see Lachin, 1977).

One-Way Contrast Between Proportions
Objective: To calculate sample size based on a large-sample assumption.

Technical Notes The sample-size calculation is based on a normality assumption. M. Chang (2007a) provides suggestions on how to determine the contrasts for various purposes.

10.3.3 Multisample Hypothesis Test for Others

One-Way Contrast Test for Exponential Survial with Uniform Enrollment and a Follow-up
Objective: To calculate sample size based on the contrast test for a dose–response relationship.

Technical Notes The asymptotic test is most powerful when the contrast shape is similar to the dose–response shape (M. Chang and Chow, 2006; M. Chang, 2007a).

Test That All k Means Are Equal with Overall Type I Error Controlled at the α Level
Objective: To calculate sample size (number of failures) based on a test for the null hypothesis that the mean survival times for all ($k \geq 2$) treatments are the same.

Technical Notes This method is developed by Makuch and Simon (1982) based on an ANOVA framework. The overall type I error rate is controlled at the α level (Fisher's LSD method). The number of failures per group increases as the number of treatment groups increases. As a result, for $k > 2$ the planned number of failures d will be somewhat greater than that obtained from the method proposed by George and Desu (1974) for a two-treatment group trial. The increase in sample size per group with k (>2) is required to preserve the overall error rate of α in light of all possible multiple comparisons. When $k = 2$, the result will degenerate to that by George and Desu (1974). The assumption of exponential survival distribution is used in the model. However, the authors point out that this method is expected to hold approximately for any proportional hazard alternatives when the maximum hazard ratio is not too large, as has been shown by Schoenfeld (1981) for the case of two treatment groups.

If the estimated ratio of the largest survival time to the smallest survival time is 2, $\alpha = 0.05$, and power = 0.9, this Makuch and Simon method gives a sample size of 53 per group, whereas the George and Desu method (1974), with a reduced nominal significant level 0.05/3 (Bonferroni adjustment) to account for the fact that three pairwise comparisons are possible, gives a sample size of 56 (see Lachin and Foulkes, 1986).

Prognostic Model with Right-Censored Data from DNA Microarrays
Objective: To calculate sample size based on a prognostic model with continuous and right-censored data from DNA microarrays.

Technical Notes DNA microarrays are arrays that provide simultaneous information about expression levels of thousands of genes and are consequently finding wide use in biomedical research. Hsieh and Lavori proposed this method for planning sample size based on a number of events: $D = (k + 1)^2/k(z_{\alpha/2} + z_{\beta})^2/(\tau \ln \delta)^2$, where τ denotes the statndard deviation of a log ratio or log intensity level of a gene over the entire set of samples, because there are no predefined classes. δ denotes the hazard ratio associated with a 1-unit change in the log ratio or log intensity x, and ln denotes the natural logarithm. Note that we are assuming that the log ratio or log intensities are based on logarithms to the base 2, so a 1-unit change in x represents a twofold change. To control the number of false positives and false negatives, α and β should not exceed 0.001 and 0.05, respectively (Hsieh and Lavori, 2000; Simon et al., 2002).

10.3.4 Multisample Confidence Interval for Others

Confidence Interval for One-Way Contrast: Large Sample
Objective: To calculate sample size based on a precision analysis for maximum mean difference among several independent samples.

Technical Notes The precision analysis for sample size is based on the maximum half-width of the confidence interval that we are willing to accept for the underlying parameter. The sample size per group is given by $n = 0.5 z_{1-\alpha/2}^2 V \sum (C_i^2/r_i) \sum r_i/E^2$, where V is the sample variance, C_i is contrast, $r_i = n_i/n_1$ is the sample size ratio, and E is the confidence interval width (Chow and Liu, 1998).

Afterword

You have learned how to design and monitor a classical or adaptive clinical trial. If you want do more research on adaptive designs, you should read the literature on this topic. For in-depth coverage of the theory and methodology, I recommend *Adaptive Design Theory and Implementation Using SAS and R* (M. Chang, 2007a). Together with ExpDesign Studio, it should act as a powerful tool in your research (e.g., simulations). You may want to visit www.statisticians.org from time to time for updates and send your questions and comments to mark.chang@statisticians.org.

One relevant aspect that has not been discussed is the IT infrastructure regarding the data query and report system used in adaptive designs. The Clinical Workbench by Biopier (www.Biopier.com) is a very impressive tool in this regard.

Classical and Adaptive Clinical Trial Designs Using ExpDesign Studio™,
By Mark Chang

APPENDIX A
Validation of ExpDesign Studio*

The validation document is intented to support pharmaceutical end users in meeting the FDA's 21 CFR part 11 requirements. However, it is important to know that it is not possible for any vendor to offer a turnkey "Part 11–compliant system." Part 11 requires both procedural and administrative controls to be put in place by the user in addition to the technical controls that a vendor can offer. At best, a vendor can offer an application containing the required technical requirements for a compliant system (www.21cfrpart11.com).

Before addressing the validation, let's quickly review the difference between ExpDesign Studio 5.0 and earlier versions. The following modules are added due to recent rapid development in adaptive trial design:

- New adaptive design module
- Adaptive trial monitoring module
- Dose-escalation trial monitoring module

Also, a random number generation module, the randomizor, has been added. The early version of an adaptive design simulator now serves as a secondary module for adaptive design. An option has been added to allow for futility-binding or nonbinding design. The default is nonbinding. In the earlier version, only futility binding is allowed.

Calculations of the number of events required for group sequential design have been added to the survival group sequential design. This has also led to an improvement in the algorithm for survival analysis. Several new methods, including Fisher's exact test for the two proportions, have been added; meanwhile, several uncommonly used methods for classical sample size calculation have been removed. A second full-scale validation for version 5.0 has been completed.

*Thanks are due Susan Shen of CTriSoft (www.CTriSoft.net) for her support in preparing the validation documents for ExpDesign Studio 5.0.

A.1 VALIDATION PROCESS FOR EXPDESIGN STUDIO

ExpDesign validation is very extensive. Usually, multiple validation approaches are used for each method. ExpDesign uses the published results and other software, such as nQuery and East, for its validations. Validation for a method is considered passed only if it passes algorithm and outcome validations. The validation documents in Section A.10 are also intented for end users to do installation and performance validations of the software, which are typically required for most companies involved in clinical trials.

A.1.1 Algorithm Validation

For algorithm validation, the following have been checked: (1) that each algorithm matches the published statistical method or procedure; (2) that numerical overflows are handled properly; (3) that appropriate numerical methods for (singularity) integrations, and the error accumulation due to recursively numerical rounding or truncations, are controlled; (4) ensuring that the local and global convergence of search algorithms (e.g., binary, fast, and shell search algorithm) are reached (if not, log out the warning massages); and (5) having tested all the logic branches.

A.1.2 Statistical Outcome Validation

Validation Using Published Results When closed-form solutions are available, we have checked ExpDesign results against the solutions under various conditions. When only numerical examples are available, we have checked results against these results, and we have checked the results under special circumstances (degenerated cases, asymptotic conditions, and/or the monotonic), under which conditions solutions can often be derived.

Validation Using the Power Curve Power or power curves (power versus treatment difference) validation is important. From the power we can check the correctness of the program. When the null hypothesis is true, the power is less than or equal to the type I error α. We have checked in ExpDesign the characteristics for all hypothesis test–based sample size calculation methods. The power is usually a monotonic function of treatment effect and sample size (power from an exact test is an exception). This property has also been used for the validation.

Validation Using Simulation Simulation is a powerful tool for validations. We have extensively used simulations in ExpDesign development and debugger and validation processes. We have used other independently published or free-domain programs in SAS, R, C, and other languages.

Validation Using Other Software We have used 95% methods in nQuery 5.0 and 6.0 to validate ExpDesign Classical Design Module (Section A.2). We have used East 4.1 and 5.0 and SAS and R source code from M. Chang 2007a) for group sequential design and adaptive design model (see Sections A.3 and A.4). We have also used the results from the book by Jennison and Turnbull (2000), Proschan et al. (2006), Wang and Tsiatis (1987), Pampallona and Tsiatis (1994), and M. Chang (2007a) to validate the group sequential design and adaptive design module (see Section A.3 and Table A.4). We have documented the numerical comparisons extensively in the tables in this appendix. Of course, this reflects only a small portion of the validation processes in ExpDesign Studio (A.2 to A.8).

A.1.3 Criteria for Passing Validation

If the difference in results is fewer than one subject or less than 0.005 in power, or within 1% for sample size, or the precision is within 0.0001 in stopping probabilities/boundary, it is considered to have passed validation.

Beta Version However, ExpDesign covers a wide range of design methods that many other software packages do not cover. Because we believe in the importance of high standard validation, we have marketed as the beta version any method that is not 100% done. There are few methods for classic design, and the ExpDesign Simulator module is deemed to be a beta version and marked "Beta" in the validation tables. Readers should take precautions in using these methods, using them for mission-critical tasks only.

A.1.4 Input and GUI Validation

GUI (graphic user interface) input validation is another way to prevent ironic results due to impropriate inputs from a user. ExpDesign implements extensive input checks to eliminate many types of input errors from the GUI. The tiptextes for the input boxes are provided to instruct user in how to enter appropriate values.

A.2 VALIDATION OF THE CLASSICAL DESIGN MODULE

All validation cases in Table A.1 power = 80%, 85%, or 90% for a one- or two-sided hypothesis testing with $\alpha = 0.05$. The ExpDesign default example in each method for the classical designs will show you the exact input parameters. You can click the example button in ExpDesign Classical Design Module to see the inputs. For simplicity, unbalanced design validations are not presented in the table.

TABLE A.1 Classical Sample Size Method Validation

ID	Short Method Title	ExpDesign	nQuery[a]
1	Two-sample t-test	64	64
2	Mann–Whitney U/Wilcoxon rank-sum test for two samples	38	38
3	Kendall's test of Independence	100	111
4	Sign test for median difference: paired sample	58	58[M]
5	Wilcoxon's signed-rank test for one or paired sample	66	66[M]
9	McNemar's test for paired sample	52	52
13	Asymptotic z-method considering variance difference	62	62[M]
14	Pearson's chi-square test (Kramer–Greenhouse)	71	72
22	Equivalence test for two proportions (large n)	132	132[CSW]
33	Test for H_0: (u_0, σ_0) vs. Ha: (u_a, σ_a): large sample	42	N.A.
34	Two-sample z-test (large sample or population variance known)	63	63[CSW]
36	Lachin's test for two treatments by two-time-point interaction	110	N.A.
37	Lachin's test for treatment by time interaction	284	N.A.
40	Exponential survival distribution with uniform patient enrollment	251	250
42	Exponential survival with uniform enrollment and follow-up	416	415
44	Test H_0: single correlation = zero using Fisher's arctan transformation	86	85
45	Test H_0: regression coefficient = zero using arctan transformation	86	85
46	Test two correlation coefficients using Fisher's arctan transformation	53	N.A.
48	Test interaction in a model with exponential survival function (two strata)	69	N.A.
49	Test interaction in a model with exponential survival function (k strata)	444	N.A.
50	One-way ANOVA for parallel groups	52	53
51	2×2 crossover study with intraclass correlation consideration	74	N.A.
52	Whitehead logistic ratio model for two groups with k categories	97	N.A.
54	One-sample t-test	34	34
55	One-sample t-test (finite population)	33	33
56	Paired-sample t-test	34	34
57	Paired-sample t-test (finite population)	54	55
58	One-sample mean confidence interval method (large sample)	61	62
59	One-sample mean confidence interval method (finite population)	58	58
60	Paired-sample mean confidence interval method (large sample)	61	62
61	Paired-sample mean confidence interval method (finite population)	58	58
62	Paired t test for equivalence of means	126	127
64	Schuirmann–Chow's two one-sided t-tests for equivalence	791	791[CR]

TABLE A.1 ***Continued***

ID	Short Method Title	ExpDesign	nQuery[a]
66	Confidence interval for difference of two means (large sample)	48	48
68	Confidence interval for one-way contrast (large sample)	123	123
69	Noninferiority test for two means based on a one-sided two-sample t-test	310	310[CR]
70	One-way repeated measures ANOVA	60	61
72	Chi-square test for one sample proportion	239	239
73	Chi-square test for one proportion with k categories	76	76
74	Confidence interval for a proportion (large n)	81	81
75	Confidence interval for odds ratio for paired proportions (large n)	512	513
76	Confidence interval for the probability of observing a rare event	15	16
77	Chi-square test for the one proportion (finite population)	147	147
79	Paired response: equivalence of p_1 and p_2 (large sample)	312	312
80	Chi-square test for two proportions with k categories	102	102
81	Confidence interval for difference in two proportions (large n)	177	177
82	Confidence interval for ln(odds ratio): unmatched case–control study	210	211
83	One-sided noninferiority for two proportions (large sample)	40	40[CSW]
84	Chi-square test for m sample proportions with k categories	101	102
85	Mantel–Haenszel test for odds ratio with k strata	2025	2026
86	Mantel–Haenszel test for odds ratio with k strata (continuity correction)	57	57
87	Cochran–Armitage test for linear/monotonic trend (dose–response)	807	808
88	Log-rank test for survival analysis	98	98
91	Logistic regression on x for binary outcome	77	76
92	Logistic regression on x for binary outcome with covariates	103	102
93	Linear regression; test for H_0: correlation coefficient = 0	82	82
94	Multiple linear regression; test for H_0: multiple correlation $R = 0$	24	24
95	Multiple regression, test 0, increased in R^2 due to extra B covariates	208	N.A.
96	Linear regression $y = a + bx$; test H_0: $b = b_0$	34	34
97	Linear regression $y_1 = a_1 + b_1x$, $y_2 = a_2 + b_2x$; test H_0: $b_1 = b_2$	36	37
98	Linear regression $y = a + bx$, confidence interval for b	384	N.A.
100	Confidence interval for Bloch–Kraemer intraclass κ coefficient	350	N.A.
101	Test for Bloch–Kraemer intraclass κ coefficient	780	780
102	Test for Bloch–Kraemer intraclass κ using z-transformation	697	N.A.
104	Two one-sided t-tests for equivalence of two means: parallel design	310	310
105	Confidence interval for repeated measures contrast	908	908
107	Two one-sided t-tests for equivalence based on ratio of means: parallel design	76	76

TABLE A.1 ***Continued***

ID	Short Method Title	ExpDesign	nQuery[a]
108	Two one-sided t-tests for equivalence based on ratio of two means: crossover design	34	34
109	Two one-sided t-tests for equivalence based on mean ratio for lognormal data	482	482
110	Exponential survival with uniform accrual, follow-up, and dropouts	120	119
112	Test all k equal survival means with overall type I error control	118	118[MS]
113	Exponential survival distribution with a Bernoulli confounding variable	118	N.A.
115	One-way repeated measures ANOVA for two groups	60	61
117	Repeated measures for two proportions	53	CL
120	Test for treatment mean difference with 2 × 2 crossover design	74	CL
121	Two-sample z-test for treatment mean difference	141	141[CR]
126	Two-way analysis of variance with interaction term	128	128
127	Two-way analysis of variance without interaction	162	Odeh
128	One-way random block design	128	Odeh
130	ANOVA with Latin square design	128	Odeh
131	William's test for minimum effective dose	335	CL
132	One-sample multiple test for zero means	60	N.A.
133	Two-sample multiple test for mean differences	122	NQ
135	One-sample exact test for proportion using binomial distribution	143	143
138	One-sample confidence interval for mean based on t-statistic	98	98[CR]
139	Paired mean confidence interval based on t-statistic	98	98[CR]
145	One-way ANOVA for parallel groups	214	215
146	Contrast test for m means (dose–response)	230	230
147	Chi-square test for m sample proportions with k categories	386	386
148	Chi-square test for equal proportions in m groups	101	102
150	Noninferior its test for survival with uniform accrual and follow-up	276	276[C]
152	Equivalence test for survival with uniform accrual and follow-up	498	498[C]
153	Equivalence test for two proportions (large n)	132	132[CC]
154	Comparing DNA expression profiles among predefined classes	58	N.A.
156	Prognostic models with right-censored data from DNA microarray	36	N.A.
157	One-way contrast between proportions	60	60[C]
159	One-way contrast test for survival with uniform accrual and follow-up	76	76[C]
161	Donner's method for mean difference using cluster randomization	403	N.A.
164	Fisher's exact test for two proportions	50	50

[a]Default source is nQuery; M, validated manually; CSW, Chow–Shao–Wang (2003); N.A., not applicable (beta version); CR, internal cross-validation using method already validated; MS, Makuch and Simon (1982); Odeh, Odeh and Fox (1991); C, Chang (2007e); CC, Chang and Chow (2006); CL, Chow and Liu (1998).

A.3 VALIDATION OF THE GROUP SEQUENTIAL DESIGN MODULE

A.3.1 Stopping Boundary and Type I Error Rate Validation

In Tables A.2 to A.4 we compare the stopping boundaries from four different sources: Jennison and Turnbull (2000) (JT); Proschan et al. (2006) (PLW), ExpDesign 5.0, and East 4.1. We can see that the stopping boundaries are virtually identical in all methods.

A.3.2 Power and Sample-Size Validation

Tables A.5 to A.10 are sample-size comparisons among different sources. In additional type I error and power, we have also validated the crossing probability at interim analyses (see Table A.11 for examples).

TABLE A.2 O'Brien–Fleming Boundary on the z-Scale at the Final Stage[a]

Number of Looks	ExpDesign Studio 5.0	PLW.(P72)	JT	East 4.1
1	1.9599	1.960	1.960	1.960
2	1.9768	1.977	1.977	1.977
3	2.0044	2.004	2.004	2.004
4	2.0243	2.024	2.024	2.024
5	2.0396	2.040	2.040	2.040
6	2.0533	2.053	2.053	2.053
7	2.0641	2.063	2.063	2.063
8	2.0717	2.072	2.072	2.072
9	2.0794	2.080	2.080	2.080
10	2.0870	2.087	2.087	2.087

[a]One-sided $\alpha = 0.025$, equal information intervals.

TABLE A.3 Pocock Boundary on the z-Scale at the Final Stage[a]

Number of Looks	ExpDesignm Studio 5.0	PLW.(P72)	JT	East 4.1
1	1.9599	1.960	1.960	1.960
2	2.1789	2.178	2.178	2.178
3	2.2892	2.289	2.289	2.290
4	2.3611	2.361	2.361	2.361
5	2.4132	2.413	2.413	2.413
6	2.4530	2.453	2.453	2.454
7	2.4852	2.485	2.485	2.486
8	2.5127	2.512	2.512	2.513
9	2.5357	2.535	2.535	2.536
10	2.5556	2.555	2.555	2.556

[a]One-sided $\alpha = 0.025$, equal information intervals.

TABLE A.4 Wang–Tsiatis Boundary (b = 0.25) on the z-Scale at the Final Stage[a]

Number of Looks	ExpDesign Studio 5.0	JT	East 4.1
1	1.9599	1.960	1.960
2	2.0380	2.038	2.038
3	2.0824	2.083	2.083
4	2.1131	2.113	2.113
5	2.1360	2.136	2.136
6	2.2544	2.154	2.154
7	2.1682	2.168	2.168
8	2.1804	2.180	2.180
9	2.1986	2.190	2.190
10	2.1988	2.199	2.199

[a]One-sided α = 0.025, equal information intervals.

TABLE A.5 Maximum Sample Size for 80% and 90% Power: of Boundary[a]

Number of Looks	ExpDesign Studio 5.0		JT[b]		East 4.1 WT (delta = 0)	
	80%	90%	80%	90%	80%	90%
1	348	466	348	466	349	467
2	351	470	351	469	352	470
3	355	475	354	474	355	475
4	357	477	356	476	357	477
5	359	479	358	478	359	479

[a]One-sided α = 0.025, equal information intervals, effect size = 0.3, four-stage sequential design comparing two means.
[b]Calculated using Tables 2.11 and 2.12 in Jennison and Turnbull (2000).

TABLE A.6 Maximum Sample Size for 80% and 90% Power: Pocock Boundary[a]

Number of Looks	ExpDesign Studio 5.0		JT[b]		East 4.1 WT (delta = 0.5)	
	80%	90%	80%	90%	80%	90%
1	348	466	348	466	349	467
2	388	514	386	513	387	514
3	407	537	406	536	407	537
4	419	552	418	551	420	553
5	429	563	428	562	429	564

[a]One-sided α = 0.025, equal information intervals, effect size = 0.3, four-stage sequential design comparing two means.
[b]Calculated using Tables 2.11 and 2.12 in Jennison and Turnbull (2000).

TABLE A.7 Maximum Sample Size for 80% and 90% Power: Wang–Tsiatis Boundary[a]

Number of Looks	ExpDesign Studio 5.0 80%	ExpDesign Studio 5.0 90%	JT[b] 80%	JT[b] 90%	East 4.1 WT (delta = 0.25) 80%	East 4.1 WT (delta = 0.25) 90%
1	348	466	348	466	349	467
2	362	483	361	482	362	483
3	368	490	367	489	368	490
4	371	495	371	494	371	495
5	374	498	373	497	374	498

[a]One-sided $\alpha = 0.025$, equal information intervals, effect size = 0.3, four-stage sequential design comparing two means.
[b]Calculated using Tables 2.11 and 2.12 in Jennison and Turnbull (2000).

TABLE A.8 Maximum Sample Size for Binary Endpoint: Four-Stage Sequential Design[a]

Boundary Type	Proportions Group 1	Proportions Group 2	ExpDesign Studio 5.0 80%	ExpDesign Studio 5.0 90%	East 4.1 (Pooled Variance) 80%	East 4.1 (Pooled Variance) 90%
OF	0.2	0.4	169	226	167	222
WT ($\Delta = 0.25$)	0.2	0.4	175	234	174	230
Pocock	0.2	0.4	198	261	197	258

[a]The differences in sample size cause less than 0.5% difference in power. It is therefore considered to be due to numerical rounding.

TABLE A.9 Maximum Sample Size (Number of Events) for Survival Endpoint: Four-Stage Sequential Design[a]

Boundary Type	ExpDesign Studio 5.0 80%	ExpDesign Studio 5.0 90%	East 4.1 (Pooled Variance) 80%	East 4.1 (Pooled Variance) 90%
OF	654 (467)	874 (624)	656 (469)	877 (626)
WT ($\Delta = 0.25$)	680 (485)	907 (647)	683 (487)	910 (649)
Pocock	768 (548)	1012 (722)	771 (551)	1016 (725)

[a]All differences in sample size < 0.5%. Therefore, it is consider due to numerical rounding. Patient accrual period $T_0 = 24.4$, study duration $T_{max} = 34.3$, median times = 10 and 13 for the two groups.

TABLE A.10 Maximum Sample Size (Number of Events) for Survival Endpoint: Three-Stage Sequential Design[a]

	ExpDesign Studio 5.0		East 4.1 (Pooled Variance)	
Boundary Type	80%	90%	80%	90%
OF	671 (517)	899 (692)	673 (519)	900 (694)
WT ($\Delta = 0.25$)	696 (536)	929 (715)	968 (538)	930 (717)
Pocock	770 (593)	1017 (783)	992 (595)	1020 (786)

[a]It has been noted that the number of events changes slightly when accrual rate changes, which should not change based on the formulation. All differences in sample size < 0.5%. It is therefore considered to be due to numerical rounding. Patient accrual period $T_0 = 8$, study duration $T_{max} = 23$, median times = 10 and 13 for the two groups.

TABLE A.11 Validation of Boundary Crossing Probabilities[a]

	ExpDesign Studio 5.0		East 4.1	
Stage	Under H_0	Under H_a	Under H_0	Under H_a
1	0.0014	0.0743	0.001	0.074
2	0.0054	0.3033	0.005	0.303
3	0.0083	0.2946	0.008	0.295
4	0.0098	0.1778	0.010	0.178

[a]Four-stage sequential design with OF boundary comparing two means.

TABLE A.12 Stopping Boundary on the *p*-Scale at the Final Stage Using Error-Spending Function

Spending Function	Information Time	ExpDesign Studio 5.0	PLW Table 5.3[a]	East 4.1[a]
OF-like	0.20	0.00000	4.877/0.00000	0.00000
	0.50	0.00159	2.963/0.00153	0.00153
	1.00	0.02454	1.969/0.02448	0.02448
Linear	0.20	0.00500	2.576/0.00500	N.A.
	0.50	0.00873	2.377/0.00873	
	1.00	0.01611	2.141/0.01614	
Pocock-like	0.20	0.00738	2.438/0.00738	0.00738
	0.50	0.00983	2.333/0.00982	0.00982
	1.00	0.01306	2.225/0.01304	0.01304

[a]Converted from the *z*-scale. One-sided $\alpha = 0.025$, equal information intervals with three looks (MINP). N.A., not applicable; PLW, Proschan, Lan, and Wittes, 2006.

A.4 VALIDATION OF THE ADAPTIVE DESIGN MODULE

A.4.1 Stopping Boundary and Type I Error Rate Validation

For MINP with OF-like, Pocock-like, and Lan–DeMets's power-spending functions, the validation results are the same as for group sequential design (Tables A.12 to A.15). Note that Cui-Hung-Wang's method is a special case of MINP (the method based on inverse-normal *p*-values).

TABLE A.13 Stopping Boundary Validation (α_2) with Two-Stage MSP: Futility Binding[a]

	α_1					
β_1	0.000	0.0025	0.005	0.010	0.015	0.020
0.05	0.5250	0.4999	0.4719	0.4050	0.3182	0.2017
0.10	0.3000	0.2820	0.2630	0.2217	0.1751	0.1225
0.15	0.2417	0.2288	0.2154	0.1871	0.1566	0.1200
0.20	0.2250	0.2152	0.2051	0.1832	0.1564	0.1200
0.25	0.2236	0.2146	0.2050	0.1832	0.1564	0.1200

[a]All values are validated using computer simulation with 1,000,000 runs and results from M. Chang (2007a, Table 4.3).

TABLE A.14 Stopping Boundary Validation (α_2) with Two-Stage MPP: Futility Binding[a]

	α_1					
β_1	0.001	0.0025	0.005	0.010	0.015	0.020
0.15	0.0048	0.0055	0.0059	0.0055	0.0043	0.0025
0.20	0.0045	0.0051	0.0054	0.0050	0.0039	0.0022
0.25	0.0043	0.0049	0.0051	0.0047	0.0036	0.0020
0.30	0.0042	0.0047	0.0049	0.0044	0.0033	0.0018
0.35	0.0041	0.0046	0.0047	0.0042	0.0032	0.0017
0.40	0.0040	0.0044	0.0046	0.0041	0.0030	0.0017
0.50	0.0039	0.0042	0.0043	0.0038	0.0029	0.0016
1.00	0.0035	0.0038	0.0038	0.0033	0.0024	0.0013

[a]All values are validated using computer simulation with 1,000,000 runs and results from M. Chang (2007a). Nonfutility binding boundaries are special cases when we force $\beta_1 = 1$.

TABLE A.15 Stopping Boundary Validation (α_2) with Two-Stage MSP: Futility Binding[a]

	α_1					
β_1	0.000	0.0025	0.005	0.010	0.015	0.020
0.05	0.5250	0.4999	0.4719	0.4050	0.3182	0.2017
0.10	0.3000	0.2820	0.2630	0.2217	0.1751	0.1225
0.15	0.2417	0.2288	0.2154	0.1871	0.1566	0.1200
0.20	0.2250	0.2152	0.2051	0.1832	0.1564	0.1200
>0.25	0.2236	0.2146	0.2050	0.1832	0.1564	0.1200

[a]All values are validated using computer simulation with 1,000,000 runs and results from M. Chang (2007a,b). Nonfutility binding boundaries are special cases when we force $\beta_1 = \alpha_2$.

The Lan–DeMets power family stopping boundary validation with MSP (>two stages) is based on simulation; therefore, the precision is dependent on the number of simulation runs. We suggest that 100,000 to 1,000,000 simulation runs are necessary to determine the stopping boundary with 0.01% precision. For K-stage designs, boundaries are verified through simulations, which is done at the time you design the trial by running a simulation under the null conditions.

A.4.2 Validation of Adaptive Design Monitoring

Two-stage results for sample-size reestimation and conditional power are verified by analytical results from M. Chang (2007) and using overall type I error rate and simulation to check (Tables A.16 and A.17). For K-stage design, simulations were used for validation and overall type I error rate and conditional power from two-stage design to check. For K-stage design with MINP, recalculation of the stopping boundaries were checked against the group sequential stopping boundaries that have already been verified.

A.5 VALIDATION OF THE MULTISTAGE DESIGN MODULE

The optimal design and MinMax design are often not unique; there could be several designs with the same expected or maximum sample size. In such cases,

TABLE A.16 Validation of Conditional Power for Two-Stage Adaptive Design[a]

Method	Effect Size	P_1	N_1	N_2	cPower from ExpDesign	cPower from M. Chang (2007a)
MSP	0.18124	0.1	100	200	0.73	0.73
MPP	0.18124	0.1	100	200	0.515	0.515
MINP	0.18124	0.1	100	200	0.626	0.626

[a]MSP boundary: $\alpha_1 = 0.0025$, $\alpha_2 = 0.2152$. MPP boundary: $\alpha_1 = 0.0025$, $\alpha_2 = 0.0038$. MINP boundary: $\alpha_1 = 0.0025$, $\alpha_2 = 0.02454$.

TABLE A.17 Validation of Sample-Size Reestimation for Two-Stage Adaptive Design[a]

Method	Effect Size	P_1	N_1	cPower	cPower from ExpDesign	cPower from M. Chang (2007)
MSP	0.18124	0.1	100	0.9	375	375
MPP	0.18124	0.1	100	0.9	569	569
MINP	0.18124	0.1	100	0.9	472	472

[a]MSP boundary: $\alpha_1 = 0.0025$, $\alpha_2 = 0.2152$. MPP boundary: $\alpha_1 = 0.0025$, $\alpha_2 = 0.0038$. MINP boundary: $\alpha_1 = 0.0025$, $\alpha_2 = 0.02454$.

ExpDesign will present all the designs in the grid and pick anyone to present the report. Examples of validations are shown in Tables A.18 to A.20.

Note that we believe that a few probabilities of early termination, PET(p_0), are incorrect in Simon's original paper. For example, for MinMax design with $p_0 = 0.2$ and the cutpoint $r_1/n_1 = 4/18$, Simon's PET(p_0) = 0.50, which is incorrect (or simply a typographical error). The PET(0.2) can easily be verified using the binomial distribution, which is 0.7164.

TABLE A.18 Two-Stage Optimal Design (MinExpSize): One-Sided α = 0.05

Simon/ExpDesign						Simon	ExpDesign
Power	p_0	p_1	R_1/n_1	r/n	EN(p_0)	PET(p_0)	PET(p_0)
0.8	0.05	0.25	0/9	2/24	14.5	0.63	0.630
0.8	0.20	0.40	3/13	12/43	20.6	0.75	0.747
0.8	0.30	0.50	5/15	18/46	23.6	0.72	0.722
0.8	0.10	0.15	2/18	7/43	24.7	0.73	0.734
0.8	0.30	0.45	9/27	30/81	41.7	0.73	0.728
0.9	0.30	0.50	8/24	24/63	34.7	0.73	0.725

Source: Simon (1989, Tables 1 and 2).

TABLE A.19 Two-Stage MinMax Design (MinMaxSize): One-Sided α = 0.05

Simon/ExpDesign						Simon	ExpDesign
Power	p_0	p_1	R_1/n_1	r/n	EN(p_0)	PET(p_0)	PET(p_0)
0.8	0.05	0.25	0/12	2/16	13.8	0.54	0.540
0.8	0.20	0.40	4/18	10/33	22.3	0.50*	0.716
0.8	0.30	0.50	6/19	16/39	25.7	0.48*	0.666
0.8	0.10	0.15	2/22	7/40	28.8	0.62	0.620
0.8	0.30	0.45	16/46	25/65	49.6	0.81	0.809
0.9	0.30	0.50	7/24	21/53	36.6	0.56	0.565

Source: Simon (1989, Tables 1 and 2). An asterisk indicates an incorrect value from Simon's original paper.

TABLE A.20 Three-Stage Optimal Design Validation[a]

Source	P_0	P_1	r_1/n_1	r_2/n_2	r_3/n_3	Alpha	Power
ExpDesign	0.05	0.25	0/8	1/13	2/19	0.049	0.805
Ensign*	0.05	0.25	0/7	1/15	3/26	0.027*	0.805
ExpDesign	0.10	0.30	0/6	2/17	5/29	0.047	0.801
Ensign	0.10	0.30	0/6	2/17	5/29	0.047	0.801

[a]Alpha and power from 1,000,000 simulation runs in SAS and numerical calculations in ExpDesign. An asterisk indicates that Ensign's (Ensign et al., 1994) Table I did not pick the optimal design, due to a conservative α value. The SAS program for validation of the three-stage design in presented in Section A.10.

TABLE A.21 Traditional 3 + 3 Escalation Design Validation

Software	Method	Mean N	Mean DLTs	Mean MTD
ExpDesign 5.0	TER	17.2	2.82	3.764
SAS Macro	TER	17.2	2.83	3.765

TABLE A.22 CRM Validation

Software	Mean MTD	Mean DLTs	Number of Patients
ExpDesign 5.0	154	3.1	11.8
SAS Macro	154	3.1	11.9

A.6 VALIDATION OF THE TRADITIONAL DOSE-ESCALATION DESIGN MODULE

A.6.1 Validation of the Traditional Escalation Rule

We have used the SAS program (Section A.10.2) to validate the traditional escalation design (Table A.21). The parameter settings are as follows: the number of simulations = 5000, the number of stages = 1, the number of dose levels = 7, the true MTD = 4 with a DLT rate of 0.2. The DLT rates for the seven dose levels are 0.01, 0.028, 0.079, 0.2, 0.423, 0.683, and 0.863. The dose-escalation rule is the 3 + 3 traditional escalation rule.

A.6.2 Validation of the Bayesian Continual Reassessment Method

We have used SAS Macro (A.10.3) to validate the CRM (Table A.22). The trial settings are specified as follows: the seven dose levels 25, 50, 82.5, 125.4, 175.6, 233.5, and 310.5, and the DLT rates 0.0098, 0.0196, 0.0475, 0.143, 0.4062, 0.7774, and 0.9683, respectively. The true MTD is 150 with a rate of 0.25. The stopping rule is defined as if the maximum number of patients at a dose level reaches six. No dose level can be avoided during the escalation.

A.7 VALIDATION OF THE TRIAL SIMULATION MODULE

The trial simulator is a beta version in ExpDesign Studio 5.0; only algorithm validations are done, and outcome results are checked for some special cases. The full outcome validations are not done because no published data are available for the validation.

A.8 VALIDATION OF THE RANDOMIZOR

The main references for implementation of the randomizor are Gentle (2003), Ross (2002), and Kokoska and Zwillinger (2000). Algorithms used to generate

TABLE A.23 Randomizor Validation[a]

Distribution	Mean		StdDev	
	Expected	Observed	Expected	Observed
Bernoulli(0.2)	0.2	0.201	0.4	0.401
Beta(0.3,0.5)	0.375	0.378	0.361	0.362
Binomial(0.2,5)	1	0.990	0.894	0.892
Caucthy(0.5,1,2)	N.A.	2.261	N.A.	0.155
Chisq(8)	8	8.011	4	3.975
Exp(3)	0.333	0.330	0.333	0.331
Gamma(3,0.5)	1.5	1.500	0.866	0.869
Geometric(0.2)	5	4.949	4.472	4.420
HalfNormal	—	0.802	—	0.602
HyperGeometric (10,5,2)	1	1.004	0.667	0.662
invGauss(4, 6)	4	3.993	3.266	3.239
Laplace(3)	0	0.0001	0.4714	0.469
Rayleigh(2.5)	3.1333	3.147	1.638	1.638
Lognormal(0.2,2)	9.025	9.041	66.67	60.664
Multinormal				
NegBinomial(1.2,0.4)	1.8	1.7743	2.121	2.096
Normal(0,1)	0	0.0089	1	0.997
Pareto(3,0.4)	0.6	0.6002	0.3464	0.334
Pascal(3,0.4)	4.5	4.5242	3.354	3.373
Poisson(20)	20	20.0163	4.472	4.454
F(6,8)	1.333	1.338	1.333	1.312
Student-*t*(5)	0	−0.005	1.291	1.283
Uniform(0,1)	0.5	0.500	0.2887	0.288
Weibull(0.5,5)	10	10.090	22.361	23.406

[a]Results based on 20,000 simulation runs. N.A., not applicable.

deviations from these distributions are well established. We have validated the quartiles and standard deviations. Examples are presented in Table A.23.

A.9 VALIDATION OF THE EXPDESIGN TOOLKITS

This distribution module has also been used for part of ExpDesign, such as sample-size calculations, and thus verified indirectly through validations of other ExpDesign modules. The cross-validations were done using ExpDesign 5.0, East 4.1, and Scientific Workplace 5.0 (SW) (see Table A.24).

We have also verified the tail part of the distribution. For example, $Z_{0.999} = 3.0902$ and $Z_{0.9999} = 3.719$ from both ExpDesign Studio 5.0 and Scientific Workplace 5.0. Validations of probability distributions and confidence intervals can be found in Tables A.25 and A.26, respectively.

TABLE A.24 Validation of Distribution Calculator: Continuous

		Percentile					
Inverse c.d.f.	Software	25%	50%	75%	95%	97.5%	99%
Chisq	ExpDesign	15.45	19.34	23.82	31.40	34.15	37.56
(20,*x*)	East 4.1	15.45	19.34	23.83	31.41	34.17	37.57
	SW 5.0	15.452	19.337	23.828	31.41	34.170	37.566
Exponential	ExpDesign	2.876	6.936	13.86	29.96	36.88	46.06
(0.1,*x*)	East 4.1	2.877	6.931	13.86	29.96	36.89	46.05
	SW 5.0	2.8768	6.9315	13.863	29.957	36.889	46.052
F(20,50,*x*)	ExpDesign	0.7555	0.9799	1.2592	1.7842	1.9932	2.2656
	SW 5.0	0.75545	0.9799	1.2592	1.7841	1.9933	2.2652
Gamma	ExpDesign	4.316	6.686	9.800	15.74	18.06	21.00
(3,2.5,*x*)	East 4.1	4.318	6.685	9.801	15.74	18.06	21.01
	SW 5.0	4.3182	6.6852	9.801	15.739	18.062	21.015
N(0,1,*x*)	ExpDesign	−0.6745	0	0.6745	1.6449	1.9599	2.3263
	East 4.1	−0.6745	0	0.6745	1.6449	1.9600	2.3263
	SW 5.0	−0.67449	0	0.67449	1.6449	1.9600	2.3263
Student *t*	ExpDesign	−0.7064	0	0.7064	1.8595	2.3058	2.8963
(8,*x*)	East 4.1	−0.7064	0	0.7064	1.8600	2.3060	2.8960
	SW 5.0	−0.70639	0	0.70639	1.8595	2.3060	2.8965
Weibull	ExpDesign	0.8042	1.2485	1.7659	2.5977	2.8848	3.2300
(2,1.5,*x*)	SW 5.0	0.80454	1.2488	1.7661	2.5962	2.8810	3.2189

TABLE A.25 Validation of the Distribution Calculator: Discrete

		N					
c.d.f.	Software	36	40	43	46	48	51
Binomial	ExpDesign	0.2386	0.5433	0.7635	0.907	0.9577	0.99
(100,0.4;*n*)	SW 5.0	0.23861	0.54329	0.76347	0.90702	0.95770	0.98999
Poisson	ExpDesign	0.2963	0.5419	0.7162	0.8479	0.9075	0.9613
(40;*n*)	SW 5.0	0.29635	0.54192	0.71622	0.84788	0.90753	0.96126

TABLE A.26 Validation of the Confidence Interval Calculator[a]

			Two-Sided 95% CI	
CI Name			ExpDesign CI	www CI
One-sample proportion	$P = 6/30$	—	(0.0771, 0.3857)	(0.0771, 0.3857)
One-sample proportion (z)	$P = 0.2$	—	(0.0569, 0.3431)	(0.0596, 0.3431)
One-sample mean (t)	$U = 1$	—	(0.2532, 1.7468)	t-distribution
One-sample mean (z)	$U = 1$	—	(0.2843, 1.7157)	(0.28, 1.72)
Two proportions (z)	$P_1 = 0.3$,	$P_2 = 0.5$	(0.0671, 0.3329)	Checked manually
Two means (t)	$U_1 = 1$,	$U_2 = 2$	(−0.0333, 2.0333)	t-distribution
Two means (z)	$U_1 = 1$,	$U_2 = 2$	(−0.0121, 2.0121)	(−0.01, 2.01)
Two-variance ratio	$S_1 = 2$,	$S_2 = 3$	(1.0706, 4.7262)	Checked manually

[a]Total sample size $n = 30$/group, the default standard deviation $S = 2$. For further information see http://www.dimensionresearch.com/resources/calculators/conf_means.html and http://www.measuringusability.com/wald.htm.

A.10 COMPUTER PROGRAMS FOR VALIDATIONS

A.10.1 SAS Macro for Three-Stage Design Validation

The following is the SAS macro for validation of α and power for three-stage designs.

```
%Macro ThreeStageDesign(p, n1, n2, n3, r1, r2, r3);

data bin; drop i nSims;
retain FSP1 0 FSP2 0 FSP3 0;
 n1=&n1; n2=&n2; n3=&n3; r1=&r1; r2=&r2; r3=&r3;
 seed=292; p=&p; nSims=1000000;
 do i=1 to nSims;
   call ranbin(seed,n1,p,x1);
   call ranbin(seed,n2-n1,p,x2);
        call ranbin(seed,n3-n2,p,x3);
        if x1<=r1 then FSP1=FSP1+1/nSims;
        if x1>r1 & x1+x2<=r2 then FSP2=FSP2+1/nSims;
        if x1>r1 & x1+x2> r2 & x1+x2+x3<=r3 then
         FSP3=FSP3+1/nSims;
 end;
 FSP=FSP1+FSP2;
 Power=1-FSP-FSP3;
 output;
run;
proc print; run;
%mend;
%ThreeStageDesign(0.05, 7, 15, 26, 0, 1, 3);
%ThreeStageDesign(0.25, 7, 15, 26, 0, 1, 3);
%ThreeStageDesign(0.05, 8, 13, 19, 0, 1, 2);
%ThreeStageDesign(0.25, 8, 13, 19, 0, 1, 2);
%ThreeStageDesign(0.1, 6, 17, 29, 0, 2, 5);
%ThreeStageDesign(0.3, 6, 17, 29, 0, 2, 5);
```

A.10.2 Traditional 3 + 3 Escalation Design Validation

```
SAS Macro for validation of 3+3 Dose-Escalation

%Macro TER3p3(nSims=50000, nLevels=10);
Data TER; Set dInput; Keep AveMTD SdMTD AveNPts
AveNRsps;
Array nPts{&nLevels}; Array nRsps{&nLevels}; Array
RspRates{&nLevels};
AveMTD=0; AveNPts=0; AveNRsps=0; nLevels=&nLevels;
```

```
Do iSim=1 to &nSims;
 Do i=1 To nLevels; nPts{i}=0; nRsps{i}=0; End;
 seedn=Round((Ranuni(281)*100000000));
 iLevel=1; TotPts=0; TotRsps=0;
Looper:
 If iLevel>&nLevels | nPts{iLevel}=6 Then Goto
Finisher;
 nPts{iLevel}=nPts{iLevel}+3;
 rspRate=RspRates{iLevel};
 Rsp=RANBIN(seedn,3,rspRate);
 nRsps{iLevel}=nRsps{iLevel}+Rsp;
 TotPts=TotPts+3; TotRsps=TotRsps+Rsp;
 If nPts(iLevel)=3 & nRsps{iLevel}=0 Then Do;
         iLevel=iLevel+1; Goto Looper;
 End;
 If nPts(iLevel)=3 & nRsps{iLevel}=1 Then Goto Looper;
 If nPts(iLevel)=6 & nRsps{iLevel}<=1 Then Do;
         iLevel=iLevel+1; Goto Looper;
 End;
Finisher:
 MTD=Min(iLevel-1, nLevels);
 AveMTD=AveMTD+MTD/&nSims;
 AveNPts=AveNPts+totPts/&nSims;
 AveNRsps=AveNRsps+TotRsps/&nSims;
End;
Output;
Run;
Proc Print Data=TER; Run;
%Mend TER3p3;

TITLE "3 + 3 TER Design";
Data dInput;
Array RspRates{7}(0.01, 0.028, 0.079, 0.2, 0.423,
0.683, 0.863);
%TER3p3(nSims=50000, nLevels=7);
Run;
```

A.10.3 SAS Program for CRM Validation

```
%Macro CRM(nSims=100, MaxNtoStop=6, MinPtsPerLevel=1,
nLevels=10, b=100, aMin=0, aMax=0.03, MTRate=0.25,
nDosesSkip=1);
Data CRM; Set DInput;
Keep MaxNtoStop MinPtsPerLevel npts DLTs AveMTD
AveMTDD;
```

```
Array nPtsAt{&nLevels}; Array nRsps{&nLevels}; Array
g{100};
Array Doses{&nLevels}; Array RRo{&nLevels}; Array
RR{&nLevels};
Array g0{100};
seed=2736; nLevels=&nLevels; MaxNtoStop=&MaxNtoStop;
DLTs=0;
AveMTD=0;AveMTDD=0; nIntPts=100; dx=(&aMax-&aMin)/
nIntPts;
MinPtsPerLevel=&MinPtsPerLevel;
Do k=1 To nIntPts; g0{k}=g{k}; End;
npts=0;
Do iSim=1 to &nSims;
 Stopping=0;
 Do k=1 To nIntPts; g{k}=g0{k};End;
 Do i=1 To nLevels; nPtsAt{i}=0; nRsps{i}=0; End;
 iLevel=1; preLevel=1;
* Do iPatient=1 TO nPts;
 Do While (stopping =0);
  npts=npts+1/&nSims;
  iLevel=min(min(iLevel, &nLevels),&nDosesSkip+preLevel
  +1);
        If nPtsAt(PreLevel) < MinPtsPerLevel Then
        iLevel = PreLevel; *
Delayed response;
        preLevel=iLevel;
        Rate=RRo{iLevel};
 nPtsAt{iLevel}=nPtsAt{iLevel}+1;
      r=Ranbin(seed,1,Rate); nRsps{iLevel}=nRsps
{iLevel}+r;
** Posterior distribution of a;
        c=0;
        Do k=1 To nIntPts;
               ak=&aMin+k*dx;
               Rate=1/(1+&b*Exp(-ak*doses{iLevel}));
               If r>0 Then L=Rate; Else L=(1-Rate);
               g{k}=L*g{k}; c=c+g{k}*dx;
        End;
        Do k=1 to nIntPts; g{k}=g{k}/c; End;
** Predict response rate and current MTD;
        MTD=iLevel; MinDR=1;
        Do i=1 To nLevels;
               RR{i}=0;
               Do k=1 To nIntPts;
                ak=&aMin+k*dx;
```

```
         RR{i}= RR{i}+1/(1+&b*Exp(-ak*doses{i}))
*g{k}*dx;
                End;
                DR=Abs(&MTRate-RR{i});
                If .<DR <MinDR Then
                      Do; MinDR = DR; iLevel=i; MTD=i;
MTDD=Doses{MTD}; End;
       End;
       MaxPtsAlevel = 0;
 Do i = 1 To nLevels;
       If MaxPtsAlevel < nPtsAt(i) Then MaxPtsAlevel
       = nPtsAt(i);
 End;
       If MaxPtsAlevel>=MaxNtoStop Then Stopping=1;
 End;
 Do i=1 To nLevels;
       DLTs=DLTs+nRsps{i}/&nSims;
 End;
 AveMTD=AveMTD+MTD/&nSims;
 AveMTDD=AveMTDD+MTDD/&nSims;
End;
Output;
Run;
Proc Print Data=CRM; run;
%Mend CRM;


Data DInput;
Array g{100}; Array
RRo{7}(0.0098,0.0196,0.0475,0.143,0.4062,0.7774,0.9683);
Array Doses{7} (25, 50, 82.5,125.4,175.6,233.5,310.5);
Do k=1 to 100; g{k}=1; End; * Flat prior. Don't have
to be normalized;
 run;
%CRM(nSims=5000, MaxNtoStop=6, MinPtsPerLevel=1,
nLevels=7, b=150, aMin=0, aMax=0.03, MTRate=0.25,
nDosesSkip=0);
Run;
```

APPENDIX B
Sample-Size Calculation Methods: Classical Design

One/Paired-Sample Hypothesis Test for the Mean

- Sign test for median difference for a paired sample
- Wilcoxon signed-rank test for one or a paired sample
- Test for H_0: (u_0, σ_0) versus H_a: (u_a, σ_a)—large sample
- One-sample t-test
- One-sample t-test: finite population
- Paired-sample t-test
- Paired-sample t-test (finite population)
- One-way repeated measures ANOVA
- One-way repeated measures contrast
- One-sample multiple test for zero means

One/Paired-Sample Hypothesis Test for Proportion

- McNemar's test for a paired sample
- Chi-square test for one sample proportion
- Chi-square test for one sample proportion: finite population
- One-sample exact test for proportion using binomial distribution

One/Paired-Sample Hypothesis Test for Others

- Kendall's test of independence
- Test H_0: correlation = zero using Fisher's arctan transformation
- Test H_0: regression coefficient = zero using arctan transformation

Classical and Adaptive Clinical Trial Designs Using ExpDesign Studio™,
By Mark Chang

- Logistic regression on x for a binary outcome
- Logistic regression on x for a binary outcome with covariates
- Linear regression; test for H_0: correlation coefficient = 0
- Multiple linear regression; test for H_0: multiple correlation $R = 0$
- Multiple regression; test zero increase in R^2 due to extra B covariates
- Linear regression $y = a + bx$; test H_0: $b = b_0$ vs. H_a: $b \neq b_0$
- Test for Bloch–Kraemer intraclass κ coefficient
- Test for Bloch–Kraemer intraclass κ using Z-transformation

Paired-Sample Equivalence Test for the Mean

- Paired t test for equivalence of means

Paired-Sample Equivalence Test for Proportion

- Paired response: equivalence of p_1 and p_2 (large sample)

One-Sample Confidence Interval for the Mean

- One-sample mean confidence method
- One-sample mean confidence interval method: finite population
- Paired-sample mean confidence interval method: large sample
- Paired-sample mean confidence interval method: finite population
- Confidence interval for repeated measures contrast
- One-sample confidence interval for a mean based on the t-statistic
- Paired mean confidence interval based on the t-statistic

One-Sample Confidence Interval for Proportion

- Confidence interval for a proportion: large n
- Confidence interval for an odds ratio for paired proportions: large n
- Confidence interval for the probability of observing a rare event

One-Sample Confidence Interval for Others

- Confidence interval for a correlation coefficient
- Linear regression $y = a + bx$, confidence interval for b
- Confidence interval for Bloch–Kraemer intraclass κ

Two-Sample Hypothesis Test for the Mean

- Two-sample *t*-test
- Mann–Whitney *U*/Wilcoxon rank-sum test for two samples
- Two-sample *z*-test: large sample or population variance known
- 2×2 crossover study
- One-way repeated measures ANOVA for two groups
- Test for a treatment mean difference with a 2×2 crossover design
- Two-sample *z*-test for treatment mean difference
- Two-sample multiple test for mean differences
- Comparing DNA expression profiles among predefined classes
- Donner's method for mean difference using cluster randomization

Two-Sample Hypothesis Test for Proportion

- Asymptotic *z*-method considering variance difference
- Pearson's chi-square test: Kramer–Greenhouse
- Lachin's test for two treatments by two-time-point interactions
- Mantel–Haenszel test for an odds ratio with *k* strata: large sample
- Whitehead logistic model for two groups with *k* categories
- Chi-square test for a two-sample proportion with *k* categories
- Mantel–Haenszel test for an odds ratio with *k* strata: continuity correction
- Repeated measures for two proportions
- Donner's method for proportion difference using cluster randomization
- Fisher's exact test

Two-Sample Hypothesis Test for Others

- Exponential survival distribution with uniform patient enrollment
- Exponential survival distribution with uniform enrollment rate and follow-up
- Test interaction in a model with an exponential survival function: two strata
- Test interaction in a model with an exponential survival function: *k* strata
- Log-rank test for survival analysis
- Exponential survival distribution with a uniform enrollment, follow-up, and dropouts
- Exponential survival distribution with a Bernoulli confounding variable

- Testing two correlation coefficients using Fisher's arctan transformation
- Linear regression $y_1 = a_1 + b_1x$, $y_2 = a_2 + b_2x$; test H_0: $b_1 = b_2$

Two-Sample Equivalence Test for the Mean

- Two one-sided t-tests for equivalence: parallel design (bivariate t)
- Two one-sided t-tests for equivalence based on a ratio of means: parallel design (bivariate t)
- Two one-sided t-tests for equivalence based on a ratio of two means: crossover design (bivariate t)
- Two one-sided t-tests for equivalence based on a mean ratio for lognormal data: parallel design (bivariate t)
- Schuirmann–Chow's two one-sided t-tests for equivalence
- Noninferiority test for means based on a one-sided two-sample t-test

Two-Sample Equivalence Test for Proportion

- Equivalence test for two proportions: large n
- One-sided noninferiority test for two proportions
- Equivalence test for two proportions using the bivariate t-distribution (large n)

Two-Sample Equivalence Test for Survival

- Noninferiority test for survival with uniform accrual and follow-up
- Equivalence test for survival with uniform accrual and follow-up

Two-Sample Confidence Interval for the Mean

- Confidence interval for the difference of two means: large sample

Two-Sample Confidence Interval for Proportion

- Confidence interval for the difference in two proportions: large n
- Confidence interval for proportional difference with minimum total size
- Confidence interval for ln(odds ratio): unmatched case–control study

Two-Sample Confidence Interval for Others

Multisample Hypothesis Test for the Mean

- ANOVA with Latin square design
- One-way ANOVA for parallel groups

- Contrast test for *m* means: dose–response
- Two-way ANOVA with an interaction term
- Two-way ANOVA without interaction
- One-way random block design
- William's test for minimum effective dose

Multisample Hypothesis Test for Proportion

- Chi-square test for equal proportions in *m* groups
- Chi-square test for *m* sample proportions with *k* categories
- One-way contrast between proportions
- Cochran–Armitage test for linear/monotonic trend: dose–response

Multisample Hypothesis Test for Others

- Prognostic model with right-censored data from DNA microarrays
- Test for all *k* equal survival means with overall type I error control
- One-way contrast test for survival with uniform accrual and follow-up

Multisample Confidence Interval for Others

- Confidence interval for one-way contrast: large sample

REFERENCES

Armitage, P. (1955). Tests for linear trends in proportions and frequencies. *Biometrics*, 11, 375–386.

Babb, J. S., and A. Rogatko (2001). Patient specific dosing in a cancer phase I clinical trial. *Stat. Med.*, 20, 2079–2090.

Babb, J. S., and A. Rogatko (2004). Bayesian methods for cancer phase I clinical trials. In *Advances in Clinical Trial Biostatistics*, N. L. Geller (Ed.), Marcel Dekker, New York.

Babb, J. S., A. Rogatko, and S. Zacks (1998). Cancer phase I clinical trials: efficient dose escalation with overdose control. *Stat. Med.*, 17, 1103–1120.

Bandyopadhyay, U., and A. Biswas (1997). Some sequential tests in clinical trials based on randomized play-the-winner rule. *Calcutta Stat. Assoc. Bull.*, 47, 67–89.

Banerjee, A., and A. A. Tsiatis (2006). Adaptive two-stage designs in phase II clinical trials. *Stat. Med.*, 25(19), 3382–3395.

Banik, N., K. Kohne, and P. Bauer (1996). On the power of Fisher's combination test for two stage sampling in the presence of nuisance parameters. *Biomet. J.*, 38, 25–37.

Bauer, P. (1989). Multistage testing with adaptive designs (with discussion). *Biomet. Inf. Med. Biol.*, 20, 130–148.

Bauer, P., and W. Brannath (2004). The advantages and disadvantages of adaptive designs for clinical trials. *Drug Discov. Today*, 9, 351–357.

Bauer, P., and M. Kieser (1999). Combining different phases in development of medical treatments within a single trial. *Stat. Med.*, 18, 1833–1848.

Bauer, P., and K. Köhne (1994). Evaluation of experiments with adaptive interim analysis. *Biometrics*, 50, 1029–1041.

Bauer, P., and K. Köhne (1996). Evaluation of experiments with adaptive interim analyses. *Biometrics*, 52, 380 (correction).

Bauer, P., and F. König (2005). The reassessment of trial perspectives from interim data: a critical view. *Stat. Med.*, 25(1), 23–36.

Bauer, P., and F. König (2006). The reassessment of trial perspectives from interim data: a critical view. *Stat. Med.*, 25, 23–36.

Bauer, P., and J. Rohmel (1995). An adaptive method for establishing a dose–response relationship. *Stat. Med.*, 14, 1595–1607.

Bechhofer, R. E., J. Kiefer, and M. Sobel (1968). *Sequential Identification and Ranking Problems*, University of Chicago Press, Chicago.

Benjamini, Y., and Y. Hochberg (1995). Controlling the false discovery rate: a practical and powerful approach to multiple testing. *J. R. Stat. Soc. Ser. B*, 57, 289–300.

Berry, D. A. (2005a). Introduction to Bayesian methods: III. Use and interpretation of Bayesian tools in design and analysis. *Clin. Trials*, 2, 295–300.

Berry, D. A. (2005b). Statistical innovations in cancer research. In *Cancer Medicine*, 7th ed., J. Holland et al. (Eds.), B.C. Decker, London, pp. 411–425.

Berry, D. A., and S. G. Eick (1995). Adaptive assignment versus balanced randomization in clinical trials: a decision analysis. *Stat. Med.*, 14, 231–246.

Berry, D. A., and B. Fristedt (1985). *Bandit Problems: Sequential Allocation of Experiments*, Chapman & Hall, London.

Berry, D. A., and D. K. Stangl (1996). *Bayesian Biostatistics*, Marcel Dekker, New York.

Berry, D. A., et al. (2002). Adaptive Bayesian designs for dose-ranging drug trials. In *Case Studies in Bayesian Statistics V*, Lecture Notes in Statistics, Springer-Verlag, New York, pp. 162–181.

Birkett, N. J. (1985). Adaptive allocation in randomized controlled trials. *Controlled Clin. Trials*, 6, 146–155.

Bloch, D. A., and H. C. Kraemer (1989). 2×2 Kappa coefficients: measures of agreement or association. *Biometrics*, 45, Mar., 269–287.

Breslow, N. E. (1981). Odds ratio estimators when the data are sparse. *Biometrika*, 68, 73–84.

Bretz, F., and L. A. Hothorn (2002). Detecting dose–response using contrasts: asymptotic power and sample-size determination for binary data. *Stat. Med.*, 21, 3325–3335.

Bretz, F., et al. (2006). Confirmatory seamless phase II/III clinical trials with hypotheses selection at interim: general concepts. *Biomet. J.*, 48(4), 623–634. DOI: 10.1002 /bimj.200510232.

Bronshtein, I. N., et al. (2004). *Handbook of Mathematics*, Springer-Verlag, Berlin.

Brophy, J. M., and L. Joseph (1995). Placing trials in context using Bayesian analysis: GUSTO revisited by Reverend Bayes. *J. Am. Med. Assoc.*, 273, 871–875.

Brown, C. C. (1981). The validity of approximation methods for interval estimation of odds ratio. *Am. J. Epidemiol.*, 113, 474–480.

Casagrande, J. T., et al. (1978). An improved approximate formula for calculating sample sizes for comparing two binomial distributions. *Biometrics*, 34, 483–486.

Chakravarty, A. (2005). Regulatory aspects in using surrogate markers in clinical trials. In *The Evaluation of Surrogate Endpoint*, Burzykowski, Molenberghs, and Buyse (Eds.), Springer-Verlag, New York.

Chaloner, K., and K. Larntz (1989). Optimal Bayesian design applied to logistic regression experiments. *J. Plann. Inference*, 21, 191–208.

Chang, M. (2006). Phase II/III seamless adaptive design. *Int. Chin. Stat. Assoc. Bull.*, Jan., 42–47.

Chang, M. (2007a). *Adaptive Design Theory and Implementation Using SAS and R*, Chapman & Hall/CRC Press, Boca Raton, FL.

Chang, M. (2007b). Adaptive design method based on sum of p-values. *Stat. Med.*, 26, 2772–2784.

Chang, M. (2007c). Clinical trial simulations in early development phases. In *Encyclopedia of Biopharmaceutical Statistics*, S. C. Chow (Ed.), Taylor & Francis, New York.

Chang, M. (2007d). Clinical trial simulations in later development phases. In *Encyclopedia of Biopharmaceutical Statistics*, S. C. Chow (Ed.), Taylor & Francis, New York.

Chang, M. (2007e). Multiple-arm superiority and noninferiority designs with various endpoints. *Pharm. Stat.*, 6, 43–52.

Chang, M., and S. C. Chow (2005). A hybrid Bayesian adaptive design for dose response trials. *J. Biopharm. Stat.*, 15, 667–691.

Chang, M., and S. C. Chow (2006). Power and sample-size for dose response studies. In *Dose Finding in Drug Development*, N. Ting (Ed.), Springer-Verlag, New York.

Chang, M., and S. C. Chow (2007). Analysis strategy of multiple-endpoint adaptive design. *J. Biopharm. Stat.*, 17(6), 1189–1200.

Chang, M., S. C. Chow, and A. Pong (2006). Adaptive design in clinical research: issues, opportunities, and recommendations. *J. Biopharm. Stat.*, 16(3), 299–309.

Chang, M., et al. (2007). BIO white paper: Innovative approaches in drug development. *J. Biopharm. Stat.* 17(5), 775–789.

Chang, M. N. (1989). Confidence intervals for a normal mean following group sequential test. *Biometrics*, 45, 249–254.

Chang, M. N., and P. C. O'Brien (1986). Confidence intervals following group sequential test. *Controlled Clin. Trials*, 7, 18–26.

Chang, M. N., H. S. Wieand, and V. T. Chang (1989). The bias of the sample proportion following a group sequential phase II trial. *Stat. Med.*, 8, 563–570.

Chapman, D. G., and J. Nam (1968). Asymptotic power of chi-square tests for linear trends in proportions. *Biometrics*, 24, 317–327.

Chen, J. J., Y. Tsong, and S. Kang (2000). Tests for equivalence or noninferiority between two proportions. *Drug Inf. J.*, 34, 569–578.

Chen, T. T. (1997). Optimal three-stage designs for phase II cancer clinical trials. *Stat. Med.*, 16, 2701–2711.

Chen, T. T., and T. H. Ng (1998). Optimal flexible designs in phase II cancer clinical trials. *Stat. Med.*, 17, 2301–2312.

Chen, Y. H. J., D. L. DeMets, and K. K. G. Lan (2004). Increasing the sample-size when the unblinded interim result is promising. *Stat. Med.*, 23, 1023–1038. DOI: 10.1002/sim.1688.

Cheng, Y., and Y. Shen (2004). Estimation of a parameter and its exact confidence interval following sequential sample-size re-estimation trials. *Biometrics*, 60, 910–918.

Chevret, S. (1993). The continual reassessment method in cancer phase I clinical trials: a simulation study. *Stat. Med.*, 12, 1093–1108.

Chevret, S. (Ed.) (2006). *Statistical Methods for Dose-Finding Experiments*. Wiley, Chichester, England.

Chow, S. C., and M. Chang (2005). Statistical consideration of adaptive methods in clinical development. *J. Biopharm. Stat.*, 15, 575–591.

Chow, S. C., and M. Chang (2006). *Adaptive Design Methods in Clinical Trials*, Chapman & Hall/CRC Press, Boca Raton, FL.

Chow S. C., and J.-P. Liu (1998). *Design and Analysis of Clinical Trials*, Wiley, New York.

Chow, S. C., and J. P. Liu (2003). *Design and Analysis of Clinical Trials*, 2nd, Wiley, Hoboken, NJ.

Chow, S. C., and J. Shao (2002). *Statistics in Drug Research*, Marcel Dekker, New York.

Chow, S. C., and J. Shao (2005). Inference for clinical trials with some protocol amendments. *J. Biopharm. Stat.*, 15, 659–666.

Chow, S. C., and J. Shao (2006). On margin and statistical test for noninferiority in active control trials. *Stat. Med.*, 25, 1101–1113.

Chow, S. C., J. Shao, and Y. P. Hu (2002). Assessing sensitivity and similarity in bridging studies. *J. Biopharm. Stat.*, 12, 385–400.

Chow, S. C., J. Shao, and H. Wang (2003). *Sample Size Calculation in Clinical Research*, Marcel Dekker, New York.

Chow, S. C., M. Chang, and A. Pong (2005). Statistical consideration of adaptive methods in clinical development. *J. Biopharm. Stat.*, 15, 575–591.

Chuang, S. C., and A. Agresti (1997). A review of tests for detecting a monotone dose-response relationship with ordinal response data. *Stat. Med.*, 16, 2599–618.

Cochran, W. G. (1954). Some methods for strengthening the common χ^2 tests. *Biometrics*, 10, 417–451.

Cohen J. (1988). *Statistical Power Analysis for the Behavioral Sciences*, 2nd ed., Lawrence Erlbaum Associates, Hillsdale, NJ.

Cornfield, J. A. (1956). Statistical problem arising from retrospective studies. In *Proceedings of the 3rd Berkeley Symposium*, University of California Press, Berkeley, California, Vol. 4, pp. 135–148.

Cox, D. R. (1972). Regression models and life-tables. *J. R. Stat. Soc.*, 34, 187–220.

Crowley, J. (Ed.) (2001). *Handbook of Statistics in Clinical Oncology*, Marcel Dekker, New York.

DeMets, D. L., C. D. Furberg, and L. M. Friedman (2006). *Data Monitoring in Clinical Trials: A Case Studies Approach*, Springer-Verlag, New York.

Devore, J. L. (1991). *Probability and Statistics for Engineering and the Sciences*, 3rd ed., Duxbury Press, Belmont, CA.

Donner, A. (1984). Approaches to sample size estimation in the design of clinical trials: a review. *Stat. Med.*, 3, 199–214.

Donner, A., N. Birkett, and C. Buck (1981). Randomization by cluster, *Am. J. Epidemiol.*, 114(6).

Efron, B. (1971). Forcing a sequential experiment to be balanced. *Biometrika*, 58, 403–417.

Efron, B. (1980). Discussion of "minimum chi-square, not maximum likelihood." *Ann. Stat.*, 8, 469–471.

Eisenhart, C. (1938). The power function of the chisq test. *Bull. Am. Math. Soc.*, 44, 32.

Ellenberg, S. S., T. R. Fleming, and D. L. DeMets (2002). *Data Monitoring Committees in Clinical Trials: A Practical Perspective*, Wiley, Hoboken, NJ.

EMEA (2002). *Point to Consider on Methodological Issues in Confirmatory Clinical Trials with Flexible Design and Analysis Plan*. The European Agency for the Evaluation of Medicinal Products Evaluation of Medicines for Human Use. CPMP/EWP/2459/02. European Medicines Agency, London.

EMEA (2004). *Point to Consider on the Choice of Non-inferiority Margin*. The European Agency for the Evaluation of Medicinal Products Evaluation of Medicines for Human Use. European Medicines Agency, London.

EMEA (2005). *Guideline on the Evaluation of Anticancer Medicinal Products in Man*. Committee for Medicinal Products for Human Use, European Medicines Agency, London. Available from http://www.emea.eu.int/pdfs/human/ewp/020595en.pdf. Accessed Aug. 10 2006.

EMEA (2006). *Reflection Paper on Methodological Issues in Confirmatory Clinical Trials with Flexible Design and Analysis Plan*. The European Agency for the Evaluation of Medicinal Products Evaluation of Medicines for Human Use. CPMP/EWP/2459/02. European Medicines Agency, London.

Emerson, S. S., and T. R. Fleming (1990). Parameter estimation following group sequential hypothesis testing. *Biometrika*, 77, 875–892.

Ensign, L. G., E. A. Gehan, D. S. Kamen, and P. F. Thall (1994). An optimal three-stage design for phase II clinical trials. *Stat. Med.*, 13, 1727–1736.

Fan, X., and D. L. DeMets (2006). Conditional and unconditional confidence intervals following a group sequential test. *J. Biopharm. Stat.*, 16, 107–122.

Fan, X., D. L. DeMets, and K. K. G. Lan (2004). Conditional bias of point estimates following a group sequential test. *J. Biopharm. Stat.*, 14, 505–530.

Faries, D. (1994). Practical modifications of the continual reassessment method for phase I cancer clinical trials. *J. Biopharm. Stat.*, 4, 147–164.

Farrington, C. P., and G. Manning (1990). Test statistics and sample size formulae for comparative binomial trials with null hypothesis of non-zero risk difference or non-unity relative risk. *Stat. Med.*, 9, 1447–1454.

FDA (1988). *Guideline for Format and Content of the Clinical and Statistical Sections of New Drug Applications*. U.S. Food and Drug Administration, Rockville, MD.

FDA (2000). *Guidance for Clinical Trial Sponsors on the Establishment and Operation of Clinical Trial Data Monitoring Committees*. U.S. Food and Drug Administration, Rockville, MD.

FDA (2005a). Guidance for clinical trial sponsors on the establishment and operation of clinical trial data monitoring committees (draft), http://www.fda.gov/cber/qdlns/clintrialdmc.htm.

FDA (2005b). Guidance for industry (draft): Clinical trial endpoints for the approval of cancer drug and biologiecs, http://www.fda.gov/cder/Guidance/6592dft.htm. Accessed Aug. 11, 2006.

FDA (2006). Innovation stagnation, critical path opportunities list, http://www.fda.gov.

FDA (2006). Draft guidance for the use of Bayesian statistics in medical device clinical trials, http://www.fda.gov/cdrh/osb/guidance/1601.pdf. Accessed May 22, 2006.

FDA (1998). Guidance for industry: Providing clinical evidence of effectiveness for human drug and biological products, http://www.fda.gov/cder/guidance/index.htm. Accessed July 20, 2005.

Feigl, P., and M. Zelen (1965). Estimation of exponential survival probabilities with concomitant information. *Biometrics*, 21, 826–838.

Fisher, L. D. (1998). Self-designing clinical trials. *Stat. Med.*, 17, 1551–1562.

Fisher, L. D. (1999). Carvedilol and the Food and Drug Administration (FDA) approval process: the FDA paradigm and reflections on hypothesis testing. *Controlled Clin. Trials*, 20, 16–39.

Fisher, L. D., and G. V. Belle (1993). *Biostatistics*, Wiley, New York.

Fisher, L. D., and L. A. Moyé (1999). Carvedilol and the Food and Drug Administration (FDA) approval process: an introduction. *Controlled Clin. Trials*, 20, 1–15

Fleiss, J. L. (1986). *The Design and Analysis of Clinical Experiments*, Willey, New York.

Fleiss, J. L., A. Tytun, and H. K. Ury (1980). A simple approximation for calculating sample sizes for comparing independent proportions. *Biometrics*, 36, June, 343–346.

Fleming, T. R., and D. L. DeMets (1996). Surrogate endpoint in clinical trials: Are we being misled? *Ann. Inter. Med.*, 125, 605–613.

Follman, D. A., M. A. Proschan, and N. L. Geller (1994). Monitoring pairwise comparisons in multi-armed clinical trials. *Biometrics*, 50, 325–336.

Freedman, L. S. (1982). Tables of the number of patients required in clinical trials using the logrank test. *Stat. Med.*, 1, 121–129.

Freedman, L. S. (1986). Tables of the number of patients required in clinical trials using the logrank test. *Stat. Med.*, 5, 97–99.

Freedman, L. S., B. I. Graubard, and A. Schatzkin (1992). Statistical validation of intermediate endpoints for chronic diseases. *Stat. Med.*, 11, 167–178.

Freidlin, B., and R. Simon (2005). Adaptive signature design: an adaptive clinical trial design for generating and prospectively testing a gene expression signature for sensitive patients. *Clin. Cancer Res.*, 11(21), Nov. 1.

Friede, T., and M. Kieser (2006). Sample size recalculation in internal pilot study designs: a review. *Biomet. J.*, 48, 537–555.

Friede, T., et al. (2003). A comparison of procedures for adaptive choice of location tests in flexible two-stage designs. *Biomet. J.*, 45, 292–310.

Friedman, B. (1949). A simple urn model. *Commum. Pure Appl. Math.*, 2, 59–70.

Gail, M. H., et al. (1984). Biased estimates of treatment effect in randomized experiments with nonlinear regressions and omitted covariates. *Biometrika*, 71, 431–444.

Gart, J. J., and D. G. Thomas (1972). Numerical results on approximate confidence limits for the odds ratio. *J. R. Stat. Soc. B.*, 34, 441–447.

Gart, J. J., and D. Thomas (1982). The performance of three approximate confidence limit methods for the odds ratio. *Am. J. Epidemiol.*, 115: 453–470.

Gallo, P., et al. (2006). Adaptive designs in clinical drug development: an executive summary of the PhRMA Working Group. *J. Biopharm. Stat.*, 16, 275–283.

Gehan, E. A. (1961). The determination of the number of patients required in a preliminary and a follow-up trial of a new chemotherapeutic agent. *J. Chron. Dis.*, 13, 346–353.

Gentle, J. E. (2003). *Random Number Generation and Monte Carlo Methods*, Springer-Verlag, New York.

George, S. L., and M. M. Desu (1974). Planning the size and duration of a clinical trial studying the time to some critical event. *J. Chron. Dis.*, 27, 15–24.

Gompertz, B. (1825). On the nature of the function expressive of the law of human mortality, and on a new mode of determining the value of life contingencies. *Philosophical Transactions of the Royal Society of London*, Vol. 115, pp. 513–585.

Gordon, I., and R. Watson (1994). A note on sample size determination for comparison of small probabilities. *Controlled Clin. Trials*, 15, 77–79.

Graybill, F. A. (1976). *Theory and Application of the Linear Model*, Wadsworth, Belmont, CA.

Hahn, G. J., and W. Q. Meeker (1991). *Statistical Intervals: A Guide for Practitioners*, Wiley, New York, Sect. 4.4.

Halperin, M., et al. (1968). Sample size for medical trials with special reference to long term therapy. *J. Chron. Dis.*, 21, 12–23.

Halpern, J., and B. W. Brown, Jr. (1987). Designing clinical trials with arbitrary specification of survival functions and for the log rank or generalized Wilcoxon test. *Controlled Clin. Trials*, 8, 177–189.

Halpern, J., and B. W. Brown, Jr. (1993). A computer program for designing clinical trials with arbitrary survival curves and group sequential testing. *Controlled Clin. Trials*, 14, 109–122.

Hauschke, D., M. Kieser, E. Diletti, and M. Burke (1999). Sample size determination for proving equivalence based on the ratio of two means for normally distributed data. *Stat. Med.*, 18, 93–105.

Herson, J., and J. Wittes (1993). The use of interm analysis for sample size adjustment. *Drug Inf. J.*, 27, 753–760.

Hsieh, F. Y. (1989). Sample size tables for logistic regression. *Stat. Med.*, 8, 795–802.

Hsieh, F. Y., and P. W. Lavori (2000). Sample size calculations for the Cox proportional hazard regression model with nonbinary coveriates. *Controlled Clin. Trials*, 21, 552–560.

Hung, H. M. J., R. T. O'Neill, P. Bauer, and K. Kohne (1997). The behavior of the *p*-value when the alternative hypothesis is true. *Biometrics*, 53, Mar., 11–22.

Hung, H. M. J., R. T. O'Neill, S. J. Wang, and J. Lawrence (2006). A regulatory view on adaptive/flexible clinical trial design. *Biometric. J.*, 48, 565–573.

Jennison, C., and B. W. Turnbull (2000). *Group Sequential Method with Applications to Clinical Trials*, Chapman & Hall/CRC Press, Boca Raton, FL.

Johnson, N. L., S. Kotz, and N. Balakrishnan (1995). *Continuous Univariate Distributions*, Wiley, New York.

Kanji, G. K. (1999). *100 Statistical Tests*, SaGE Publications, Thousand Oaks, CA.

Kastenbaum, M. A., D. G. Hoel, and K. O. Bowman (1970). Sample size requirements: one-way analysis of variance. *Biometrika*, 57, Aug., 421–430.

Kendall, M. G., and A. Stuart (1967). *The Advanced Theory of Statistics, Vol.2: Inference and Relationship*, 2nd ed., Hafner Publishing, New York.

Kokoska, S., and D. Zwillinger (2000). *Standard Probability and Statistics Tables and Formulae*, CRC Press, Boca Raton, FL.

Kolassa, J. E. (1995). A comparison of size and power calculations for the Wilcoxon statistic for ordered categorical data. *Stat. Med.*, 14, 1577–1581.

Kupper, L. L., and K. B. Hafner (1989). How appropriate are popular sample size formulas? *Am. Stat.*, 43, May, 101–105.

Lachin, J. M. (1977). Sample size determinations for $r \times c$ comparative trials. *Biometrics*, 33, June, 315–324.

Lachin, J. M. (1981). Introduction to sample size determination and power analysis for clinical trials. *Controlled Clin. Trials*, 2, 93–113.

Lachin, J. M., and M. A. Foulkes (1986). Evaluation of sample size and power for analyses of survival with allowance for nonuniform patient entry, losses to follow-up, noncompliance, and stratification. *Biometrics*, 42, Sept., 507–519.

Lakatos, E. (1988). Sample sizes based on the log-rank statistic in complex clinical trials. *Biometrics*, 44, Mar., 229–241.

Lakatos, E., and K. K. G. Lan (1992). A comparison of sample size methods for the logrank statistic. *Stat. Med.*, 11, 179–191.

Lan, K. K. G., and D. L. DeMets (1983). Discrete sequential boundaries for clinical trials. *Biometrika*, 70, 659–663.

Lan, K. K. G., and D. Zucker (1993). Sequential monitoring of clinical trials: The role of information in Brownian motion. *Stat. Med.*, 12, 753–765.

Lee, E. T. (1992). *Statistical Methods for Survival Data Analysis*, 2nd ed., Wiley, New York.

Lee, S.-Y. (1996). Power calculation for a score test in the dependent censoring model. *Stat. Med.*, 15, 1049–1058.

Lehmann, E. L. (1975). *Nonparametric: Statistical Methods Based on Ranks*. Holden-Day, San Francisco, California.

Lin, L. I.-K. (1992). Assay validation using the concordance correlation coefficient. *Biometrics*, 48, June, 599–604.

Lin, S. C. (1995). Sample size for therapeutic equivalence based on confidence interval. *Drug Inf. J.*, 29, 45–50.

Lin, Y., and W. J. Shih (2001). Statistical properties of the traditional algorithm-based designs for phase I cancer clinical trials. *Biostatistics*, 2, 203–215.

Liu, K.-J. (1992). Sample size determination under an exponential model in the presence of a confounder and type I censoring. *Controlled Clin. Trials*, 13, 446–458.

Liu, K.-J. (1996). Sample size for the exact conditional test under inverse sampling. *Stat. Med.*, 15, 671–678.

Liu, K.-J. (1997). Exact equivalence test for risk ratio and its sample size determination under inverse sampling. *Stat. Med.*, 16, 1777–1786.

Makuch, R. W., and R. M. Simon (1978). Sample size requirements for evaluating a conservative therapy. *Cancer Treatment Rep.*, 62, July, 1037–1040.

Makuch, R. W., and R. M. Simon (1982). Sample size requirements for comparing time-to-failure among *k* treatment groups. *J. Chron. Dis.*, 35, 861–867.

May, W. L., and W. D. Johnson (1997a). Confidence intervals for differences in correlated binary proportions. *Stat. Med.*, 16, 2127–2136.

May, W. L., and W. D. Johnson (1997b). The validity and power of tests for equality of two correlated proportions. *Stat. Med.*, 16, 1081–1096.

McCullagh, P. (1980). Regression model for ordinal data. *J. R. Stat. Soc. Ser. B*, 43, 109–142.

Miettinen, O. S. (1968). The matched pairs design in the case of all-or-none responses. *Biometrics*, June, 339–352.

Miettinen, O. (1976). Estimability and estimation in case-referent studies. *Am. J. Epidemiol.*, 103, 226–235.

Muller, K. E., and C. N. Barton (1989). Approximate power for repeated-measures ANOVA lacking sphericity. *J. Am. Stat. Assoc.*, 84, June, 549–555.

Nam, J. (1987). A simple approximation for calculating sample sizes for detecting linear trend in proportions. *Biometrics*, 43, 701–705.

Nam, J.-M. (1992). Sample size determination for case-control studies and the comparison of stratiified and unstratified analyses. *Biometrics*, 48, June, 389–395.

Nester, M. R. (1996). An applied statistician's creed. *Appl. Stat.*, 45, 401–410.

Newcombe, R. G. (1998). Improved confidence intervals for the difference between binomial proportions based on paired data. *Stat. Med.*, 17, 2635–2650.

Noether, G. E. (1987). Sample size determination for some common nonparametric tests. *J. Am. Stat. Assoc.*, 82, June, 645–647.

Obuchowski, N. A., and D. K. McClish (1997). Sample size determination for diagnostic accuracy studies involving binormal roc curve indices. *Stat. Med.*, 16, 1529–1542.

Odeh, R. E., and M. Fox (1991). *Sample Size Choice*, Marcel Dekker, New York.

O'Neill, R. T. (1984). Sample sizes for estimation of the odds ratio in unmatched case–control studies. *Am. J. Epidemiol.*, 120, 145–153.

O'Quigley, J., M. Pepe, and L. Fisher (1990). Continual reassessment method: A practical design for phase I clinical trial in cancer. *Biometrics*, 46, 33–48.

O'Quigley, J., and L. Shen (1996). Continual reassessment method: A likelihood approach. *Biometrics*, 52, 673–684.

Owen, D. B. (1965). A special case of a bivariate non-central t-distribution. *Biometrika*, 52, 437–446.

Owen, D. B. (1968). A survey of properties and applications of the noncentral t-distribution. *Technometrics*, 10, Aug., 445–478.

Pampallona, S., and A. A. Tsiatis (1994). Group sequential designs for one-sided and two-sided hypothesis testing with provision for early stopping in favor of null hypothesis. *J. Statist. Plann. Iinference*, 42, 19–35.

Patnaik, P. B. (1949). The non central chisq and F distributions and their applications. *Biometrika*, 36, 202–232.

Peterson, B., and S. L. George (1993). Sample size requirements and length of study for testing interaction in a $1 \times k$ factorial design when time-to-failure is the outcome. *Controlled Clin. Trials*, 14, 511–522.

Phillips, K. F. (1990). Power of the two one-sided tests procedure in bioequivalence. *J. Pharmacokinet. Biopharm.*, 18, 137–145.

Proschan, M. A. (1996). On the distribution of the unpaired t-statistic with paired data. *Stat. Med.*, 15, 1059–1063.

Proschan, M. A., K. K. G. Lan, and J. T. Wittes (2006). *Statistical Monitoring of Clinical Trials: A Unified Approach*, Springer-Verlag, New York.

Ratkowsky, D. A., M. A. Evans, and J. R. Alldredge (1993). *Cross-over Experiments: Design, Analysis, and Application*, Marcel Dekker, New York.

Robinson, L. D., and N. P. Jewell (1991). Some surprising results about covariate adjustment in logistic regression models. *Int. Stat. Rev.*, 59, 227–240.

Ross, S. M. (2002). *Simulation*, 3rd ed., Academic Press, London.

Rubinstein, L. V., M. H. Gail, and T. J. Santner (1981). Planning the duration of a comparative clinical trial with loss to follow-up and a period of continued observation. *J. Chron. Dis.*, 34, 469–479.

Sahai, H., and A. Khurshid (1996). Formulae and tables for the determination of sample sizes and power in clinical trials for testing differences in proportions for the two-sample design: a review. *Stat. Med.*, 15, 1–21.

Sandvik, L., J. Erikssen, P. Mowinckel, and E. A. Rodland (1996). A Method for determining the size of internal pilot studies. *Stat. Med.*, 15, 1587–1590.

Schoenfeld, D. A. (1981). The asymptotic properties of nonparametric tests for comparing survival distributions. *Biometrika*, 68, 316–319.

Schoenfeld, D. A. (1983). Sample-size formula for the proportional-hazards regression model. *Biometrics*, 39, June, 499–503.

Schuirmann, D. J. (1987). A Comparison of the two one-sided tests procedure and the power approach for assessing the equivalence of average bioavailibility. *J. Pharmacokinet. Biopharm.*, 15, 657–680.

Self, S. G., and R. H. Mauriitsen (1988). Power/sample size calculations for generalized linear models. *Biometrics*, 44, Mar., 79–86.

Self, S. G., R. H. Mauritsen, and J. Ohara (1992). Power calculations for likelihood ratio tests in generalized linear models. *Biometrics*, 48, Mar., 31–39.

Shao, J., M. Chang, and S. C. Chow (2005). Statistical inference for cancer trials with treatment switching. *Stat. Med.*, 24, 1783–1790.

Shih, J. H. (1995). Sample size calculation for complex clinical trials with survival endpoints. *Controlled Clin. Trials*, 16, 395–407.

Shuster, J. J. (1993). *Practical Handbook of Sample Size Guidelines for Clinical Trials*, CRC Press, Boca Raton, FL.

Simon, R. (1989). Optimal two-stage designs for phase II clinical trials. *Controlled Clin. Trials*, 10, 1–10

Simon, R., M. Radmacher et al. (2002). Design of study using DNA microarray. *Genet. Epidemiol.*, 23, 21–36.

Smith, J., J. Connett, and R. McHugh (1985). Planning the size of a matched case–control study for estimation of the odds ratio. *Am. J. Epidemiol.*, 122, 345–347.

Thall, P. F., R. Simon, and S. S. Ellenberg (1988). Two-stage selection and testing designs for comparative clinical trials. *Biometrika*, 75, 303–310.

Thall, P. F., R. Simon, and S. S. Ellenberg (1989). A two-stage design for choosing among several experimental treatments and a control in clinical trials. *Biometrics*, 45, 537–547.

Thall, P., R. Millikan, and H. G. Sung (2000). Evaluating multiple treatment courses in clinical trials. *Stat. Med.*, 19, 1011–1028.

Thomas, R. G., and M. Conlon (1992). Sample size determination based on Fisher's exact test for use in 2×2 comparative trials with low event rates. *Controlled Clin. Trials*, 13, 134–147.

Walker, G. A. (1997). *Common Statistical Methods for Clinical Research*, SAS Institute, Cary, NC.

Wang, L., et al. (1977). *Mathematic Handbook* (in Chinese), Advanced-Education Press, Beijing, China.

Wang, S. K., and A. A. Tsiatis (1987). Approximately optimal one-parameter boundaries for group sequential trials. *Biometrics*, 43, 193–199.

Wei, L. J. (1978). The adaptive biased-coin design for sequential experiments. *Ann. Stat.*, 9, 92–100.

Wei, L. J., and S. Durham (1978). The randomized play-the-winner rule in medical trials. *J. Am. Stat. Assoc.*, 73, 840–843.

Whitehead, J. (1993). Sample size calculations for ordered categorical data. *Stat. Med.*, 12, 2257–2271.

Whitehead, J. (1994). Sequential methods based on the boundaries approach for the clinical comparison of survival times (with discussions). *Stat. Med.*, 13, 1357–1368.

Whitehead, J. (1996). Sample sizes calculations for ordered categorical data. *Stat. Med.*, 15, 1065–1066.

Whitehead, J. (1997a). Bayesian decision procedures with application to dose-finding studies. *Int. J. Pharm. Med.*, 11, 201–208.

Whitehead, J. (1997b). *The Design and Analysis of Sequential Clinical Trials*, rev. 2nd ed., Wiley, Chichester, England.

Whitehead, J., and I. Stratton (1983). Group sequential clinical trials with triangular continuation regions. *Biometrics*, 39, 227–236.

Whitmore, G. A. (1983). A regression method for censored inverse-Gaussian data. *Can. J. Stat.*, 11, 305–315.

Whitmore, G. A., M. J. Crowder, and J. F. Lawless (1998). Failure inference from a marker process based on a bivariate Wiener model. *Lifetime Data Anal.*, 4, 229–251.

Williams, D. A. (1971). A test for difference between treatment means when several dose levels are compared with a zero dose control. *Biometrics*, 27, 103–117.

Williams, D. A. (1972). Comparison of several dose levels with a zero dose control. *Biometrics*, 28, 519–531.

Wittes, J., et al. (2005). Stopping the randomized aldactone evaluation study early for efficacy. In *Data Monitoring in Clinical Trials*, D. L. DeMets, et al. (Eds.), Springer, New York.

Woolf, B. (1955). On estimating the relation between blood group and disease. *Ann. Hum. Genet.*, 19, 251–253.

Woolson, R. F., J. A. Bean, and P. B. Rojas (1986). Sample size for case-control studies using Cochran's statistic. *Biometrics*, 42, 927–932.

Xu, Z. J. (1985). *Monte Carlo Method* (in Chinese), Chinese Academic Press, Shanghai, China.

INDEX

Classical and Adaptive Clinical Trial Designs Using ExpDesign Studio™,
By Mark Chang

System Requirements, Software Installation, and Software License Agreement

SYSTEM REQUIREMENTS

- IBM or compatible PC with 80486, 50 MHz or higher
- CD-ROM drive
- 50 MB of free disk space
- 64 MB of RAM or higher
- Microsoft Windows 95 or higher

SOFTWARE INSTALLATION

- Insert the ExpDesign Studio CD into the CD-ROM drive on your computer.
- Click on the **Start** button 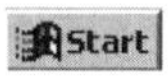

 to begin the installation procedure. The Windows Start menu will appear.
- Select **RUN** in the Start menu. The Run dialog box will appear.
- If ExpDesign Studio is in E: drive, enter **E: setup** in the **Open** edit box.
- Click the **OK** button.
- Follow the instructions on the computer screen for the remaining steps.
- If a file being copied is not newer than the file currently on your computer system, it is recommended that you keep your existing file.

CTriSoft SOFTWARE LICENSE AGREEMENT

The following constitutes the terms of the License Agreement between a single user (User) of this software package, and the producer of the package, CTriSoft. By opening the package, you (the User) are agreeing to become bound by the terms of this agreement. If you do not agree to the terms of this agreement, do not open the package, and contact the CTriSoft Customer

Classical and Adaptive Clinical Trial Designs Using ExpDesign Studio™,
By Mark Chang

Service in order to obtain an authorization number for the return of the package. This License Agreement pertains also to all third-party software included in or distributed with CTriSoft products.

License

Unless explicitly stated on the program media (CD or disks), the enclosed software package is sold to be used on one computer system by one user at a time. This License Agreement explicitly excludes renting or loaning the package. Unless explicitly stated on the program media, this License Agreement explicitly excludes the use of this package on multiuser systems, networks, or any time-sharing systems. (Contact CTriSoft concerning multiuser license programs.) The user is allowed to install the software package on a hard disk and make a backup copy for archival purposes. However, the software will never be installed on more than one hard disk at a time. The documentation accompanying this software package (or any of its parts) shall not be copied or reproduced in any form.

Disclaimer of Warranty

Although producing error-free software is obviously a goal of every software manufacturer, it can never be guaranteed that a software program is actually free of errors. Business and scientific application software is inherently complex (and it can be used with virtually unlimited numbers of data and command settings, producing idiosyncratic operational environments for the software); therefore, the User is cautioned to verify the results of his or her work. This software package is provided “as is” without warranty of any kind. CTriSoft and distributors of CTriSoft software products make no representation or warranties with respect to the contents of this software package and specifically disclaim any implied warranties or merchantability or fitness for any particular purpose. In no event shall CTriSoft be liable for any damages whatsoever arising out of the use of, inability to use, or malfunctioning of this software package. CTriSoft does not warrant that this software package will meet the User’s requirements or that the operation of the software package will be uninterrupted or error free.

Updates, Corrections, Improvements

The User has a right to purchase all subsequent updates, new releases, new versions, and modifications of the software package introduced by CTriSoft for an update fee or for a reduced price. CTriSoft is not obligated to inform the User about new updates, improvements, modifications, and/or corrections of errors introduced to its software packages. In no event shall CTriSoft be liable for any damages whatsoever arising out of the failure to notify the User about a known defect of the software package.